14"

99λ

Nurses' Guide
to
Cancer Care

Nurses' Guide
to
Cancer Care

Constance S. Kirkpatrick, RN, MS
Pacific Lutheran University

Rowman & Littlefield
Publishers

ROWMAN & LITTLEFIELD

Published in the United States of America in 1986
by Rowman & Littlefield, Publishers
(a division of Littlefield, Adams & Company)
81 Adams Drive, Totowa, New Jersey 07512

Library of Congress Cataloging-in-Publication Data

Kirkpatrick, Constance S.
  Nurses' guide to cancer care.

  Bibliography: p. 287
  Includes index.
  1. Cancer—Nursing. I. Title.
[DNLM: 1. Neoplasms—nursing.   WY 156 K59n]
RC266.K57   1986   610.73'698   86-17666
ISBN 0-8476-7500-9
ISBN 0-8476-7501-7 (pbk.)

89 88 87 86
10 9 8 7 6 5 4 3 2 1
Printed in the United States of America

Contents

Tables

Figures

Preface

Cancer is the second most common cause of death in the United States today, surpassed only by cardiovascular disease. At present incidence rates, cancer is affecting three out of four American families. These facts attest to the need for a specialty component devoted to the implementation of current, comprehensive cancer nursing care. Bringing together information from authoritative sources and clinical experience, this book offers nurse practitioners a guide to the complete, integrated practice of nursing for cancer patients. Although intended primarily for the nurse who functions as a clinical specialist or primary provider of cancer screening services, the information included in this volume can make an important contribution to the skills and knowledge of the medical-surgical nurse responsible for the care of the many oncology patients who are placed on general hospital floors.

Ranked Cause of Death, United States, 1980, Older Adults (over 65)

Heart disease	1
Cancer	2
Arteriosclerosis	5
Influenza and pneumonia	4
Stroke	5
Diabetes mellitus	6
Accidents (except automobiles)	7
Bronchitis, emphysema, asthma	8
Cirrhosis of the liver	9
Motor vehicle accidents	10

Since the field of cancer nursing incorporates concepts from the disciplines of epidemiology, accounting, sociology, psychology, medicine, and biology, it requires the primary practitioner to be knowledgeable in a number of areas that are not covered in a basic nursing program. This guidebook provides both the broad coverage and detailed information and procedures that serve as the basis for comprehensive cancer nursing care at a primary provider or management level. Appropriate for use as a study guide, it also encompasses the content specified for inclusion in the Oncology Nursing Certification examination of the Oncology Nursing Certification Corporation.

Acknowledgments

Many people have contributed to the completion of this work. In particular, I would like to acknowledge the contributions of Mary Jo Aspinall, Nursing Editor for Rowman & Littlefield; Mary Ann Daly, Nurse Manager in Medical–Surgical Nursing; Judy Hanada, Nurse Coordinator in Oncology at University Hospital in Seattle; and Beverly Vincent, Oncology Clinical Nurse Specialist at University Hospital in Seattle. Ann M. McElroy, Oncology/Medical Educator with Multicare Medical Center in Tacoma, and Cathy Eddinger, Oncology Nurse Manager with the same organization, also provided valuable help. Layne Nordgren, Director of Media Services, Pacific Lutheran University Library, was of major help in designing illustrations. My husband, Michael, deserves special acknowledgment for his active help and support.

1

Issues in Management and Delivery of Services in Cancer Care

Historical Perspectives

Paleopathologists have demonstrated that dinosaurs were afflicted with neoplastic disorders even before *Homo sapiens* existed. It is known today that vertebrates, invertebrates, and plants are all capable of developing neoplastic diseases. It is also believed that all cells in the body carry the potential for malignancy. Thus, the picture develops of a disease that has been a part of virtually all forms of life over the span of millions of years. By the fourth century B.C., Hippocrates had coined the term "carcinoma" for the various neoplastic diseases that were then recognized and described, and thought due to an excess of black bile. In the second century A.D., Galen suggested the similarity between the neoplastic diseases and the form of a crab, and the term "cancer" came into use. By the seventeenth century, surgeries were being done to treat malignant diseases. During the nineteenth century, with the advent of the cellular theory, the study of cancer became more systematic. In 1829, Recamier introduced the term "metastasis" to describe the spread of cancer. Waldeyer, working during the same period, demonstrated that cancers spread primarily through the blood and lymphatic vessels in the metastatic process. In 1855, Virchow promoted the theory that each cell arises from a preexisting cell. By 1900, experimental animal studies of cancer were well under way. Of course, over the last eighty-five years, the discoveries have been monumental, and the nature of cancer treatment has undergone intensive scrutiny and evolution. Halsted devised his extensive surgical procedure for breast cancer during the 1890s; today, such surgery has been questioned, as the systemic nature of cancer becomes clearer and alternative treatments prove effective.

Surgery is the oldest of the currently employed forms of treatment for various cancers. Some of the surgical approaches have not changed greatly since the early 1900s. When the cobalt–60 unit became available in the 1950s, radiation therapy became an integral

1

part of cancer treatment, used in conjunction with surgical techniques. After World War II, chemotherapy trials started, first with nitrogen mustard as a palliative measure. In 1966, combination chemotherapy developed as a result of a better understanding of cell kinetics in malignant diseases.

Oncology nursing may be considered to have formally begun with the establishment of the first contagious disease hospital for cancer established in Rheims, France in 1740 (Hilkemeyer 1982). The Royal Marsden Hospital in England was established for the care of the cancer patient in 1951; in this case, the focus was on the patient's well-being, not on controlling the spread of the dreaded disease.

Education of nurses for this specialty developed from informal on-the-job training to the establishment of formal education programs in the 1950s. Hilkemeyer (1982) recalls that it would have been "unthinkable" for nurses to administer chemotherapy in the early 1950s, yet some thirty years later it is an essential part of the functions of the cancer nurse. The competencies expected of the oncology nurse were delineated for the first time on a national level with the 1979 publication of the Outcome Standards for Cancer Nursing by the Oncology Nursing Society and the Division of Medical Surgical Nursing Practice of the American Nurses Association. Through higher educational standards in nursing and the proven competency of nurses to provide the patient services, cancer nursing has evolved into a distinct, highly respected nursing specialty area. With the advent of a certification program in oncology nursing in 1986, this specialty area takes another leap forward in establishing competencies of the individual practitioner.

Research in cancer nursing has expanded enormously in the last ten years. The journals devoted to the specialty, *The Oncology Nursing Forum* and *Cancer Nursing: An International Journal for Cancer Care*, have provided nurses a forum to share research and created an element of encouragement for attempting innovations in care. The increasing number of master's-prepared nurses in the role of clinical oncology nurse specialist is an impetus to expanding the amount of clinical research done by oncology nurses in the future.

Economic Perspectives

In August 1982, with the passage of the federal Tax Equity and Fiscal Responsibility Act (TEFRA), the foundation was established for a new concept of health care delivery in the United States. Through Medicare and Medicaid, the federal government pays 40 percent of all hospital bills; these expenditures comprised 4.5 percent of the gross national product in 1950 and 9.4 percent by 1982. TEFRA was designed to cut back services or conditions that were not critical to adequate health care in order to contain costs, which were escalating out of control. Later in 1982, Richard Schweiker, Secretary of the Department of Health and Human Services, saw his proposal for a prospective payment system for Medicare based on diagnostic related groups (DRGs) adopted by Congress. The following year, Title IV of the 1983 Social Security Amendments adopted by Congress established prospective payments based on DRGs as law. Essentially, what these regulations do is establish exact payments for specific diagnoses based on length of stay. If hospitals keep Medicare patients beyond the limits set by the new laws, they must pick up the additional costs themselves. Hospitals may not bill a patient for any costs beyond the federal reimbursement amount unless the patient requests the additional stay and understands the costs involved. Of course, there are built-in safeguards to cover complications and extraordinary expenses. Should a hospital discharge a patient prior to the standard length of time, reimbursement is still at the full amount for the DRG involved.

It is interesting to note nursing's involvement in these regulations. John Thompson, a nurse researcher with Yale University, did much original work in the 1960s to define expected length of hospitalization for quality-of-care studies that later provided the structure for the DRGs. The federal agency responsible for the implementation, interpretation, and development of the new Medicare regulations, the Health Care Financing Administration (HCFA), was headed until 1985 by Carolyn Davis, R.N., Ph.D., F.A.A.N..

Oncology nurses need to understand the basics of the new legislation as it will directly impinge on their practice and prospectives for development in the overall health care delivery system. Certain aspects of the regulations that affect oncology nursing particularly are described below.

1. Specific payments for hospice care are established.
2. Reimbursement of hospital-based training programs such as diploma nursing programs and nurse anesthesia programs will be phased out or significantly reduced by 1987.
3. Hospitals exempted from the DRG prospective payment system include cancer hospitals. To date, M. D. Anderson Hospital, Fox Chase Cancer Center, and the City of Hope Hospital qualify for this exemption.
4. Outpatient services, skilled nursing homes and home care

agencies, presently exempted, will have specific prospective payment schedules.

5. Some comprehensive cancer centers, including research units, are exempted. However, because the costs involved in patient care for cancer patients in clinical trials have been found to be greater than costs for general cancer patients, nonexempted cancer centers are finding it difficult to support research.

Currently, research is being done at the federal level to determine the feasibility of establishing prospective payment schedules for physicians' fees. This is being sharply opposed by organized medicine, which prefers to control curtailments within the profession. This development, along with the regulations related to DRGs, has created three areas of significance for nurses in cancer care.

First, an overwhelming concern of hospital administrators and nursing administrators is cost containment. Of the approximately 7,000 hospitals in the nation, 1,000 are expected to close by 1990 (Yasko 1984). To avoid this eventuality, actual nursing care costs are being scrutinized on a widespread basis for the first time. In the past, nursing costs have been an elusive figure, hidden within the per diem room rate, and not a major administrative concern. Now nursing supervisors are being evaluated by upper management in good measure according to their ability to control staff costs. The cost of nursing care is often as much as 50 percent of a hospital's operating budget, and most hospital administrators concur that staff reductions are the single most effective way to decrease the institution's expenses. As a consequence, decreased full-time staff and increased per diem staff has been a growing trend nationwide.

Secondly, hospital services that produce no revenue are being curtailed or eliminated. Social workers, occupational therapists, psychologists, dieticians, respiratory therapists, and similar health-related professionals are finding that their functions are being returned to the nursing department.

Thirdly, the autonomy of the nursing role is the focus of conflicting pressures. Because of the general oversupply of physicians nationwide, and particularly in the specialties of radiation therapy and medical oncology, some physicians are expanding their practice to include what was once strictly nursing territory or taking positions once considered nursing jobs. Today, there are cases of physicians applying for nursing supervisory positions as well as for clinical nurse specialist positions. Patient education, infection control, and central supply supervision are examples of areas that physicians in some parts of the country are bringing under their control. The master's-prepared oncology clinical nurse specialist who commands a greater salary than the entry level nurse may find competition for this role from unexpected sources.

On the other hand, the need for greater nursing care of patients in their own homes subsequent to earlier hospital discharges is opening up opportunities for independent nursing practitioners. Even in the hospital setting, nurses may find that their power to provide sophisticated nursing care, including family and patient teaching, that will result in early discharges, and increased revenue for the hospital will allow them to expand the independent practice of nursing.

Nurse managers of the oncology unit will need to consider all these factors carefully in determining how to allocate budget dollars or propose new positions to hospital and nursing administration.

Distribution of Cancer Care Services

Today, the major providers of cancer care to individuals are ambulatory cancer clinics. For example, M. D. Anderson Hospital in Houston has approximately 400 cancer patient beds, but sees an average of 1,200 outpatients each month in cancer clinics. The role of these clinics in the future is likely to continue to increase due to a number of factors. To begin with, economic constraints on health care costs in general dictate that utilization of hospital facilities be limited whenever possible. Furthermore, the increasing sophistication of technology employed in delivering cancer care, such as external and internal pumps and long-term venous access devices, has allowed patients to continue with their daily routines rather than be admitted to a hospital for therapy. Furthermore, home health agencies and nursing homes may be expected to increase their share of the cancer care market. These trends in cancer care are of major significance in defining the clientele a hospital unit will support.

The Hospital-Based Cancer Unit

Unique Characteristics

The nursing care requirements of patients on an oncology unit are significantly greater on the whole than those of patients on general medical-surgical units. Tillman (1984) found that the average required nursing care hours per patient day was 6.16 for oncology patients on a cancer unit as opposed to 4.88 hours for medical-surgical patients. Other researchers approximate the same figures. Such data do not suggest that caring for cancer patients on a cancer unit is more or less costly than caring for them on general service units. Cancer patients in all settings have been found to require more nursing hours than other types of patients. Acuity, not diagnosis, is the traditional basis for determining the nursing care hours required for patients. Although medical patients with such conditions as paralysis or out-of-control diabetes require many hours of direct care, the mix of patients in medical nursing balances the scale in such a way that cancer units have patients who overall require significantly more direct care.

The nursing care required does not generally involve monitoring equipment or other intensive care measures that are easily understood by administrators to require adequate nursing staff support. Oncology patients require more nursing support in activities of daily living, medication administration, nutrient support, intravenous fluid administration, and scheduled treatments and specimen collection (Tillman 1984). The required nursing activities to support these patient needs must be carefully documented to justify adequate staff.

Nurses on an oncology unit also must spend significantly more time supporting patients or family members who are anxious about the cancer diagnosis and prognosis.

Differences Between Oncology Units and Hospice Units

Hospice care has been defined as an integrated program of appropriate hospital and home care for the patient with limited life expectancy. Emphasis is on psychosocial support for the patient and family and control of pain and symptoms in the patient. Generally, the individual eligible for hospice care is defined as one who has six months or less to live. The staff works to make the patient's last days as meaningful and enjoyable as possible, while minimizing treatments. Hospice care is made cost effective by keeping procedures, laboratory studies, and hospitalization at a minimum and using volunteers when possible. There are over a thousand hospice programs in the United States today and they exist in many forms, including free-standing units, units of a general acute care hospital, and home-care agencies. In order to continue to exist, these programs must rely on grants, federal reimbursement, and the conservative use of resources.

Because cancer is overwhelmingly a disease of the elderly, the designated cancer unit is largely comprised of Medicare-eligible patients. Therefore, reimbursement of expenses under the DRG system by the federal government is applicable to most patient utilizers of the unit. Reimbursement rates for specific cancers do not allow for reimbursed extension of stay for psychosocial factors or family issues. The cancer unit, then, as opposed to hospice units, must include quality-of-life issues in the care of patients within the parameters of time allotted for medical treatments in order to remain economically viable.

Characteristics of Cancer Unit Clientele

Current utilization of designated cancer beds is primarily by the aged with multiple medical problems, the incapacitated who cannot be cared for at home, and those undergoing multiple diagnostic tests or extensive treatments for whom hospitalization is more convenient. Although some patients are still hospitalized for chemotherapy, especially those who require close monitoring due to age or concomitant disease, most chemotherapy is administered on an out-patient basis.

Patients requiring surgery as part of their cancer treatment may be cared for on a cancer unit, but are often placed on a general surgical floor and discharged within a few days when their surgical course of treatment has sufficiently progressed. A large medical center or designated cancer hospital will have a surgical oncology floor. Most community hospitals, however, find that the nursing treatment required by these cancer patients is similar to that needed by other surgical patients, and expediency and economy dictate their inclusion on the general surgical floor. An exception to this general rule is the patient undergoing palliative surgery or one who requires cancer treatments subsequent to surgery during the same hospital admission. Persons admitted for uncomplicated surgery for cancer or laparotomies generally recover on general surgical floors in most community hospitals.

In light of these factors, the nature of the patient population on an oncology unit has changed substantially in the last decade. In order to justify the existence of a designated cancer unit, many community hospitals are using some of the beds not in use for cancer treatment on the oncology unit for hospice care. When a patient is admitted for hospice care, the charge for the room and the nature of the treatment are significantly changed. It may be difficult for staff nurses to shift gears and modify their practice to meet differing needs of the cancer patient and hospice patient. There may be a tendency to consider hospice patients as minimal care patients, an attitude which defeats the purpose of the specialized designation.

Organization and Operation of Cancer Units

There is very limited information in the general literature on the organization and operation of cancer units. The most comprehensive information stems from data compiled by the Oregon Comprehensive Cancer Program (OCCP) in 1979 from forty-four cancer units and a 1981 national conference they sponsored for one hundred cancer experts. In 1985, Moseley and Brown assembled much of the information from these sources for publication. They established guidelines in the Standards for Special Care Units of the Joint Commission for Accreditation of Hospitals (JCAH). These guidelines organize recommendations around ten concepts, which will be looked at individually in terms of selected information unique to cancer units derived from this source and more recently published information.

1. *Planning*
   • An oncology unit should arise from a preexisting hospital cancer program. A cancer program includes a cancer committee, tumor board, tumor registry, multidisciplinary patient services program and cancer education programs.
   • A minimum of 15 percent of the total admissions should have cancer diagnoses to justify costs. The number of beds designated for the cancer unit should be calculated so that an occupancy rate of at least 80 percent is maintained to allow the unit to be self-sustaining.
   • Approval of the cancer program by the American College of Surgeons' Commission on Cancer is beneficial for establishing credentials for the community.
   • Planning should be a multidisciplinary effort that includes oncologists, oncology nurses, administration, pharmacy, tumor registry, and dietary and rehabilitation services.

2. *Space Requirements*
   • Private rooms are most desirable to provide for the physical, emotional, and family needs of the cancer patient.
   • Isolated space for patients with radioactive implants should be provided.
   • Adequate professional meeting space and separate lounge space should be provided for the staff.

3. *Admissions*
   • Admission of nononcology patients should occur only if the space is not needed by cancer patients.

- Oncology patients should have the option of being treated in other areas of the hospital or in other programs if they so desire.

4. *Plans of Treatment*
   - Standardized patient care guidelines should be developed.
   - Individual patient care plans should be maintained.

5. *Services*
   - Diagnostic, acute care, and rehabilitative services should be available.
   - An integrated treatment approach should be provided, including surgery, chemotherapy, radiation, medical management, and immunotherapy.
   - Support services, including rehabilitative services, dietary, and social services and pastoral care should be available.
   - Discharge planning should be initiated upon the admission of the patient to the unit.
   - Patient education should be a multidisciplinary responsibility and have high priority. The Oncology Nursing Society's Outcome Standards for Cancer Patient Education should serve as a guide.

6. *Organization of Services*
   - A cooperative, integrated relationship should exist between the cancer unit and other hospital components.
   - The cancer committee should oversee and offer guidance for the operation of the cancer unit. Direct supervision of the unit should be through the medical director of the unit.

7. *Staff*
   - Weekly team conferences on patient care issues and monthly operational issues meetings should be held by representatives from all members of the multidisciplinary team.
   - Nursing staff should have expertise and competence in clinical management of cancer patients.
   - An adequate nurse/patient ratio should be maintained. A minimum of seven hours per patient day of nursing support is recommended.
   - Baccalaureate nurses should be utilized in staff positions to maximize the comprehensive nursing role.

8. *Orientation and Education of Staff*
   - An orientation program for staff nurses should be established based on the the Oncology Nursing Society's Standards for

Cancer Nursing Education and the American Nurse's Association's Standards of Practice.
• Ongoing formal and continuing education should be strongly supported for all staff.

9. *Certification*
• Development of a certification process for oncology nurses should be supported.

10. *Evaluation*
• Satisfaction of patients and families should be evaluated routinely.
• Avenues for the channeling of staff concerns should be well understood by all staff and their use supported.
• Quality of care evaluation tools should be established by the multidisciplinary team and routinely utilized.

Determining Cancer Nursing Costs

With the advent of the prospective payment method of reimbursement for Medicare-Medicaid patient expenses, nurses can no longer expect future great gains in salaries or growth in staff nursing ranks. Instead, nursing must justify its worth by determining the cost of services provided the patient. Then payment systems can be developed using nursing units as revenue-producing cost centers for the hospital.

Cost accounting may be discussed in terms of direct and indirect costs. Direct costs are expenses associated with a specific procedure or service; nursing salaries, for example, are ordinarily a cost associated with room rate charges. Indirect costs include expenses that cannot be directly applied to specific events or services. Staff orientation, time-off benefits for education, and in-service programs are examples of indirect costs.

Stanfill and McDonnell (1985) described strategies for separating out nursing costs. First, the room rate must be broken down into its component parts so that nursing costs can be clearly identified. Secondly, the smallest functional unit to which cost control and accountability can be assigned and revenue allocated must be identified as a cost center. A nursing unit, such as an oncology unit, is frequently considered a cost center. With these two strategies accomplished, variable billing can be introduced with nursing a separate and distinct entity.

Most hospitals are now using a patient classification system (PCS) to differentiate nursing costs among unit patients. An example of a form used in one such system is shown in Figure 1.1. The validity and reliability of these systems are not uniformly established across the nation. Nonetheless, a well-defined PCS establishes management productivity objectives on a daily basis so that nurse managers can determine base costs and adjust staffing in response to these costs. Other methods of determining nursing costs include the traditional per diem method, and costs per DRG or nursing diagnosis.

Most hospitals determine the nursing cost per patient day, then apply information from the PCS to find the average number of nursing hours per patient per day. The cost of one hour of nursing care is multiplied by the number of hours of care received by patients at different levels of acuity according to the PCS, and a rational base is established for costing out nursing services.

Once the cost of nursing care is documented, charges can be generated in the form of variable billing. Variable billing is currently in use for many departments in institutions such as dietary, laboratory, and central supply. A cost center (that is, the cancer unit) would establish its expense base and then bill for expenses plus profit for the resources consumed by each patient separately. Nursing costs would show up on billings customized for each patient and based on the PCS level of acuteness determined by nursing for the patient.

The future direction nursing must take is toward fee-for-service. Only a handful of hospitals are currently billing for nursing services separately, but many are conducting in-house trials on the system and will go public in the near future.

What the Cancer Unit Is Expected to Provide

First, a clear understanding of the expectations of the different groups utilizing the cancer unit needs to be established. Hospital administrators expect a cost-effective, well-utilized unit that will attract physicians and the community to the hospital. Generally, an average census count of 80 percent or more is required for a viable unit. Nursing administration expects a smooth-running unit with a capable, stable staff who will not create malpractice problems for the hospital and will evidence flexibility to meet hospital needs beyond the cancer unit.

Staff nurses desire strong, knowledgeable leadership with an emphasis on quality patient care and staff development. The American Academy of Nursing studied magnet hospitals of the United States and found that most had decentralized departmental structures, had a heavy nursing involvement in hospital committees, and in many cases employed clinical specialists. A positive nursing image was

DATE: _____ (at 11:59 PM)

NURSING UNIT: _____

SUMMARY DATA:

Census _____

Category V: _____
Category IV: _____
Category III: _____
Category II: _____
Category I: _____

TOTAL

ADMISSIONS, DISCHARGES, TRANSFERS, DEATHS
12M–11:59 PM

No.	NAME	A(√)	D(√)	T(√)	DEATHS(√)
1					
2					
3					
4					
5					
6					
7					

PATIENT NAMES AND HISTORY NUMBERS

CATEGORY

THERAPEUTIC INDICATOR

Life Support V
Acute renal failure requiring peritoneal dialysis
Acute major hemorrhage
Cardiac tamponade
Cardiorespiratory arrest
Potential for violence/suicidal
Respiratory failure requiring ventilator support
Severe graft versus host disease/infectious process
Shock requiring pressors

Intensive IV
Acute cord compression
Electrolyte disorders, severe
Pulmonary edema requiring diuresis
Seizures/increased intracranial pressure
Self care deficit 2° to age
Sepsis/uncontrolled fever
Unstable cardiac status/MI or major arrhythmia
Unstable hematological status/blast crisis/DIC
Unstable respiratory status requiring intensive intervention

Modified Intensive III
Aplasia, potential for infection

Clinical status requiring intensive parenteral therapy

Compromised respiratory status requiring respiratory therapy

Electrolyte disorder, mild to moderate

Graft versus host disease, chronic/stable

Impaired physical mobility/severe pain

Impaired skin integrity/decubitus ulcer

Infectious complication requiring strict isolation

Knowledge deficit requiring intensive patient/family education

Nutritional deficit requiring enteral/parenteral nutrition

Potential/adverse reaction(s) requiring intensive monitoring

Renal failure requiring hemodialysis

Severe gastrointestinal disturbance(s)

Superior vena cava syndrome

Unstable neurological signs/disorientation/emotional disturbance

Urinary and/or bowel incontinence

Sensory deficits (hearing, vision, speech)

Intermediate II
Clinical status requiring parenteral therapy

Fever, potential for infection

Hematological status requiring blood transfusions

Infectious complications requiring enteric isolation

Potential post-operative complications/BMT donors

Minimal I
Anxiety, mild to moderate requiring support/observation

Therapy requiring radiation precautions/isolation/self care

Staffing (R.N.):

Days	Evenings	Nights

Figure 1.1   The Johns Hopkins Oncology Center Patient Classification System Form

Reprinted by permission from Linda M. Arenth, "The Development and Validation of an Oncology Patient Classification System," *Oncology Nursing Forum* 12, no 6 (1985), p. 19. © 1985, Oncology Nursing Society.

considered important by staff nurses as well as a focus on education supporting improved nursing care. Frequent in-service programs, support of formal academic education, and emphasis on career development were cited as key factors in making a hospital a magnet for professional nurses (Rogers 1985).

Patients, as well, have expectations of the cancer unit. Although nurses base their care on what they perceive as the patients' needs, some studies suggest that the two perspectives may be quite dissimilar. In a study by Larson (1984), oncology nurses indicated that listening to patients was the most important nursing behavior they felt they evidenced. On the other hand, patients perceived the most important nursing behaviors as the ability to manage equipment, give shots, respond quickly, and know when to call the physician. Of fifty nursing behaviors from which to choose, patients selected as least important items that included sitting with the patient, asking what name he or she would prefer to be called, offering reasonable alternatives, helping the patient establish goals, and telling the patient of available support systems. It may be that cancer patients feel that the best they can receive from nurses would be care that is organized, on time, and competently implemented. Nurses need to validate that what they do to demonstrate caring is important to the patients they serve.

Families of cancer patients have been studied regarding their areas of concern about nursing care. Dyck and Wright (1985) published data showing that almost 40 percent of families felt that more adequate care could have been provided their loved ones. Twenty-nine percent of those surveyed indicated that obtaining information from nurses was difficult and 18 percent felt there was a lack of professionalism among nurses. Other previous research generally follows the same pattern. One important conclusion made by Dyck and Wright and corroborated by a number of other researchers was that "families . . . perceived their needs as best being met when the patients' needs for good care were being met by competent nurses" (ibid., 56).

General Management Concerns

In order for the cancer unit to remain economically workable and attractive to physicians and patients, nursing management must integrate numerous factors to assure the smooth running of the unit. The factors can be considered within the framework of two main categories: competency of staff and attitude of staff.

STAFF COMPETENCY

As described above, patients prize competency in nurses as the most important means of expressing caring, and administration prizes competency in order to assure the most efficient care so as to conserve expenses for viable operation of the hospital. There are specific actions nursing management can take in order to assure competency of the staff. First, the hiring of nurses for the cancer unit should be done with an eye to their capacity for clinical dexterity or established clinical expertise. The ability to communicate with others, to document activities, and to display a cooperative spirit, while useful attributes, cannot substitute for the ability to handle equipment and various nursing activities in an organized, timely manner.

Frequent use of in-services, allowing time off the unit to attend educational offerings, and encouraging continuing formal education are other means of promoting competency. Staff must feel they are part of a dynamic organization that is responsive to new methods of nursing care and that values education in its many forms.

Promoting continuity of care is another means of establishing competency. Patient assignment schedules which change from day to day do not allow nursing staff to streamline rountines and treatments.

It may be useful to consider the advantages of committing part of the salary budget to a position for a clinical nurse specialist. One of the hallmarks of this professional is clinical competency. Hiring a leadership-level employee in the fiscally constrained atmosphere of today does require rigorous justification. However, the benefits in terms of increased competency of the staff through the teaching, example-setting, and practice of the clinical specialists have been found to be well warranted. This has been most clearly demonstrated in the case of magnet hospitals. A high quality clinical nurse specialist can create an environment of efficient, progressive, and sophisticated standards of practice.

Evaluations of staff nurses should be based on their management of specific outcome criteria established for the clientele. This process of evaluation based on the product the nurse produces (ideally a well-managed, well-informed patient) rather than the attributes or behaviors of the nurse as a person will enable the staff to become more self-directed and goal-oriented. Of course, not all patients will evidence satisfactory progress or good adjustments to diagnosis, prognosis, therapy, or nursing care. The staff nurse who responds appropriately to patient behavior, whether the behavior is appropriate or not, would be managing nursing care reasonably. The goals may not be reached, but nursing actions are directed toward them as patient outcomes.

For example, nursing management could select the Outcome Standards for Cancer Nursing Practice compiled by the Oncology Nursing Society and American Nurses' Association as the standard expected outcome for the unit's clientele (see bibliography for publishing information). Then, a reasonable case load could be determined, based on level of acuteness and numbers, on a monthly basis for each of the nursing staff. During the year, audits of performance based on ability to carry sufficient numbers of patients and documentation of approriate patient outcomes could be done. Staff would correlate documentation of care with pertinent goals of the unit and be able to determine their relative productivity during the year.

STAFF ATTITUDE

The attitude of an oncology nursing staff cannot be entirely separated from the concept of competency. Nurses who feel that they epitomize the best in standards of care will generally show a concomitant positive attitude. Even so, there are specific conditions that can help create a positive attitude among the staff.

The encouragement of the individual nurse to grow professionally should be a foremost consideration. Efforts to increase competency, such as those mentioned above, also let the nurse know that the organization cares about him or her as an individual. The clinical nurse specialist can be instrumental in helping staff nurses progress in their professional role and can administer education programs.

In addition, there are physical considerations that will increase the morale of the nursing staff. Shift reports should be given in a room conducive to professional communications. Standing at counters, or seated in a locker room, or around a coffee table with half the staff on the floor is inappropriate, although still common. The casualness of the reporting circumstances conveys an unspoken message to nurses about their value and professionalism.

Professional workers have a private workspace available to them in virtually all fields except registered nursing. Clearly, the large number of nurses and limited space available curtail individual desk space; however, the unit should provide space for a small library and writing area specifically for the registered nursing staff. Some space— a cubbyhole or at least a separate file folder—should be provided for each individual nurse. Nurses willingly concede the need to provide patients with some measure of privacy in their room space, but may neglect their own needs for private space to allow a sense of control in some small measure.

Other Methods of Delivering Cancer Nursing Services

Because so much of future cancer nursing care will be delivered in outpatient clinics, nursing homes, and patients' homes, these practice areas need to be considered. The elements discussed in the previous section for the management of a cancer unit are pertinent to these other delivery systems, but some specific considerations need to be addressed.

Outpatient Clinics

A main feature of an ambulatory care service is a high patient-volume-to-time ratio, which keeps per-patient costs relatively low. The need to maintain or increase cost constraints will continue into the future with the economic realities of health care regulations. Thus, many nurses practicing in these settings will find that their time is spent primarily in organization of patient flow, administration of chemotherapy, paperwork, and assisting physicians. This general pattern leaves little time for the administration of nursing care, that is, treating human responses to actual or potential health problems. Staffing of nurses is not likely to increase so that such nursing activities can be rendered in an structured, institutionalized manner. Therefore, nurses must respond to these realities by incorporating nursing care into the routine of the clinic in which they practice.

If nurses can delineate responsibilities within the nursing staff on a rotating basis so that the functional activities are done by some nurses while one or more nurses focus on nursing care, satisfaction with the nursing role may be increased. Smaller clinics or doctors' offices generally do not provide for this type of staffing, however. At least one very large cancer clinic uses a checklist on which patients indicate their concerns while waiting for their appointment. In a busy center, this has proved an effective means of improving the delivery of nursing services by allowing nurses to focus quickly on areas concerning which patients have indicated interest or anxiety.

Home Care

Cardiac conditions and malignancies are the two most frequent diagnoses encountered in home health agencies. There are some studies suggesting that cancer patients treated at home require more frequent visits than those with other diagnoses. The functions of the nurse treating the home patient are mainly in the area of symptom management, but also include teaching, counseling, and ongoing assessment of needs. Nurses prepared to deliver home care should be as highly educated as possible, for ingenuity, independence, and self-direction are basic requirements for delivering a total program to cover patient and family needs. Some services employ only clinical nurse specialists with masters-degree preparation in nursing. Generally, a minimum of a baccalaureate degree is required for health department-based services.

One phenomenon that is becoming apparent in home health care is the proliferation of a wide variety of agencies, small and large, which have very different infrastructures and are competing for the same market. There are nurse-owned corporations, national firms, independent local agencies, health department sections, hospital-based home health agencies and HMO-affiliated groups all seeking to gain patients on a fiscally sound basis. Not all of these systems will survive, and small agencies may be the first to disappear because of their limited marketing ability or limited reserves. In each of these groups, nurses play the key role as the primary providers of the services offered. Management and ownership are functions that nursing could reasonably assume with much greater frequency in the future.

Nursing Homes

Perhaps the greatest disadvantage cancer patients encounter in many nursing homes is the lack of staff specially trained to provide cancer nursing services. This is a situation that can be rectified. Selected staff nurses can be trained in cancer care, an inclusive library of books and journals can be maintained on current techniques and issues, and consultant nurses can be employed to provide teaching or direct services. Nursing homes constitute an expanding area for the delivery of cancer nursing care and, due to increasing numbers of these patients in this setting, may be able to specialize care more frequently in the future.

Families are sometimes shocked to hear that their loved one who has cancer is not "sick" enough for the hospital, but is to be placed in a nursing home. In the past, the hospital took in patients for chronic care, and many families continue to expect this; the need for new management of patient placements to contain rising costs is not yet fully appreciated by the public. This new strategy of placing cancer patients is a reality to be faced and may prove a benefit to nurses who wish to increase nursing's role in the balance of services provided the cancer patient. Medical management is less emphasized in the extended care facility than in the hospital, allowing nursing services to predominate. It is in nursing homes that nursing may have its greatest effect on the quality of overall care provided the cancer patient.

It would be beneficial to the field of cancer nursing if nurses who manage cancer patients in these various settings would coordinate within communities to collaborate on techniques, research, referrals, and practice. Nursing is at the threshold nationwide of a new era in patient care delivery—one in which the nurse's role will be paramount in determining the effectiveness of various delivery systems. Nursing management will be the key to many future success stories; how patients will be treated for cancer, if not how they will be cured, is the future business of the cancer nurse.

Referral Resources

A diagnosis of cancer creates tremendous coping challenges for the person and family concerned. The illness is usually lengthy, often very expensive, and associated with psychological and social stresses. There are many resources available with help; however, they are sometimes never used by the people who need them the most because the resource is unknown to the individual, is not available locally, or involves too much red tape.

National Level Resources

Comprehensive cancer centers are available in sixteen states across the country and in the District of Columbia (see Appendix). These centers are exclusively dedicated to cancer research, diagnosis, treatment, and teaching. Although neighborhood hospitals are normally adequately equipped to treat common cancers, cancers requiring complicated therapy, monitoring, or specialty nursing are best treated at comprehensive centers, if they are accessible. New protocols in cancer treatment are frequently available only at these centers, for patients who choose to participate in them.

A tremendous resource for the individual with cancer is the American Cancer Society (ACS). This voluntary organization is concerned with support of research, public and professional education, and service. At a national level, an individual may wish to use the ACS as a source of referral information on physicians with a particular specialty in cancer care, or to provide information about questionable therapies.

The National Cancer Institute (NCI) is another resource for information on a wide variety of cancer topics. In addition, they support cancer research and professional education endeavors. They are particularly helpful in providing literature on cancer topics for patients and health professionals.

The NCI funds the Cancer Information Service (CIS), which is affiliated with the ACS and Comprehensive Cancer Centers around the United States. The CIS serves the public and professionals by answering questions about cancer through a nationwide telphone system. Questions on support, treatment alternatives, and available resources are addressed by trained professionals. All calls are strictly confidential and are toll free.

There are also a number of national organizations with local chapters offering specialized information on various cancers or cancer-related topics. The Leukemia Society of American, Inc., and the United Ostomy Association are examples. The ACS is an excellent resource for information on how to contact local chapters of these and similar organizations. Some specific organizations, like the International Association of Laryngectomees and Reach to Recovery, are supported by the ACS. The laryngectomee organization offers support and rehabilitation help for people with laryngectomies; Reach to Recovery assists women who have had mastectomies.

There are also a variety of organizations involved in psychological and social support for cancer patients and their families. The Candlelighters, an organization of parents of young cancer patients, and Make Today Count are examples. New chapters of these organizations are being formed in various cities around the country each year. CanSurmount and I Can Cope are two mutual support programs of the ACS; chapters are available throughout the country.

Regional Level Resources

The ACS has divisional offices in each state of the nation. This level of the ACS organization offers individuals information about regional facilities available for cancer treatment, administers and/or supports educational programs for the public and professionals, and funds research for statewide projects. The ACS is the only organization offering a wide range of services for cancer patients at the regional level.

Local Level Resources

Once again, the ACS is an excellent resource for information and support of cancer patients. Although the charter of the ACS precludes their financial support of treatment for individuals, they can often offer substantial support for home care, nursing supplies and transportation for individuals. The ACS also funds local projects for the detection and treatment of some cancers. Counseling services are available from the ACS in some areas, as well as substantial rehabilitation services. Another source of local support is through informal organizations of cancer patients and families sponsored by neighborhood hospitals, health maintenance organizations, or churches. Community mental health centers may also be utilized to provide psychological support on an outpatient basis. The United Cancer Council is a federation of voluntary cancer agencies funded by United Way that offers nursing services, housekeeping services, prostheses, and rehabilitation aid.

Financial Resources

Costs directly related to the treatment of cancer can ultimately reach into tens or hundreds of thousands of dollars. In the majority of cases, costs related to hospitalization and medical care are financed through individual or group health insurance plans, or through the government programs, Medicare and Medicaid. For patients under age sixty-five, Blue Cross and private insurers are the source of payment for cancer care in more than 77 percent of cases. For patients over age sixty-five, Medicare pays expenses of cancer care for nearly 88 percent of cases. Associated costs for private nursing at home, supplies, transportation, and medications sometimes are not covered by insurance plans and must be financed through personal resources. About 90 percent of cancer patients have insurance coverage for 50 to 100 percent of costs. Those without any health insurance are most likely to be young (ages eighteen to twenty) and to reside in the South or western parts of the United States. Occasionally, charity organizations, church groups, or small, local organizations will provide financial aid to individuals. For the large majority of individuals, however, such philanthropic support does not develop.

Some working people or those who privately maintain health insurance may not be at risk of financial collapse in meeting cancer treatment costs because they are covered by comprehensive health insurance or have adequate financial reserves. The very poor, who are supported by government programs, are likewise not subject to financial burdens of cancer care. However, there is a growing class of people, sometimes referred to as the medically indigent, who are self-supporting when well, but when ill with cancer are unable to meet the associated costs by themselves. Each state and community has a different capacity to help these individuals. Sometimes these individuals must spend all their individual resources before they are eligible for government aid. Welfare departments may offer help to many of these people. In some areas, there are tax-supported hospitals available for free or low-cost medical care. Some people become eligible for financial help from Medicare or Medicaid when they need financial help to meet cancer treatment costs. The Community Services Administration finances services for cancer patients through welfare agencies, agencies for the aged, and other local organizations. The Rehabilitation Services Administration can pay for services designed to return cancer patients to a productive life.

Veterans who are eligible for care in the Veterans Administration network of hospitals can receive free care for cancer at these facilities. The military provides full care for those in the armed forces as well as eligible dependents or retired personnel. Sometimes hospitals have a fund available to support indigent care; the patient should be informed early in treatment about this possibility and apply directly to the hospital's finance office.

Because the arrangements for financial assistance can be complex and vary from community to community, the best resource for help is a social worker associated with the treatment hospital, the ACS, local health departments, or nurse community care coordinators associated with the treatment facility.

Social Issues

Sometimes an individual must leave employment in order to complete treatments and recovery from cancer. Although most employed cancer patients return to their jobs (78.8 percent of women and 70.6 percent of men), in some cases, returning to the workplace may be difficult, even for those who are completely recovered (McKenna 1984). Mellette (1985) found that some 75 percent of cancer patients found adjusting to a return to work to be better than or about what was expected, while only 25 percent found more problems than they had expected. The more a person earned prior to the cancer diagnosis, the more likely the patient was to return to work after cancer treatment. Over 93 percent of those earning over $25,000 returned to work after treatment, while 93 percent of the $15,000 to $25,000 group did so, and 89 percent of those earning less than $7,500 (McKenna 1984). Employers may fear that people who have had cancer will take excessive sick leave, be unable to keep pace, require special concessions, or cause company insurance premiums to rise.

The federal government, in response to the needs of individuals who are in this predicament, passed the Rehabilitation Act of 1973, including those who have been treated for cancer among the handicapped. In so doing, the government made it illegal for any company with contracts or subcontracts to the federal government of $50,000 or more, and with fifty or more employees, to discriminate against someone who has had cancer. Companies that fall under these parameters must maintain an affirmative action program for the handicapped, which may include rehabilitative training. Although those who have had cancer in the past may not consider themselves handicapped, if they are limited in their opportunities for employment because of their past medical history, they are in fact socially handicapped. If a company receives any funds from the Department of Health and Human Services, it may not discriminate against the handicapped, regardless of the firm's size or the amount of money it receives from the federal source. The person who has had cancer and is looking for work might consider the many local governmental, educational, and health-related businesses that receive federal funding as a good starting point for a job search.

Individuals who feel that they have been unfairly denied employment by a firm with government contracts coming under the umbrella of the Rehabilitation Act should file a complaint under Section 503 of the Act with the Office of Federal Contract Compliance Programs of the U.S. Department of Labor. If a firm that receives money from the Department of Health and Human Services (DHHS) has discriminated against an individual who has had cancer, that individual has recourse through the DHHS Office of Civil Rights, under Section 504 of the Act.

Some thirty-five states have passed statutes prohibiting discrimination against cancer patients. Each state's department of labor or office of civil rights can advise individuals about the law of that particular state. Other sources of information and assistance in discrimination matters are the Rehabilitation Services Administration, the Equal Employment Opportunities Commission, the National Labor Relations Board and the American Civil Liberties Union (NCI 1985).

Nurses can work through local political organizations, professional organizations, and legislative representatives to assure that their states do not discriminate unfairly against those who have had cancer. As people extend the length of their working careers, and as more individuals who would once have died are being returned to society, the need to assure that these people can participate equally in the workplace is critical. Some 24 percent of past cancer patients have reported difficulty getting health insurance after cancer, although 10 percent of these individuals became eligible for Medicaid or Medicare (McKenna 1984). Many individuals with a past history of cancer also find it difficult or impossible to get life insurance. About 27 percent of new employees with a past history of cancer reported denial of life insurance through group programs (McKenna 1984). If the person who has had cancer is a major financial supporter of a family, this can be a particularly difficult situation. Nurses may consider this an issue worth pursuing with state legislatures.

Another social issue nurses may consider important to act on is the prevention of cancer and promotion of healthy lifestyles through legislative action. Local professional organizations may consider developing an agenda of issues that affect society, and nurses in particular as direct care givers. Examples of issues for which nurses in various states have lobbied are provisions for nonsmoking public areas and the provision of cancer screening services for disadvantaged groups.

Cancer Quackery

Unproven, or unorthodox, methods of cancer treatment are methods that have not been shown to be active in animal models or clinical trials, but that nonetheless are promoted as effective means of cure, palliation, or control of cancer. Sponsors of these methods may be outright charlatans dispensing harmless compounds for profit, or persons of sound scientific accomplishment who persist in promoting a method which research has not shown to be effective. Such a person may present as a persecuted messiah fighting against the medical-industrial complex. The hallmarks associated with cancer quackery are secrecy about ingredients or procedures, unwillingness to communicate research findings, and claims that the sponsor is being denied access to regular methods of drug distribution and evaluation. Proponents of cancer quackery are often unwilling or unable to comply with Food and Drug Administration guidelines and regulations on the use of investigational drugs.

The Food and Drug Administration estimates that the public spends more than two billion dollars yearly on unproven cancer treatments (Mooney 1984). The American Cancer Society and the Food and Drug Administration keep files on ineffective or unproven methods of cancer therapy, which they will share with professionals and the general public. Three organizations are listed with the American Cancer Society as proponents of unproven therapies: the

Independent Citizens Research Foundation for the Study of De-generative Diseases, the International Association of Cancer Victims and Friends, Inc., and the National Health Organization (Horton and Hill 1977).

Dealing with patients who are convinced of the effectiveness of a cancer cure that they cannot get from their physician can be an emotionally charged situation. In a preliminary study, some 41 percent of cancer patients indicated that they would be willing to try, or had tried, unproven cancer treatments (Mooney 1984). Therefore, it is seen that this is by no means an insignificant problem. Nurses can refer patients to the American Cancer Society and Food and Drug Administration for information on specific unproven therapies or to the Cancer Information Service of the National Cancer Institute. Nurses may need to describe the treatment evaluation process used to assure that Americans are not subjected to therapies without clear justification for their use. Sometimes patients may need to get a second opinion from a reputable physician in order to assure them-selves that they are doing the best for themselves. Sometimes patients are simply looking for a sense of personal involvement from their health care providers, and particularly need to sense warmth and personalized attention in the management of their cancer treatment.

2

The Cancer Process and Cancer Epidemiology

Carcinogenesis and the Cancer Process

The Transformed Phenotype

There are some one hundred neoplastic disorders that have been identified up to the present time. The characteristic they share is that each of the cancerous cells typical of the various disorders has an altered morphology and biochemical properties distinct from the comparable normal cell. The chance that any one cell will undergo the sequence of events required for malignant transformation is extremely small. The fact that cancer is so common attests to the fact that cells are commonly exposed to factors in the process of carcinogenesis. Cancer is not simply a rapid, disorderly proliferation of immature cells, but is revealing itself to be a logical, coordinated process in which cancer cells acquire specialized capabilities.

Altered Morphological and Biological Properties

The altered genetic makeup of the cancer cell is responsible for the abnormal properties seen in neoplastic disorders. One important morphological difference in cancer cells as opposed to normal cells is the cell membrane structure. Kamata and Feramisco (1984) and other investigators have shown that the membrane is altered so that growth factors can adhere to the transformed cell in greater quantities than normal. This may involve a change in receptor sites for the growth factors that are normally present. These growth factors signal cells to enter mitosis so the cancer cells have an advantage over normal cells for local growth as they preferentially use the available supply of growth factor compounds. Cancer cells go through the same cell cycle as nonmalignant cells, but they are much less likely to enter the GO (resting) phase of the cell cycle than are normal cells. It has also been suggested that some cancer cells may use autocrine secretion of growth factor to produce their own growth factor and thus further

26

their growth independently. It is suggested by research that most oncogenes may act through growth factor receptor pathways (Cochran et al. 1984). Because of other changes in the genetic structure of the cancer cell, it no longer responds to normal growth control mechanisms and continues to divide without impedence.

A biochemical alteration that is important to cancer cells is the increased rate of uptake of glucose, which allows an increased rate of synthesis of proteins. Because they utilize the anabolic pathway of protein synthesis very efficiently, cancer cells are extremely effective producers. Anatomically, the cancer cell is seen to have a larger nucleus than the normal cell, and its chromatin often clumps in an abnormal manner.

Carcinogenesis, Initiators, and Promotors

Carcinogenesis is a process that can occupy the better part of an individual's lifespan. It is generally thought that susceptibility factors set the stage for malignant transformations, while carcinogens and promotors actively transform a cell from one stage to another along a causal pathway. This causal pathway is a progressive one for which scientists are working to define distinct stages that would be useful for understanding cancer. Two concepts are currently being explored most actively, the multistage model and the two-stage model. The two-stage model offers the advantages of adhering closely to a biological interpretation (initiation and promotion) and parsimony in interpreting observations. As two cellular transitions in carcinogenesis have been demonstrated and can be reasonably described, the two-stage model most accurately reflects the carcinogenesis process as it is understood to date, and is most widely accepted.

Factors are broadly considered initiators if they act at an early stage in the carcinogenesis sequence and are considered promotors if their effect is later in the process. Promotors are compounds that are themselves noncarcinogenic, but that can induce tumors from cells previously exposed to an initiator. If a factor acts as a promotor, then after its effect is sufficient, the cancer is established. Initiators, on the other hand, may exert their effect, but the cancer might not become established for an extended period of time, depending on when or if promotors were introduced to the system. A complete carcinogen is both an initiator and promotor, so will cause cancer on its own.

Sometimes initiators are ingested in a form that is not carcinogenic (precarcinogenic), but are transformed in the liver to a malignant form. Liver detoxifying enzymes, which normally act to detoxify all foreign substances transported through the blood system, sometimes convert precarcinogens to highly carcinogenic, activated substances. Unfortunately, as the liver detoxifying enzyme systems break compound substances into smaller units for consumption or excretion, they cannot determine if larger or smaller units would be safer for the body. The detoxifying enzyme systems act in different ways; it has been suggested that some inheritable combinations of systems may increase the susceptibility of individuals to cancer because of the way they convert substances that are precarcinogenic. Profiles of liver detoxifying enzyme systems are being developed in an effort to discover a means of predicting individual susceptibility to cancer. Initiators and promotors can each induce the expression of latent oncogenes, which may be the dominant means by which malignant cell properties are established (Freedman et al. 1973).

Public health professionals in particular, but all health professionals should be aware of the different cancer impact on society produced by promotors and initiators. If an identified cancer-initiating factor were removed from society, the effect on the incidence of that cancer would not become apparent for a long time, as the population already exposed would continue to be subjected to promoting factors and subsequently express the disease. If promotors were eliminated from society, however, the reduction in population incidence would be apparent within a relatively short period of time.

Inhibitors of the Carcinogenic Process

A variety of factors that tend to inhibit the progression of the carcinogenic process have been identified. They include dietary factors such as antioxidants, inducers of metabolic deactivation, and inhibitors of metabolic activation; host resistance factors; scavengers of electrophiles; error-free DNA repair mechanisms; and hormones that induce differentiation.

Activated carcinogens, certain viruses, and radiation are factors that are known to be capable of reactivating oncogenes, or modifying their expression, which causes the malignant properties of cancer cells. They do this by modifying the host DNA in such a way that the oncogene sequences are "exposed" for their expression. For example, recently it has been shown that there are "viral enhancer elements," which are DNA sequences of a virus that increase the efficiency of a promotor of oncogene expression. These enhancers are thought to be very important in initiating oncogene expression (Brady et al. 1984). Most activated carcinogens do not permanently bind to the host cell's DNA, however, to be incorporated in daughter cells. Several protective mechanisms work to preclude this devastating change to the cell.

One protective factor is thought to be the need for at least two separate oncogenes in the right combination to be activated for the cell to express malignancy (two changes from a carcinogen, the second made more probable by promotors). There are also built-in DNA repair mechanisms in normal cells which cut out defective or modified DNA segments and replace them with correct nucleotides (DNA subunits) from the nucleus. In addition, some DNA changes are lethal to the cell, so malignancy is halted with the death of the cell. Should daughter cells inherit a gene with a mutation, the stage may be set for a future expressed malignant change. However, a mutation may occur on any of a cell's roughly 50,000 genes, most of which have nothing to do with cancer, so most transformed cells do not go on to become cancerous. It is interesting that approximately 20 percent of cancers are thought by some geneticists working in the field to be associated with conditions of faulty DNA repair (Rensberger 1984).

It should be noted that even when a disease such as cancer is established, it may not be clinically detected. The period from the time of the actual onset to the point at which the disease can be clinically detected is called the latency period. This period differs depending on the particular condition and the methods available for detecting it. Figure 2.1 describes the progression of the carcinogenic process.

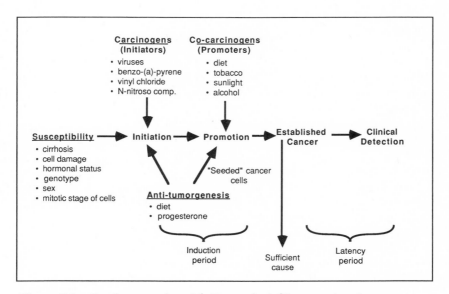

Figure 2.1   Carcinogenesis, with Examples of Intervening Agents

Summary of Carcinogenesis

A summary of how initiators, promotors, and oncogenes may interact in at least some cancers is as follows: The first cellular mutation—initiation—by a carcinogen sensitizes the cell to the actions of a relevant promotor, through the new expression of an oncogene. The promotor allows the preferential proliferation of the initiated cell over neighboring cells, so more initiated cells are available for a second mutation. As more time passes, the pool of transformed cells available for a second mutation increases, so with increasing time, the probability of an ultimate cancerous mutation increases. If a promotor is removed, the rate of increase in the number of sensitized cells is slowed, decreasing the likelihood of cancer. Unfortunately, the initiated cells may look and behave like normal cells, so there is no way yet possible to detect their presence. A second mutation, which escapes the defensive mechanisms present in the cell, completes the malignant transformation. Only if the required combination of oncogenes are exposed, however, will a cancer develop.

This suggested scenario explains why the tissues that have rapidly proliferating cells, such as the gastrointestinal tract, the skin, endometrium, and lung, tend to have higher rates of cancer incidence, and why slowly replicating tissues such as the nerves and brain rarely become malignant.

Oncogenes

Tumor cells contain reactivated genes that probably evolved to operate during embryonic development but that were supposed thereafter to shut down permanently. These cancer genes, referred to as oncogenes, or onc genes, have recently been receiving wide attention. Their reactivation is considered to be one means, at least, by which a cell is transformed from normal to malignant. These reactivated oncogenes regulate certain cell processes that cause the characteristic properties of cancer cells.

Oncogenes have been found in all human cells, where they are sometimes referred to as cellular oncogenes, and in certain viruses, where they are called viral oncogenes. A number of specific human oncogenes have been identified. Several have been classified as part of the "ras" gene family because of their relatedness to certain viral oncogenes with the ras designation. The activated oncogene has only one amino acid change from the normal or "protooncogene" DNA form (Kamata and Feramisco 1984).

Metastasis

The mechanism that allows cancer cells to divide and spread throughout the host body to establish new pockets of growth is not yet well understood. This spreading of cancer cells from the original point of development is called metastasis. Metastasis is not haphazard. The genetic makeup of the cancer cell is altered in specific ways depending on the corresponding normal cell type, so that the altered cell has an affinity for certain areas of the body over others, and relatively consistent patterns of metastasis develop that are distinct for each cancer type. Metastasis is the major cause of death from cancer. Unfortunately, many times in clinical oncology it happens that the metastasic cancer cells are resistent to therapies that were effective in removing the primary cancer. This is due to the fact that, in general, metastases do not result from the random survival of cells released from the primary tumor; rather, they result from the selective survival and growth of specialized malignant cells that preexist in the parent tumor. Metastasis is the selective emergence of preexistent subpopulations of tumor cells endowed with special properties that allow them to survive throughout the body. It has been shown that at least some tumor masses have cells that are biologically diverse, and it is becoming more certain that this genetic heterogeneity is responsible for many of the treatment failures seen in metastatic cancer care (Rensberger 1984). The cancer process, from its inception, is shown in Figure 2.2.

Current Concepts in Cancer Epidemiology

Over the last few decades, epidemiology has progressed from a largely common sense-based research discipline into a distinct research field with clear methodology and a set of formal ideas. The organization of epidemiology into a refined research discipline coincided with the concomitant rise of the field of oncology as a distinct medical specialty and the birth of the computer age. These three separate phenomena are currently coordinated into the modern field of cancer epidemiology.

Nurses in almost any practice deal with cancer patients or individuals who will one day be diagnosed with cancer. An understanding of current theories from the field of cancer epidemiology will allow them to speak knowledgeably with other professionals on related topics and to offer health teaching that includes information designed to modify cancer risk. Current baccalaureate nursing programs teach

1. Carcinogenic substances are breathed into lungs. They may also enter in food and by absorption through the skin.

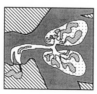

2. Carcinogens enter cells that contain detoxification enzymes.

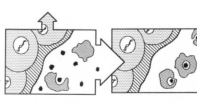

2a. Vast majority of carcinogen molecules are detoxified and put into a form that can be excreted in urine.

3. Activated carcinogen binds to many sites in cell. If it binds at a specific site on DNA, it can cause a mutation when cell divides.

3a. Normally, DNA repair mechanism removes bound carcinogen and repairs damaged gene.

4. Cancer requires more than one altered gene. Chance of second mutation is increased by promoter molecules that favor proliferation of altered cells over normal cells. Thus more altered cells are exposed for repeat of steps 2 and 3.

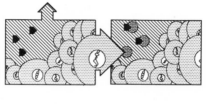

4a. Evidence suggests some anticancer substances work by blocking action of promoters and other substances that transform normal cells into cancer cells.

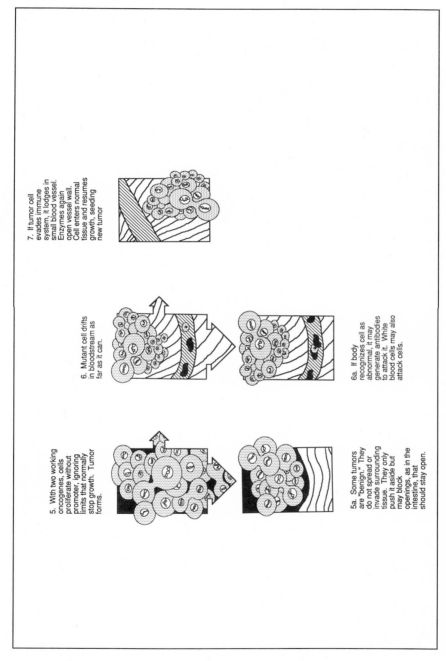

Figure 2.2 How Cancer Works

Reprinted by permission from Boyce Rensberger, "Cancer: The New Synthesis," *Science 84*, pp. 30–31. © 1984, American Association for the Advancement of Science. Modified from illustration by R. Gettier-Street.

5. With two working oncogenes, cells proliferate without promoter, ignoring limits that normally stop growth. Tumor forms.

5a. Some tumors are "benign." They do not spread or invade surrounding tissue. They only push it aside but may block openings, as in the intestine, that should stay open.

6. Mutant cell drifts in bloodstream as far as it can.

6a. If body recognizes cell as abnormal, it may generate antibodies to attack it. White blood cells may also attack cells.

7. If tumor cell evades immune system, it lodges in small blood vessel. Enzymes again open vessel wall. Cell enters normal tissue and resumes growth, seeding new tumor

basic epidemiological principles as part of their curriculums; the cancer nurse needs more specialized information to be thoroughly grounded in the subject of cancer care.

Less than forty years ago, cancer was considered to be a natural part of aging. When epidemiological research began to implicate factors from the environment in the production of the disease, a profound change in the field of cancer care occurred. The possibility that prevention of cancer was possible took hold. This major conceptual change regarding the nature of cancer production among researchers occurred in the 1950s with the accumulation of evidence implicating cigarette smoking in lung cancer. Today, it is becoming increasingly apparent that (1) the environment is responsible for at least part of the cancer burden on society, and (2) the relationship is not a simple one.

At the national level, cancer researchers have embarked on projects aimed at reducing the cancer burden 40 to 50 percent by the year 2000. To accomplish this, scientists expect cancer control to stem from four major areas: reduction in smoking, improved diet, wider use of screening, and improved treatment methods. The reduction in the incidence of cancer expected to result from less smoking is 15 percent; from improved diet, 10 percent; and from screening and treatment, 5 and 20 percent respectively. These estimates, which appear dramatic, reflect a profound change in the way cancer research is being funded at the national level. In the 1920s, emphasis was on diagnosis and treatment. Physician education and case-finding were the methods engaged to curb cancer mortality. In the 1960s emphasis shifted to cancer cures. Enormous sums of money were expended in an effort to find the treatment that would prove effective against cancer. In addition, basic "bench" scientists were tasked with finding the key to cancer causation that would alleviate this disease altogether. In the early 1980s, Congress still persisted in emphasizing a curative approach to cancer research funding, but scientists successfully lobbied for sizable sums to be earmarked for preventive research. This shift was based on the recognition that if etiologic factors in cancer causation were identified and eliminated, then cancer could be prevented even if its exact mechanism was never fully understood. This type of research is the epidemiologic approach. Current recommendations for cancer prevention are summarized in Table 2.1.

Causation, Susceptibility, and Carcinogens

In reviewing causation, first a consideration of what the word means is necessary. Epidemiologists have formulated a general model

Table 2.1   Primary and Secondary Elements in Cancer Prevention

Primary

Smoking	Cigarette smoking is responsible for 85% of lung cancer cases among men and 75% among women—about 83% overall. If the number of smokers was reduced by half, 75,000 lives would be saved each year. Smoking accounts for about 30% of all cancer deaths.
Nutrition	Risk for colon, breast and uterine cancers increases for obese people. High-fat diet may be a factor in the development of certain cancers such as breast, colon and prostate. High-fiber foods may help reduce risk of colon cancer. Foods rich in vitamins A and C may help lower risk for cancers of larynx, esophagus and lung. Eating cruciferous vegetables may help protect against certain cancers. Salt-cured, smoked and nitrite-cured foods have been linked to esophageal and stomach cancer. The heavy use of alcohol, especially when accompanied by cigarette smoking or chewing tobacco, increases risk of cancers of the mouth, larynx, throat, esophagus, and liver. (See below)
Sunlight	Almost all of the 400,000 cases of nonmelanoma skin cancer developed each year in the U.S. are considered to be sun-related. Recent epidemiological evidence shows that sun exposure is a major factor in the development of melanoma and that the incidence increases for those living near the equator.
Alcohol	Oral cancer and cancers of the larynx, throat, esophagus, and liver occur more frequently among heavy drinkers of alcohol.
Smokeless Tobaccos	Increased risk factor for cancers of the mouth, larynx, throat, and esophagus. Highly habit forming.
Estrogen	For mature women, certain risks associated with estrogen treatment to control menopausal symptoms, including an increased risk of endometrial cancer. However, estrogen can be given safely under careful physician control.
Radiation	Excess exposure to X ray can increase cancer risk. Most medical X rays are adjusted to deliver the lowest dose possible without sacrificing image quality.
Occupational Hazards	Exposure to a number of industrial agents (nickel, chromate, asbestos, vinyl chloride, etc.) increases risk. Risk factor greatly increased when combined with smoking.

Secondary

Colorectal tests	The ACS recommends three tests for the early detection of colon and rectum cancer in people without symptoms. The digital rectal examination, performed by a physician during

Table 2.1   Continued

	an office visit, should be performed every year after the age of 40; the stool blood test is recommended every year after 50; and the proctosigmoidoscopy examination should be carried out every 3 to 5 years after the age of 50 following two annual exams with negative results.
Pap test	For the average risk person, a Pap test is recommended annually until two consecutive satisfactory tests are negative, and then once every three years. The Pap test is highly effective in detecting cancer of the uterine cervix, but is less effective in detecting endometrial cancer.
Breast cancer detection	The ACS recommends the monthly practice of breast self-examination (BSE) by women 20 years and older as a routine good health habit. Physical examination of the breast should be done every three years from ages 20–40 and then every year. The ACS recommends a mammogram every year for asymptomatic women age 50 and over, and a baseline mammogram between ages 35 and 39. Women 40 to 49 should have mammography every 1–2 years, depending on physical and mammographic findings.

Source: American Cancer Society, *1985 Cancer Facts and Figures,* 17.

of causation to facilitate the conceptualization of problems. They distinguish between sufficient causes and components of sufficient causes. A *sufficient cause* is one that will inevitably produce the effect. In biological models and cancer models in particular, a sufficient cause is very difficult to identify. Components of sufficient causes, however, increase the probability of the effect by their presence but require the presence of other components to produce it. The causes that epidemiologists study as causal risk factors are component causes. Although these causal risk factors are not sufficient to exert the effect by themselves, blocking their action will prevent the outcome, at least through one mechanism.

Components of sufficient causes have been described as either active or passive. *Passive component causes,* which establish the fertile soil in which other components may grow, are often called susceptibility factors. *Susceptibility factors* are generally considered to be specific genetic characteristics, lifestyle, and physical conditions. In common parlance, *active component causes* are referred to as carcinogenic factors and may be promotors or initiators. *Carcinogenic factors* include chemicals in many forms, taken for pleasure, by accident, or unknowingly; radiation; certain viruses; contaminated foodstuffs;

dietary factors; hormones in certain cases; and other elements of the environment. The distinction between susceptibility factors and carcinogenic factors, in areas such as "physical conditions," is somewhat arbitrary.

An example of how removal of a sufficient cause component affected the incidence of a cancer in the United States recently is the story of exogenous estrogen and uterine cancer. In an effort to address the distress of women experiencing "hot flashes" post-menopausally, physicians began, in the late 1960s, routinely prescribing estrogen, which was effective in alleviating the discomfort and postponing other distressing body changes. By the middle 1970s, epidemiologists became aware of an epidemic of uterine corpus cancer and were able to show that its increase coincided with the use of post-menopausal estrogen over a number of years. Once the relationship was identified, physicians stopped the prescription of estrogen for extended periods of time, and within several years the incidence rate began decreasing. Today, it is suggested that long–term use of exogenous estrogen acts as a promotor for uterine cancer. Thus, although the hormone acting alone was certainly not responsible for causing uterine cancer, progression of the carcinogenic process was slowed or halted by its withdrawal from the population at risk.

For a variety of reasons, researchers concerned with public health are concentrating efforts on eliminating promotors rather than initiators. In terms of producing the greatest good for the greatest number of people, this strategy makes good sense because of the way these two classes of carcinogens operate. While initiation results from a limited exposure to the carcinogen and is considered irreversible, promotors usually require repeated exposure at frequent intervals and their carcinogenic effect is often reversible. Thus, limiting the promotor's effect in the population could prevent the occurence of disease and also reverse malignant changes in individuals even if efforts were not 100 percent effective. In the case of initiators, however, efforts would have to be much more effective to curb disease incidence.

The post-initiation phase occurs over a long period of time. The factors which influence it are perhaps the most important subject we need to understand to reduce cancer risk effectively.

How the Body Handles Carcinogens

Dangerous substances have been around ever since the time of the cave man—mushrooms, hydrocarbons in smoke and broiled meat, and the natural insecticides in plants, for example. The fact that modern society has caused a tremendous explosion in the number of chemicals to which we are exposed daily does not mean that we are inherently unable to cope with this new threat. Every time an individual smokes a cigarette, eats fruit laced with traces of insecticides, eats a food artificially colored, or absorbs a solvent through the skin, the liver gears up to rid the body of the chemicals ingested or absorbed. This is partly accomplished by an amazing and powerful enzyme system of the liver referred to as cytochrome P–450, a mixed-function enzyme system.

Whether a person eats an apple, swallows a pill or drinks contaminated water, the body reacts in the same way. It breaks down the substance in the liver, utilizes any part it can, and excretes the rest through the kidneys. In order to be excreted through the kidneys, a substance must first be made water soluble. Substances that are water soluble when ingested, like penicillin, are excreted intact. Many substances dissolve only in fat, however, and so must be processed by the liver before being used or excreted. The mixed function enzyme systems of the liver, which are activated by many carcinogenic chemicals, serve as the body's main line of defense against many kinds of poisons and chemicals and are partly responsible for the survival of the human race. They also play a role in the prevention of many cancers. Why, then, are certain chemicals carcinogenic to man when the enzyme systems dismantle them? Studies have shown that some human carcinogens are really precarcinogens that require several biotransformations before being able to cause cancer. For example, a common carcinogen, benzo(a)pyrene is transformed in the liver to about forty different metabolites, some of which are highly reactive substances. Other studies have indicated that certain individuals have a combination of detoxifying liver enzymes that tends to produce harmful metabolites rather than inert ones for excretion.

The complexity of the liver detoxifying enzyme systems is only just beginning to be appreciated. Stimulation of the system affects the body's store of natural vitamins and steroid hormones by increasing the rate of their metabolism as well as that of the triggering substance. Some 200 chemicals have been shown to speed up biotransformation by inducing the synthesis of cytochrome P–450s. Thus, while increasing the rate of removal of carcinogens, activation of the P–450s may increase the body's need for fat-soluble vitamins. Many substances, on the other hand, slow down biotransformation by inactivating or inhibiting the P–450s. Lead is such a substance.

By far the greatest influence on the efficiency of an individual's cytochrome P–450 system is genetic inheritance. A specific gene called "Ah locus" controls the induction of cytochrome P–450s upon exposure to aromatic hydrocarbons (carcinogens) and thus may play a role in individual susceptibility to cancer. Rapid induction of the P–450s in response to aromatic hydrocarbons releases reactive metabolites so rapidly that the body may not be able to excrete them quickly enough to prevent their effect on cells. Slower induction of the P–450 system would be an advantage in this case. The cruciferous vegetables have been shown to activate the P–450 system and are associated with a decrease in the risks of many cancers studied. Therefore, it seems likely that a highly reactive P–450 system is advantageous in the vast majority of situations. The role of genetic differences in liver detoxifying systems is unclear at this time.

As scientists now have to take into account the interactions of diet, chemicals, environment, living habits, and genetics in determining cancer risk, the complexity of the task is seen to be enormous.

The Epidemiological Method

The goal of epidemiology is to establish causation, and the establishment of an association and its quantitative estimation are the hallmark of epidemiologic studies. Statistical determination of confidence limits is made to establish the relative importance of chance in the numbers generated. To quantify the relationship between cases and populations, epidemiologists primarily use three methods: measures of incidence, prevalence, and mortality. They also study descriptive elements of cancer in terms of agent, host, and environment or person, time, and place. Table 2.2 illustrates how mortality rates show important trends in the cancer experience of the United States.

Incidence

The number of new cases of cancer in a specified period of time and in a defined population is the cancer incidence. This frequency measure can be expressed in two basic ways, as a probability or as an instantaneous rate of occurrence. Incidence expressed as a probability would be a fraction between 0 and 1.0. For example, the probability that a person of age seventy will develop cancer is about 0.015 over one year. Much more frequently, the incidence is expressed as a rate. For example, the incidence rate of stomach cancer among Japanese males is 91.4 per 100,000 men. Because specific cancers occur rarely in the population relative to many infectious diseases, rates are usually expressed per 100,000 in order to yield case numbers large enough for useful comparisons to be made. In practice, rates may

Table 2.2   Thirty-Year Trends—Age-adjusted Cancer Death Rates per 100,000, 1949–51 to 1979–81

Sex	Site	1949–51	1979–81	Percent change
M	All sites	168	217	+29
F	All sites	148	136	−8
M	Prostate	21	23	+9
F	Breast	26	26	N.S.
M	Colorectal	26	25	N.S.
F	Colorectal	25	19	−27
M	Lung	22	71	+224
F	Lung	5	21	+331
M	Pancreas	8	11	+29
F	Pancreas	6	7	+27
M	Stomach	25	8	−66
F	Stomach	14	4	−71
F	Ovary	8	8	N.S.
F	Uterus	22	8	−64
M	Leukemia	7	9	+19
F	Leukemia	5	5	N.S.

Source: American Cancer Society, *1985 Cancer Facts and Figures.*

sometimes be noted as a single figure, and a standard 100,000 reference population is assumed. When reading epidemiologic literature, care should be taken to note the size of the reference population, however, as rates per million, or cases as a function of some other figure, are also used.

Prevalence

The number of cases, both old and new, that are present at a point in time in a defined population is the cancer prevalence. Figures on cancer prevalence are not regularly available in any population, as they are derived from surveys that are difficult to conduct. The difficulty arises from the lack of agreement on when a person may be considered no longer to have cancer, if treatment is completed and no active disease seen. Rather than attempting to determine the prevalence of cancer, sometimes a "cancer load" is measured. The cancer load is defined as the number of persons in a population with either present cancer or a past history of cancer. Incidence data is the best frequency measurement for use in the study of disease etiology, as it the incidence that will directly change as a factor of different exposures to initiators or promotors of cancer.

Mortality

The number of deaths due to cancer in a specified time period and in a defined population is the cancer mortality. Cancer mortality is the most widely available frequency measurement. Similar conceptually to incidence, mortality can be expressed as a probability or as an instantaneous rate. The comments concerning incidence data apply equally to mortality data. Because of the way that deaths are reported, cancer mortality figures have an element of inaccuracy in them. If an ill cancer patient succumbs to pneumonia, the death might be attributed to either the cancer or the pneumonia, depending on the way the physician completed the death certificate. This is a rather simplified example of how inaccuracies can occur; more complex difficulties with reported cancer mortality figures also exist. Figure 2.3 illustrates the cancer experience in the United States from 1930 through 1981. The changes in rates for stomach and lung cancer are dramatically apparent.

Epidemiologists are most concerned with disease etiology, therefore cancer incidence is the most appropriate frequency measurement to apply. Many times, however, mortality data is what is available to use. Because mortality data and incidence data do not correlate exactly, that is, each cancer case does not result in a cancer death, mortality rates must be carefully applied to epidemiologic problem solving. The presentation of information in Table 2.3 is useful for conceptualization of the relative importance of various cancers as a function of incidence.

The Epidemiologic Triad

Agent, host, and environment are a triad of concepts sometimes used by epidemiologists to study cancer causation. Although the epidemiologic triad is more frequently applied to studies of infectious processes, the concepts can be adapted to the study of cancer etiology. Factors that are derived from the innate properties of the agent (for example, viral oncogenes) are studied in order to define methods more effectively to control their expression in the population. These factors include morphology, antigenic character, growth requirements, ability to survive outside a host, spectrum of hosts, and the

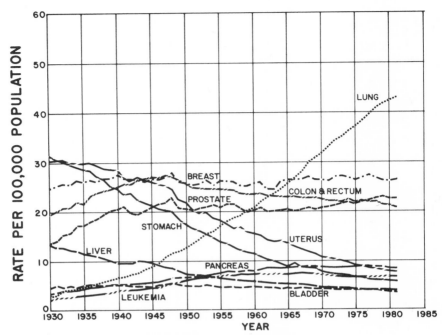

*Rate for the population standardized for age on the 1970 U.S. population
Sources of Data: National Center for Health Statistics and
Bureau of the Census, United States.
Note: Rates are for both sexes combined except breast and uterus female population only
and prostate male population only.

Figure 2.3   Cancer Death Rates by Sites, United States, 1930–81
Reprinted by permission from *1985 Cancer Facts and Figures*, p. 11. © 1985, American Cancer Society.

Table 2.3   United States Cancer Incidence—1986 Estimates

	Males	Females
melanoma	3%	2%
oral	4%	2%
pancreas	3%	3%
urinary	9%	4%
leukemia/lymphoma	8%	7%
ovary	—	4%
uterus	—	11%
colorectal	14%	16%
prostate	19%	—
breast	—	26%
lung	22%	11%
other sites	18%	14%

Source: National Cancer Institutes.

ability to become resistant to antineoplastic drugs or to produce toxins.

Host factors that influence resistance or susceptibility to the effects of an agent include age, race, sex, genetic makeup, immune status, physical state, and behavioral factors. Many differences in host resistance and susceptibility exist for various cancer types.

The environment influences the existence of the agent and opportunities for exposure. Carcinogens and promotors are particularly important aspects of the environment considered in the study of cancer etiology.

Person, Time and Place

Person, time, and place are classic descriptive epidemiologic variables that serve as a major source of clues to cancer etiology. Age pattern, sex, and racial differences observed in rates for various cancers are fundamental in descriptive cancer epidemiology. Time trends often offer clues to cancer etiology. Epidemiologists may study changes in the environment that coincide with changes in cancer mortality rates to generate hypotheses of causative factors involved. Variations observed in the occurrence of cancer in different geographical locations have been extremely important in generating hypotheses of cancer etiology. Because the globe offers the scientist an immense pool of highly variable conditions to study, geographic comparisons have been a very successful modality employed to help determine influences on cancer rates. Trends in survival rates may reflect risk factor exposure changes, treatment changes, or a combination of both. Figure 2.4 illustrates survival changes for major cancer sites.

Study Designs

In epidemiology, case-control studies are most frequently employed to study cancer etiology. In this study design, individuals with the cancer under consideration are compared to controls from the population regarding the factor hypothesized to exert an effect on cancer incidence. An estimation of the relative risk of acquiring the cancer when exposed to the factor is generated. A better design in terms of establishing the relationship between cancer and a factor is the cohort study. In this design, the researcher first picks a group of people who do not have the cancer being considered but who are exposed to the implicated factor, and also picks a group without the cancer who are not exposed to the factor. Then the two groups are

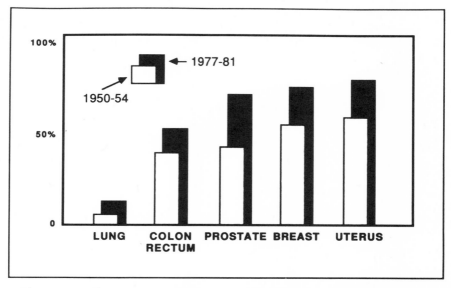

Figure 2.4   Five-Year Cancer Survival Rates: Trends for Selected Sites, 1950–54 and 1977–81

Reprinted by permission from *1985 Cancer Facts and Figures,* p. 11. © 1985, American Cancer Society.

followed through time, and differences in the occurence of the cancer are noted for each group. In this case, a direct relative risk can be established between the factor and cancer type. Although there are other study designs used in epidemiology, the case-control study and cohort study are the two most widely employed. Variations in these two designs are used to fit different situations encountered by the epidemiologist.

Factors in Cancer Etiology

The factors selected for inclusion in this work—diet, chemicals and drugs, pollution, radiation, tobacco, viral oncogenes, and hormones—are those that are currently under intense scrutiny and for which there is established evidence of their role in cancer etiology. Readers interested in more complete coverage of the role of specific factors in cancer etiology are referred to the selected bibliography at the end of this chapter.

Dietary Factors

In the fall of 1985 at the Second National Conference on Diet, Nutrition and Cancer, a panel of experts responded with a resounding silence when pressed to suggest specific dietary recommendations on schedules and quantities of vitamins and nutrients discussed during the conference. The data are so new, and replications so few, that to go to the public with such recommendations would have been premature. A number of different agencies, including the National Cancer Institute (NCI) and American Cancer Society (ACS), have provided professionals and the public with dietary recommendations that take into account the diet and cancer research to date. Based on the available information, the ACS's position is that the modifications represent a healthy, medically sound diet that is appropriate for the general public irrespective of its potential for reducing cancer risk. Evidence does exist that dietary factors influence cancer risk, but specific doses, schedules, and contraindications that would be appropriate are not yet available.

This section provides information from biochemical and epidemiological research on the relationship of nutrients and cancer incidence. However, a cautionary note must be made initially; that is, the laws of probability indicate that some of what is purported today will ultimately prove woefully incomplete when further research is done. The danger in embracing new information before the mechanism of action or circumstantial differences in effects of the substance are understood is illustrated by the case of vitamin C.

Vitamin C has been shown to inhibit the action of many carcinogens and is especially effective in detoxifying nitrosamines and nitrosamides in the stomach. This sounds very good and may suggest that it would be a useful dietary tool against cancer. It is useful; however, one would want to caution against recommending large doses of vitamin C to a bladder cancer patient. Recent studies show that, in some animal models, vitamin C actually promotes bladder cancer, and the research may prove applicable to humans. With so much unknown about the effects on various tissues of vitamin C taken in quantities beyond those considered part of a good, general diet, prudent use is indicated.

Self-medicating or taking supplements of a substance based on initially promising research data could prove unwise. The interaction of nutrients with each other and with various body enzyme systems and changes in the in-vivo environment all need to be considered before a nutrient can be recommended with adequate accompanying cautionary information.

It may be recalled that the reduction in cancer incidence by the year 2000 from changes in dietary habits is projected at around 10 percent. Doll and Peto (1981) compiled information suggesting that diet may be responsible for 10 to 70 percent of the environmental cancer risk. The wide range in the risk estimates cited indicates the current uncertainty about the importance diet will ultimately be found to have in the population-attributable risk of cancer. Some researchers suggest that diet will have the greatest significance in overall cancer risk second only to tobacco use in years to come.

With these caveats noted, the following information is presented for use in helping individuals understand how to modify their diet to minimize cancer risk and to inform the health provider about the direction research is taking regarding some diet-related issues.

MUTAGENS AND CARCINOGENS IN THE FOOD SUPPLY

Within the limits of current testing ability, the risk from mutagens and carcinogens in the average diet of Americans is probably very small. Most of the known mutagens that contaminate foods are seen in undeveloped countries. Aflatoxin B1, the most potent liver carcinogen known, is produced through the metabolism of molds. It is usually seen in warm humid areas of Africa and the Far East, and is carefully regulated in U.S. food supplies. Unfortunately, it cannot be entirely eliminated from foods, only carefully controlled. It is a contaminant of grains, peanuts, tree nuts, and beans.

Several spices, including oil of sassafras and tarragon, have known carcinogens in their chemical make-up, but are not used in large amounts in the typical American diet. Mushrooms, including the commercial variety, contain hydrazines, which are carcinogenic, but are not a major part of typical diets and thus pose minimal risk.

Twenty-five percent of the background radiation Americans receive is from food, as soil and ground water are contaminated from natural processes. This is an entirely insignificant amount of radioactivity from a mutagenic perspective. It is also impossible to regulate. The irradiation of foods, discussed recently as a means of sterilization, is not a process which results in radioactivity in foods.

Nitrosamines, which were once plentiful in cheese, beer, and preserved meat, have been reduced to a great extent subsequent to legislation (primarily the Delaney Act) and popular concern. The meat industry is currently using a liquid curing process, rather than the traditional smoking process, which reduces the burden of nitrosamines, which are carcinogens.

The role of pesticides in cancer risk is largely unknown but considered small. Despite widespread exposure of the general public to low levels of pesticides for a considerable period of time, no trends of increased cancer incidence attributable to this factor have been clearly identified.

The carcinogen polyvinyl chloride is widely used for food storage containers. It has been detected in alcoholic drinks, vinegar, margarine, and finished drinking water. Although it has been shown to cause cancer when ingested in large amounts in animals, no studies have been done to date on its effect as a contaminant of foods.

It is currently felt that most cancer risk in nutrition comes not from the contamination of foods, but from deficiencies or excesses of specific nutrients or nonnutrient factors in the general food supply.

DIETARY FAT

Of all the dietary components studied to date, fat is the one for which there is the most extensive and compelling evidence for an association with cancer. The original implication of dietary fat in the etiology of various cancers came from international studies showing that nations with a low per capita intake of fat also showed a lower incidence of several cancer types. Cancers of the breast, colon, endometrium, ovary, prostate, and perhaps kidney are today considered to be linked to dietary fat. The most complete evidence links fat with breast and colon cancer. As the data become more refined, different types of fats are being shown to alter cancer risk dissimilarly.

Unsaturated vegetable fats have been shown to be more closely linked to some cancers than the highly saturated oils, such as olive or coconut oil. This difference between the effect of saturated and unsaturated oils on cancer promotion tends to disappear when the total fat in the diet exceeds 20 percent. Of course, it has been well documented that polyunsaturated oils are more protective against heart disease than saturated oils. However, when fat intake is maintained between 5 and 20 percent of total calories, saturated oils have been shown to result in fewer cancerous tumors in animals. Menhaden oil, a polyunsaturated fish oil, may prove to be an exception to the rule of saturated oils being more protective in tumorigenesis. In animal models, it acts to actually suppress some cancers. The inclusion of fish in American diets may prove helpful in reducing the risk of some cancers and is consistent with a generally healthy diet. Fish eaten twice a week has been shown to reduce cancer risk.

Two very different populations with similar low incidence rates of breast cancer are the Eskimos and the Japanese. The Eskimos' very high fat diet would predispose them to an increased risk of breast cancer. Their actual low rates may be attributable to the regular, plentiful inclusion of fish in their diet. By contrast, the Japanese normally have a diet containing about 10 percent fat. Compared to the usual American diet, which contains some 40 percent fat, this is a very austere consumption pattern. These two populations demonstrate that different dietary patterns can yield favorable results in terms of reducing cancer risk.

There is general agreement that obesity is correlated with endometrial cancer. Because of a close association between fat consumption and obesity, the cancers associated with fat consumption are also more common in the obese. The endometrium is a highly estrogen-responsive organ; it is considered possible that fats and hormonal regulation may play a role together in the development of endometrial cancer in susceptible persons.

Fat studies in animals have shown that when a high fat diet is reversed to a low fat diet, the incidence of cancer decreases rapidly in the animal population. In humans, it is suggested from population studies that the risk of cancer changes in such cases in a period of one to two years (DeWys 1985). It has been demonstrated, however, that there is a point of no return in regard to fat consumption and cancer incidence. If a high fat diet is consumed beyond a certain period, reversal proves ineffective. Whether this threshold effect applies to humans is presently unknown, but it is considered very likely. If fat acts as a promotor in carcinogenesis, this threshold model would fit very well.

Appropriate guidelines that may be suggested for fat consumption are: first, reduce fat to 30 percent of calories (the best goal would be to achieve 20 percent of calories from fat, but that would probably prove unpalatable to most Americans); secondly, include high fiber foods in the diet, as low fat and high fiber seem to act synergistically.

COOKING METHODS

Practices that could reduce the carcinogenic potential of foods include modifying cooking methods that are commonly employed. When proteins (primarily meats) are grilled over open flames or coals, benzo(a)pyrene, a powerful carcinogen and cancer initiator, is produced by the smoke generated from fat dripping onto the heat source. Charcoal broiling also produces other powerful mutagens besides benzo(a)pyrene. The blackened portion of meats prepared this way contains the carcinogens. Placing a barrier such as aluminum foil between the heat source and meat can reduce the risk of generating benzo(a)pyrene in the food. Recent research also suggests that cooking proteins at high temperatures creates carcinogens that are not produced with low-temperature cooking. Whether the same burning mechanism is responsible or some other process produces the effect is uncertain. Since frying fish or meat in fat that has been used repeatedly can also produce benzo(a)pyrene, it is advisable to discard oil once it has been used for frying.

The overall importance of carcinogen-producing cooking methods to the total population's burden of cancer is considered very small. At the same time, changing cooking habits to reflect safer methods may prove a relatively easy way to chip away at cancer incidence.

FIBER

There is epidemiological evidence that suggests a negative correlation between colorectal cancer incidence and total fiber intake. Most studies on fiber and cancer risk have looked at total fiber rather than at the impact of specific components. The fiber component of foods may be in the form of cellulose, lignin, hemicelluloses, pentosans, gums, and/or pectins. These substances provide the bulk in the diet and are found in vegetables, fruits, and whole-grain cereals. Fiber in the diet produces larger, softer stools, more frequent defecation and more rapid intestinal transit time. The mode of action of fiber in inhibiting colon cancer is not yet understood, although large studies have indicated that there is no relationship between constipation and colon cancer, so fiber may not exert its inhibitory effect through this mechanism.

Populations that have a high fiber diet are at low risk for colon cancer, while those with a low fiber, high fat diet tend to show high incidence rates for this malignancy. High fiber diets are also associated with lower risks for appendicitis, diverticulosis, and colonic polyps.

Some evidence exists that pectin may be an important fiber source protecting primarily the upper intestinal tract, while bran protects the lower gastrointestinal tract. Some scientists dispute the protective value of fiber, suggesting that other qualities of the high fiber foods, particularly fruits and vegetables, are responsible for cancer risk reductions. Even if fiber itself does not prove protective against cancer, the high fiber foods are protective and can be recommended as wholesome substitutes for fatty foods.

CRUCIFEROUS VEGETABLES

Cruciferous vegetables belong to the mustard family, whose flowers have four parts that form the pattern of a cross. They include brussel sprouts, cabbage, broccoli, kohlrabi, rutabagas, turnips, and cauliflower. These plants probably exert their anticancer effect by inducing increased activity of enzyme systems that detoxify carcinogenic agents (cytochrome P–450 liver enzyme systems described earlier). These vegetables contain indole–3–acetonitrile, which is quite stable and the active anticarcinogenic ingredient. The cruciferous vegetables, by acting through the liver detoxifying enzyme systems pathway, would be effective only against cancer initiation and would not affect initiator–activated body cells. Therefore, its *regular* consumption would be most useful in reducing cancer risk. Epidemiologic studies suggest that consumption of these vegetables may reduce cancer risk, particularly of the colon and lung. Although optimal amounts to include in a diet are not yet known, these vegetables could be included at one or more meals at least twice a week as part of a generally healthy diet.

VITAMINS AND MINERALS

One of the reasons that vitamins and minerals may prove very useful against cancer in the future is because it is easier to get members of the public to add useful elements to their diets than to eliminate harmful ones. Those micronutrients that have shown the most promise in reducing cancer risk so far are vitamins A, C, and E, and selenium.

It has been clearly demonstrated that cancer risk is increased with a deficiency of vitamin A in the diet. The role of this vitamin as a supplement in excess of that necessary for good general health is not yet known. Current trials using physicians as subjects are underway to study this question. Most of the data to date come from animal studies since human trials take long periods of time and are difficult to control. Vitamin A in two of its most common forms, retinol (preformed) and beta–carotene (precursor form), was recently studied for anticancer properties. Generally it was found that the beta–carotene form was most active in a cancer protective role (Thomas 1985). Beta–carotene acts as an antioxidant in the body. Found to have low toxicity even with long–term use, it may prove useful as a cancer preventive agent.

Vitamin C inhibits the formation of N–nitroso compounds from nitrites. Nowadays, vitamin C is added to preserved meats to counter the mutagenic effects of the nitrites used in the preservation process. Nitrosamines and nitrosamides have been found to be factors in the induction of human gastric, esophageal, and nasal cancers, and the incidence rates for these cancers are negatively correlated with intake of fresh fruits and vegetables rich in vitamin C. Interestingly, fruits and vegetables are rich in nitrosamines and nitrosamides that they pick up from chemically contaminated soil and water. However, their high vitamin C content more than offsets any potential carcinogenic effect of the N-nitroso compounds. As with vitamin A, a deficiency of vitamin C has been associated with increased cancer risk.

Animal models have shown that very large doses of vitamin C promote the induction of bladder cancer by carcinogens in rats. Thus, vitamin C taken in excess of amounts necessary for good general health should probably not be recommended to those who are at high risk for bladder cancer, such as workers in dye, pest control, paint, rubber, and textile industries.

Vitamin E blocks the formation of carcinogenic nitroso compounds in the body in a manner similar to vitamin C. Because vitamin E is available in a wide variety of foods, and as identifying groups of people with substantially different levels of intake has been difficult, no epidemiology studies have been done on this vitamin.

Death rates for cancers of the head and neck are lower in areas where the soil and foliage contain higher levels of selenium. Animal studies have shown that selenium supplements can reduce the incidence of tumors subsequent to exposure to carcinogens or ultraviolet light. Selenium is toxic when taken in high doses. Therefore, until more exact data is available, deficiencies should be corrected, but supplements are not recommended.

ADDITIVES

Ninety-three percent of all food additives in this country consist of sugar, salt, corn syrup, and dextrose, all of which are quite harmless as they pertain to cancer, except perhaps as promoters of obesity. The two artificial sweeteners in common use today are saccharine and aspartame. Saccharine has shown no ill effects in human trials, although animal studies have suggested a relationship to bladder cancer. Aspartame is made up of two very simple compounds that are eaten daily in large amounts in a typical diet. Scientists are not in accordance on the effect of aspartame on cancer risk, but it is considered generally to be of insignificant risk with moderate consumption.

BHA and BHT are antioxidants and preservatives in common use. BHT has shown both tumor-inhibiting activity and tumor-promotion activity under different circumstances. BHA has shown no promotion of cancer and may, in fact, inhibit neoplasia (DeWys 1985). Further studies are presently underway to clarify the mode of action of these two compounds. They are generally considered to act on the detoxifying enzyme systems of the liver.

In 1960, there were some 200 dyes on the market for use in foods and cosmetics, but by 1984, 63 had been banned by the Food and Drug Administration. Food colorings and flavor enhancers have not all been completely evaluated to date, but are currently under study. Based on animal studies, red dye number 3 is now being considered for removal from food sources by the Food and Drug Administration.

Alcohol

Heavy drinkers of alcohol, especially those who also smoke, are at very high risk for cancers of the oral cavity, larynx, and esophagus. Furthermore, alcohol contributes to cirrhosis, which is linked to liver cancer. Moderation in drinking is an important cancer risk reducing activity. Alcohol appears to act by making epithelial tissues more susceptible to the action of contact carcinogens, particularly those associated with tobacco.

Since these habits may be difficult to inhibit in individuals, it is important that those with these habits establish good nutritional practices, particularly increasing vitamin C and beta-carotene in their diets. Although diet cannot totally eliminate increased risk from exposure to alcohol and tobacco, it may reduce the incidence of esophageal and oral cancers in these individuals.

Chemicals and Drugs

Recent data implicating environmental exposure to chemicals as a factor in the etiology of some cancers have contributed another notion; that is, that these cancers may be preventable. Various authors in the field of environmental carcinogenesis estimate that from 60 to 90 percent of human cancer is environmental in origin. The American Chemical Society lists over 4 million organic and inorganic chemicals, most of which have identified structures. Of the 442 chemicals evaluated in volumes 1 to 20 of the IARC Monographs, 143 were shown to have "sufficient" evidence of carcinogenicity in experimental animals, and there are more than 50,000 chemicals in common use today with hundreds more added each year for which no toxicologic data are available. Evidence for the carcinogenicity of chemicals is obtained from animal models, the Salmonella typhimurium-microsome mutagenicity test and other short-term assays, as well as epidemiological studies, none of which can offer perfect accuracy or keep up with all the chemicals in use or being developed. The list of known human chemical carcinogens is very short and clearly incomplete (see Table 2.4). The list of suspected human carcinogens is much longer and growing steadily.

When one thinks of environmental carcinogens, occupational exposures often first come to mind, but the source for chemical exposures extends to lifestyle habits, such as smoking, the use of cosmetics, or gardening pesticides; drugs for medical use; home heating methods; as well as contamination of the air and water supplies and other exposures.

It is simplistic to expect that reducing exposure to chemicals that clearly or probably cause cancer is a matter of curbing individual choices or stopping their production by industry. We rely on many of the products that result in the generation of carcinogens, and people routinely continue behaviors shown to be hazardous (such as smoking).

A sampling of drugs that have proved to be carcinogenic include hormones, which will be discussed later, and the compounds shown in Table 2.5. It is apparent from this table that the treatment of cancer itself presents a risk for future malignancies—a risk, it is agreed, that is clearly justified. The list of drugs currently being investigated for carcinogenicity is fairly extensive. The use of some of these drugs has

---

Table 2.4 Industrial Processes and Chemicals Judged Carcinogenic for Humans

4-aminobiphenyl
Arsenic and certain arsenic compounds
Asbestos
Manufacture of auramine
Benzene
Benzidine
N,N-bis(2-chloroethyl)-2-naphthylamine (chlornaphazine)
Bis (chloromethyl)ether and technical grade chloromethyl methyl ether
Chromium and certain chromium compounds
Diethylstilbestrol (DES)
Underground hermatite mining
Manufacture of isopropul alcohol by the strong acid process
Melphalan
Mustard gas
2-naphthylamine
Nickel refining
Soots, tars and mineral oils
Vinyl chloride

Note: Authority quoted is the International Agency for Research on Cancer.
Source: Office of Technology Assessment, 1982, 141.

Table 2.5   Examples of Carcinogenic Drugs

Drug	Use	Site of cancer
Arsenicals	In Fowler's solution	Skin
Chlornaphazine (from aniline dye)	Cancer chemotherapy	Bladder
Alkylating agents	Cancer chemotherapy	Leukemia, lymphoma
Immunosuppressives, antimetabolites	Organ transplants, cancer chemotherapy	Reticulum cell sarcoma
Radiopharmaceuticals	Cancer therapy, Diagnostic Tests	Osteosarcoma, liver

Source: Derived from Schottenfeld and Fraumeni 1982, 305.

been largely curtailed informally by physicians or formally by the Food and Drug Administration, even though conclusive evidence implicating them has not yet been established. Others exert important therapeutic effects that justify their continued use.

Reserpine, used for hypertension and some forms of mental illness, has been the subject of controversy over its possible role in breast cancer. Case control studies weigh in on both sides of the issue, with findings against the relationship marginally stronger. Animal studies support the breast cancer association and implicate reserpine in some cancers in males. Phenacetin use in heavy doses over prolonged periods is associated with renal cancer. Its use is being widely restricted. Chloramphenical, clinically associated with leukopenia and aplastic anemia, has been linked to leukemia, although studies are limited. The intramuscular injection of iron has been related to local occurences of fibrosarcoma since the 1960s. Very limited data are available to prove or disprove a causal relationship, however. Phenylbutazone, hydantoin derivatives, amphetamines, and phenobarbitone have each been associated with increased cancer risk in limited studies. Hydantoin deriviatives and phenobarbitone are both currently used in the treatment of epilepsy, and all of these drugs are being actively studied for their carcinogenicity. Coal tar products have been associated with skin cancer, particularly when combined with ultraviolet radiation. Dermatologists, however, have found them to be overwhelmingly safe substances and research continues to determine whether they pose a hazard.

Pollution

AIR POLLUTION

Pollution of the air by industry and home heating measures has been extensively explored for its relationship to human cancers. In 1272, King Edward of England banned the use of smoking coal in order to reduce the tremendous air pollution around London in an early public health protective measure. In recent years, the composition of the pollution generated by various sources has been carefully analyzed and studies have been repeatedly done to ascertain the relationship of cancers and industrial pollutants.

Air pollution can be considered to be composed of two general components: particulates (largely tar and soot), and major gases (carbon monoxide from automobiles and sulfur dioxide from coal and oil use). Sulfur dioxide combined with water produces sulfuric acid, the active component of acid rain. Repeated studies of the relationship of air pollution to increased cancer rates, particularly lung cancer, have shown marginally positive correlation. There has been shown to exist an urban-rural gradient in lung cancer rates; however, studies are inconclusive because smoking tends to be more prevalent in urban areas. The noted result of excess lung cancer beyond that attributable to smoking in urban areas has been small. Furthermore, the excess could be explained by occupational exposures rather than air pollution. To date, air pollution has not been shown to be a significant threat to health in terms of promoting carcinogenesis.

WATER POLLUTION

The quality of drinking water in the United States is considered to be the finest in the world. Nonetheless, finished drinking water throughout the nation has been found to contain microbiologic particulates, radionuclides, solid particulates, inorganic solutes, and organic chemicals in various mixtures.

Studies of asbestos contamination of water have failed to show any excess cancer incidence in high-asbestos contaminated water supply areas—positive studies have been dismissed as too poorly controlled in terms of dietary factors and smoking to support their correlations. Thus the role of asbestos-contaminated water in cancer etiology is still in doubt.

Fluoridation of water has proven innocuous in terms of cancer causation after analysis of epidemiological data. Although major cities with fluoridated water showed higher cancer rates than those without fluoridation in early studies, when socioeconomic risk factors were controlled, the differences disappeared.

Today, synthetic organic chemicals are the focus of much attention by epidemiologists studying water pollution and cancer. Of the hundreds of chemicals known to contaminate water supplies, at least forty have been shown to be carcinogenic, and, to date, most of the others have unknown carcinogenesis potential. Very general ecological studies have shown that various contaminants, primarily chlorine, were associated with gastrointestinal cancers and bladder cancer.

Inorganic arsenic and possibly other trace metals have been implicated in increased skin cancer rates when introduced to water supplies. Animal models have not supported this association, but it is under study in other epidemiologic projects.

The summary evidence is that except in the case of high contamination, such as arsenic in Taiwan water supplies, no waterborne substances pose a significant cancer hazard to Americans. Preliminary evidence for an association with certain cancers exists, but is not expected to prove of high magnitude. The National Cancer Institute is presently conducting a large study of bladder cancer determinants and is including water quality as a factor to be considered.

Radiation

IONIZING RADIATION

The greatest population exposure to ionizing radiation comes from natural background sources and amounts to about 0.130 rad per year. Studies attempting to link background radiation to cancer have all been negative. The second largest source of radiation on populations after background radiation is medical X-rays (not mammographies), which amounts to about 0.077 rad per year average. Occupational exposures, nuclear weapon testing, and nuclear power contribute negligible radiation to the environment (about 0.008 rad per year). Nuclear workers at both the Hanford works in Washington and New Hampshire Naval Shipyard have been studied for excess cancer rates. No excess cancer incidence has been shown to date in these populations.

Ionizing radiation is responsible for less than 3 percent of cancer cases in the United States today. The only significant way of reducing that mortality rate is by eliminating a portion of the medical X-rays that are routinely used in the United States.

In the 1930s and 1940s, before the dangers associated with radiation were fully understood, many children were exposed to radiation at significant doses to treat enlarged thymus glands, tonsilitis, ringworm, and other conditions. A subsequent excess of cancer has been seen in the subpopulations thus exposed.

It is well known from past experiences with radiation, such as the atomic bomb explosions in Japan and other historical incidents, that radiation is a complete carcinogen. It can cause various cancers by itself, particularly leukemia; but the cancer burden from radiation today in the United States is minimal because of very low exposure.

SOLAR RADIATION

The ultraviolet light from the sun has been characterized as UV-C, with the most energy; UV-B with a moderate energy spectrum; and UV-A, with the least energy of the three. UV-C radiation never reaches the earth's surface. UV-A radiation is the portion of the ultraviolet spectrum that produces tanning and that lately has been shown to contribute to the production of cataracts. Large quantities of UV-A are required to produce a biological effect. It is the UV-B part of the spectrum which is of major concern in terms of health risks.

There is good evidence that skin cancer may arise from UV-induced changes in DNA. UV-B is implicated in sunburning, skin aging, and cancer. The ozone layer of the atmosphere is the primary determinant of how much UV-B radiation hits the earth's surface. Protecting the ozone layer is an ecologic necessity.

Sunlight is responsible for the vast majority of squamous and basal cell carcinomas of the skin. It has also been implicated in the incidence of melanoma, although the relationship is not as clear-cut. There is evidence that nonmelanoma skin cancer is associated with cumulative UV-B exposure, while melanoma is associated with intermittent exposure to high intensity UV-B radiation. A big risk factor for melanoma has been found to be blistering sunburn during childhood or adolescence, particularly among poor tanners.

In recent years, there has been a schizophrenic attitude toward sunlight and skin cancer. On the one hand, sunscreens have gained much attention and they are recommended by health care providers. On the other hand, the seriousness of nonmelanoma skin cancers has been largely dismissed in the media. These skin cancers are considered to be inconsequential and entirely curable. However, the American Cancer Society's data indicate that in 1985, nearly 2,000 people were expected to die of nonmelanoma skin cancer in the United States, with melanoma accounting for 5,500 deaths in 1985 (ACS data). Although these numbers are small compared to the total number of cancer cases, nonmelanoma death rates could be lowered by taking the risk seriously and maintaining protection from sunlight; and melanoma incidence might also be reduced significantly.

Populations closest to the equator experience the most exposure to UV-B radiation. Since UV-B is at its highest intensity between the hours of 10 a.m. and 2 p.m., when the sun's rays pass through the least ozone, outdoor activities should be carried on in the early morning and middle-to-late afternoon.

The incidence of both melanoma and nonmelanoma skin cancers has been increasing in recent years. Those at highest risk for developing these cancers are individuals with light skin complexion who sunburn easily and who have red hair with freckles. Melanoma is also more frequent among those with dysplastic nevi syndrome. Melanoma is seen among women most frequently on the legs, while men most frequently experience melanoma on the trunk. Nonmelanoma skin cancers occur generally on those body areas most frequently exposed to the sun, such as the nose, ears, lower lip, and cheeks.

The etiology of melanoma is not dependent solely on total ultraviolet exposure. The best explanation for the distribution of melanoma is that intermittent exposure is most dangerous, particularly during childhood. The total dose of sunlight needed to produce a melanoma lesion is far less than that required for nonmelanoma skin cancers and does not seem to be related to total accumulation. Some recent research has correlated fluorescent lights with melanoma incidence. When fluorescent lights are not enclosed behind plastic diffusers, they emit energy from the UV-B spectrum that may cause biological activity. This would be consistent with the observation that individuals in the upper socioeconomic classes are more likely to get melanoma than those in lower classes, who may be more likely to be exposed to the sun on a regular basis. The office worker may be exposed to much more fluorescent lighting and be more likely to acquire a sunburn over the weekend, both possible risk factors for melanoma.

The total number of moles present on a person's skin is also correlated to the risk of melanoma. The more moles present, especially on the arms, the higher the melanoma risk. Researchers are moving rapidly in the study of melanoma, but right now the evidence indicates that the complete etiology will prove complex and not easily interpreted.

Tobacco

In 1985, lung cancer officially became the biggest cancer killer of both men and women and is overwhelmingly attributable to tobacco smoke inhalation. After three decades of major epidemiologic studies of cigarette smoking and lung cancer, the causative role of tobacco in the etiology of this largely incurable disease is no longer in doubt. Tobacco use is the major public health problem of the world today, contributing enormously to the incidence of various cancers, heart disease, and chronic lung disease.

The cancers that are more frequent among those who use tobacco products are cancers of the larynx, lung, oral cavity, esophagus, pancreas, kidney, and bladder. Some general principles apply to the relationship of tobacco use and cancer. One principle is that the greater the exposure, the greater the risk. The length of time of the habit, amount of produce used, depth and mode of inhalation, and type of produce used are all factors in determining actual exposure. A second principle is that cessation of the habit does not immediately confer a reduced risk. Because there is a long latency period in tobacco-caused cancers, disease risk falls gradually over a fifteen-year period before it approaches that of a nonsmoker. Finally, the relative risk of developing a tobacco-related cancer depends on the susceptibility of specific organ sites to different concentrations of tobacco constituent metabolites. For example, oral cancer incidence is increased with the use of snuff, but lung cancer risk rises less dramatically with the use of this form of tobacco. The greatest carcinogenic effect of tobacco is on those organs with which it comes in direct contact. In some cases, after the enzyme detoxifying systems of the liver metabolize tobacco compounds, but before the kidney can excrete them, organs such as the pancreas, kidney, and bladder are exposed to the active metabolites of tobacco with carcinogenic potential. In these cases, tobacco has a direct carcinogenic effect as well as an indirect one (see Table 2.6).

The use of cigars and pipes results in fewer lung cancer cases than found among cigarette smokers, but is still associated with significantly more lung cancer than is found among nonsmokers. Although cigar and pipe smokers do not inhale as much smoke, they are exposed to sidestream smoke of the burning product.

Passive smoking, or the inhalation of tobacco used by others in one's vicinity, may result in increased lung cancer risk if the amount of smoke present is heavy and encountered over substantial periods of time. Although research on passive smoking is limited, initial studies do not show increased risk with most forms of passive smoking—that is, occasional exposure to a smoke-filled room.

The popularity of chewing tobacco is increasing, possibly due to the substantially increased advertising of this tobacco product by the tobacco industry. With increased use, the incidence of oral cancers is also rising. These oral cancers arise in the areas of the mouth with which the tobacco is in direct contact, indicating that there are carcinogens within the tobacco itself.

Epidemiological evidence supports the notion that the newer filtered, low tar cigarettes are less carcinogenic than the older high tar varieties. Jewish males and persons with higher levels of education tend to smoke less, and those who do smoke use filtered cigarettes.

Table 2.6   Major Environmental Factors Associated with Cancer

Factor	Cancer sites	Risk (percent)
Diet	Colon, breast, endometrium, ovary	35–50
Tobacco	Lung	75–90
Tobacco	Upper respiratory tract, bladder, esophagus, kidney, pancreas	22–30
Occupation, asbestos	Thorax	3–18
Alcohol	Upper respiratory tract, larynx, liver	3–5
Infection, viral, etc.	Cervix, prostate, other sites	1–15
Sexual practices and patterns	Breast, endometrium, ovary, cervix, testis	1–13
Pollution	Lung, bladder, rectum	Less than 5
Medicines and radiation	Leukemia, bone, lung, thyroid, ovary, breast, endometrium	1–4
Background radiation	Skin, thyroid, leukemia, bone, breast, lung	Less than 3

Source: Modified from *Cancer Risk.* (Washington, D.C.: Office of Technology Assessment, 1982).

Their lung cancer rates are lower than those of black males, who tend to smoke more and use more nonfiltered cigarettes. Compensation for reduced tar and nicotine exposure in filtered cigarettes by increased inhalation and/or amounts of tobacco product used is seen among some individuals who switch from high to low tar cigarettes. This can offset the benefit of using the low tar product.

Although tobacco companies resist the notion that cigarette smoking is directly linked to lung cancer, over the years they have changed the formulations of their products to decrease the number of known carcinogens that are delivered. Before 1960, the amounts of many such chemicals present in tobacco were several times greater than the amounts present in 1979. Low tar cigarettes have substantially reduced amounts of the same chemicals. Thus, many of the products now available confer less risk than those of twenty-five years ago; nonetheless, increased consumption and the long-term use of these products still is entirely sufficient to induce lung cancer and associated cancers.

Because of differences in choices of tobacco product type used, as well as total amount of smoking done, dissimilarities are emerging in lung cancer rates among various segments of the population. Tobacco–related disease is becoming increasingly a disease of lower income males. Smoking is overrepresented among gays, blacks, the mentally ill, the poor, and males. Although the female rates are increasing, they will probably not reach that of males because women tend to choose low tar products. In considering why patients use products proven to be detrimental to health, it is useful to recall that beliefs and behavior do not necessarily correlate well, as shown in Figure 2.5.

The use of alcohol and tobacco together multiplies the risk of mouth and pharyngeal cancer and cancers of the larynx and esophagus. Unfortunately, heavy drinkers tend to be smokers. Moderation of alcohol intake among smokers would help decrease the rates of these cancers.

Viral Oncogenes, Human Oncogenes

The ability of some viruses to transform normal cells into malignant ones is no longer disputed. Among humans, two viruses have been firmly linked to cancers: the Epstein-Barr virus (EBV) to

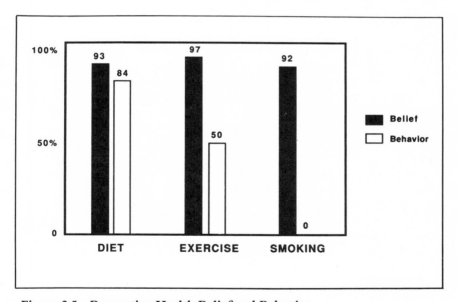

Figure 2.5   Preventive Health Belief and Behavior
Reprinted by permission from Barbara Stewart, Carol Lietar, and Barbara Demers, "Smoking Among Nurses: A Health Role Model Problem," *Proceedings of the Fourth National Conference on Cancer Nursing–1983,* p. 55. © 1984, American Cancer Society.

nasopharyngeal cancer and Burkitt's lymphoma, and hepatitis B virus (HBV) to hepatocellular carcinoma. Herpes simplex 2 virus (HSV–2) is linked to cervical cancer, but the evidence is much weaker than for the two previously mentioned cases. The importance of the papilloma virus in cervical cancer is currently being explored. Genital warts, which are caused by this virus, are strongly suspected as a risk factor for cervical cancer. Human T-cell Lymphotropic Virus-III (HTLV-III) has been shown to cause acquired immune deficiency syndrome (AIDS) in recent years, sparking tremendous attention to viruses and disease in humans. HTLV–1, the first human retrovirus discovered, causes one form of adult leukemia. Cytomegaloviruses (CMV) have been linked to Kaposi's sarcoma and have been found in the tissues of persons with various cancers. In the past, the importance of viruses in the overall risk of cancer was considered slight; as more is understood about these relationships, however, this is changing.

Because Burkitt's lymphoma and nasopharyngeal and hepatic cancers are not major cancers in the United States, attention to viral oncogenes was not emphasized in past research on cancer control. Today, with the discovery of naturally occuring viral oncogene counterparts in human cells and the presence of AIDS, interest is high.

The properties of mammalian cells can become permanently changed following infection by DNA and RNA viruses. The relevant viral genome, called a viral oncogene, can become integrated into the host cell chromosomes, sometimes causing cancerous changes (McClure et al. 1984). At present, two types of viral oncogenes have been discovered; one immortalizes cells and the other turns immortalized cells malignant. These viral oncogene types are very common and have been shown to be capable of causing cancer in humans. Viral oncogenes have been implicated in the induction of acute lymphocytic leukemia, acute myelogenous leukemia, acute nonlymphocytic leukemia, and chronic myelogenous leukemia. The viral oncogenes involved, which have been termed "B-lym," code for polypeptide growth factors.

Naturally occurring human oncogenes that are not exposed for expression, called cellular oncogenes or onc genes, are present in all mammalian cells. They probably play a role in normal growth and development, being "switched off" when no longer needed. Something occurs to switch these genes back on inappropriately and lead to immortality of the cell line. Translocations between chromosomes, sometimes seen in cancer patients, may be one way in which these oncogenes are activated. Promotors in the environment then may act to turn an immortal cell malignant.

The prospect of genetic engineering in the future of cancer control is exciting. The role of oncogenes and viruses in cancer needs to be fully elucidated before the information can be used for patient benefit, however, but the potential can now be seen.

Hormones

Both estrogens and androgens have been shown to have carcinogenic potential in humans. By 1940, the carcinogenic potential of diethylstilbesterol (DES) had been shown in animal models, but it was not until 1971 that the evidence of human carcinogenicity became clear. DES was used prior to the 1970s for a variety of gynecological conditions that responded to exogenous estrogen. It was also included in the animal feed of livestock to hasten weight gain.

During the 1940s and 1950s, Boston obstetricians used high doses of DES in women during the first trimester of pregnancy in hopes of decreasing the incidence of spontaneous abortions. Some 15 to 20 years later, a small epidemic of vaginal cancers in young women occurred in the Boston area. The vaginal adenocarcinoma seen had previously been virtually unheard of in young women. Epidemiologic studies discovered the relationship between maternal ingestion of DES and subsequent vaginal cancer in daughters. Even though DES has been shown in large clinical trials to be ineffective in preventing miscarriages and is no longer used for this purpose, it is still widely used for treating menopausal symptoms and for post-coital contraception (the morning-after pill) (Stolley 1982). There is evidence that DES increases the risk of breast cancer slightly in women who use DES themselves, and preliminary studies have implicated it in endometrial and ovarian cancer.

Estrogen supplements used to treat menopausal symptoms are associated with an increased uterine cancer risk. The National Institutes of Health in 1979 summarized the evidence of an association between estrogen use and endometrial cancer as follows:

> In the absence of exogenous estrogens, the incidence rate of endometrial cancer is approximately 1 per 1,000 post-menopausal women per year. It was recognized that this rate increases severalfold beginning after approximately two to four years' use of 0.625 or 1.25 mg of conjugated estrogens per day . . . Estrogen use is most strongly associated with lesions of the lowest grade and earliest stage. [NIH 1979]

Oral contraceptives containing a high proportion of estrogen promote endometrial cancer, whereas combination preparations with a high progesterone content may protect against this cancer. Women who have used combined oral contraceptives have only 50 percent of the incidence of endometrial cancer of nonusers (Stolley 1982). Today, almost all of the oral contraceptives offered include a large proportion of progesterone, and thus pose no hazard of increased risk of endometrial cancer and, indeed, may serve as a preventive.

The relationship of estrogen use and breast cancer remains unclear, however. Many human trials have failed to show a relationship, but animal models show that DES, for example, can cause breast tumors. This question continues to be closely studied.

Androgens (male hormones) are structurally related to the estrogens. They are used in treating various cancers, sexual behavior disorders, anemias, osteoporosis, hypopituitarism, and to induce pubertal changes. Transsexuals and athletes seeking to increase muscle bulk are subpopulations who may be exposed to androgens over extended periods of time. Various studies have implicated androgen use with an increased risk of liver cancer. Many of these studies, however, were on individuals with congenital anemias who may have been at increased risk for liver cancer through some other mechanism. Therefore, the relationship is by no means certain.

3

Treatment Modalities for Cancer and Nursing Implications

Principles of Surgery in Cancer Management

Surgery represents the first, and for many years the only, cancer treatment. Today, surgery is used to prevent, detect, treat, and palliate cancer—quite a leap from its humble beginnings.

Curative resections are those in which all obvious tumor is removed, along with a margin of healthy tissue, and organs or tissues that are likely sources of microinvasion of tumor cells. Palliative resections are made when curative resections are found to be impossible at operation; in these cases, cancer that cannot be removed remains in the body. Palliative resections also refer to surgery undertaken for symptom relief rather than for cure.

Tumors that are so large, so widely disseminated, or in such an awkward position that they defy removal are categorized as inoperable. Furthermore, if the tumor's removal would not result in any improved prognosis, or if the patient could not physically tolerate the procedure, the tumor is considered inoperable. If the surgery would create unacceptable psychological ramifications in the patient, it should be avoided if other alternatives exist, and the patient should be involved in the decision on whether or not to proceed in any case. Options of acceptable therapy now exist for almost all types of cancer, and assessments of the entire clinical situation are made prior to the undertaking of a surgical alternative.

Sometimes, surgery is used to prevent cancer in high risk populations. Examples are a prophylactic subcutaneous mastectomy performed on a woman at very high risk for breast cancer, or establishment of a colostomy in a patient who has severe familial polyposis coli.

Surgery may also be used solely to stage a cancer properly; this is the case with staging laparotomy in Hodgkin's disease to ensure that proper therapy is undertaken. Surgery is also being used as an adjunct to chemotherapy, as when blood vessels are isolated for regional perfusion or to position implantable infusion pumps.

Nursing responsibilities for cancer surgeries are not dissimilar to those for other general surgeries. Although most patients fear surgery, the patient with cancer faces surgery with fears not only about the outcome of the procedure, but also about what the surgeon will find. It takes sensitivity to provide emotional support for these patients in great need, who frequently face further treatments once the surgery is over, as well as a tremendous disruption of their lives.

One of the main goals of surgery is to aid in the staging and grading of cancer. Figure 3.1 shows how this is accomplished by

---

STAGING

T: Primary tumor
N: Regional lymph nodes
M: Distant metastasis

TX- Cannot assess
TO- No evidence of primary tumors
Tis- Carcinoma in situ
T1, T2, T3, T4 -   Increasing tumor size or involvement

NX- Cannot assess
NO- No evidence of regional node involvement
N1, N2, N3, N4-   Increasing degree of abnormality
       of regional nodes

MX- Cannot assess
MO- No evidence of distant metastasis
M1- Distant metastasis present (sites specified)

GRADING

GX- Cannot assess
G1- Well-differentiated
G2- Moderately well-differentiated
G3, G4-   Poorly to very poorly differentiated

Figure 3.1   Staging and Grading of Cancer
Systems of the American Joint Committee on Cancer; compiled from Beahrs, 1983

means of the so-called TNM system. Figure 3.2 displays the Host Performance Scale which is used by physicians to systematically describe any debility that may occur as a result of cancer. Both these assessment scales result in comparability of descriptions of the cancer experience of patients.

Principles and Administration of Chemotherapeutic Agents

Mechanism of Action of Chemotherapeutic Agents

Most chemotherapeutic agents in use today appear to have their effect primarily on cell multiplication and tumor growth. Because cell multiplication is a characteristic of normal cells as well as cancer cells, these agents are also toxic to normal body tissues, particularly those with rapid rates of turnover. The ideal antineoplastic agent would eradicate all cancer cells, while preserving normal marrow and allowing body organs to return to normal function. Because so little is understood of the biochemical differences between cancer and normal cells, it has not yet been possible consistently to design antineoplastic drugs based on these differences; instead, empirical experimentation with animal models is the means by which most effective cancer drugs are discovered today.

Nearly all agents in use today act on macromolecular synthesis and functions of cancer cells (Skeel 1982). Exceptions are the newer biological response modifiers (BRM), which are considered to be part of immunotherapy. Unlike BRM agents, which act on the cytoplas-

---

H-   Physical state of the patient, considering all factors

    HO- Normal activity
    H1- Symptomatic, ambulatory, self-care
    H2- Ambulatory > 50% of time; occasionally needs assistance
    H3- Ambulatory < 50% of time; nursing care needed
    H4- Bedridden; may need hospitalization

Figure 3.2   Host Performance Scale
Systems of the American Joint Committee on Cancer. This simplified scale is the one preferred for current use. Compiled from Beahrs, 1983

mic organization of cancer cells, most chemotherapeutic agents interfere with synthesis of DNA, RNA, or proteins; or act by interfering with the appropriate function of cell products. When an agent's effect is sufficient, a proportion of cells die. Each time a dose of the drug is given, the same proportion of cells die. To act successfully, an antineoplastic agent must cause cell death proportionally greater than cell growth. Unfortunately, clinical experience indicates that a number of factors interfere with such a straightforward model. All cells in a tumor are not equally sensitive to most drugs; tumor cell heterogeneity has been shown to exist in many tumors, and mutations in cancer cells continue to contribute new cell forms over time. Furthermore, the location of cells probably has an effect of their sensitivity to a drug.

It is now believed that most cancer cells do not in fact grow faster than normal cells, but enter a resting phase less often than normal cells. It is also believed that cancer cells complete cell cycles qualitatively the same as those of normal cells. Cells begin a cell cycle in Gap 1 (G1), during which time enzymes, proteins, and RNA are manufactured. This is followed by the DNA synthesis (S) phase, when all DNA synthesis is accomplished. Then a Gap 2 (G2) phase begins, when more protein and RNA synthesis occurs. After G2, a mitosis (M) phase occurs, when daughter cells are produced, with each one entering G1. Body organs develop an equilibrium between cells in G1 and those in an inactive, or resting phase (G0). Cells in G0 are particularly insensitive to chemotherapeutic agents.

PHASE-SPECIFIC DRUGS

Some chemotherapeutic agents act primarily during a particular phase in the cell cycle. Asparaginase and prednisone act on cells during G1; the antimetabolites and hydroxyurea act during S phase; bleomycin and etoposide act during G2; and mitotic inhibitors act during the M phase.

CYCLE-SPECIFIC DRUGS

Drugs in this class act primarily on cells that are active in some phase of growth (not in G0). They are active on cells during any growth phase, although some may act more aggressively against cells in a particular phase. Some activity against cells in G0 is seen with most of the drugs, but not as much as when cells are in active growth. The alkylating agents chlorambucil, cyclophosphamide, melphalan, busulfan, dacarbazine, and cisplatin, and the antibiotics dactinomycin, daunorubicin, and doxorubicin act in this manner.

CYCLE-NONSPECIFIC DRUGS

Cycle-nonspecific drugs act against cells that are in either a growing phase or resting phase. They include the alkylating agent mechlorethamine, and the nitrosoureas carmustine, lomustine, and semustine.

Effectiveness of Chemotherapeutic Agents

Since antineoplastic agents kill a proportion of tumor cells, rather than a set number, debulking a tumor by surgery or radiotherapy is theoretically advisable and is often seen to be useful in clinical situations. This is particularly true for the antimetabolites.

Combination chemotherapy uses the principle of employing agents that act by different means so that less toxic amounts of any one drug can be given to achieve a similar overall effect to very high doses of a single agent. In addition, combination chemotherapy confers an advantage in counteracting the emergence of resistant clones of tumor cells. Using agents that are active during several growth phases as well as the resting phase can increase the proportion of cells killed, for an overall greater cell kill rate. Drugs may also act synergistically, or one may rescue the host from toxic effects of another.

Whether anticancer agents are given singly, simultaneously, or in sequence can determine their effectiveness or limiting toxicity. The term "schedule dependency" refers to the phenomenon of therapeutic changes based on changes in dosage and/or scheduling of one or more drugs. Synergistic or antagonistic interplays are observed with various drug combinations. For example, methotrexate and 5–fluorouracil, which are frequently used in concert, have been shown in tissue culture test and animal models to have either synergistic or antagonistic effects depending on the dosage, sequence, and time interval between drug administrations (Capizzi 1985). As more is understood about schedule dependency of drug action, the precision of administration will become more and more critical.

Response to therapy may be considered in terms of increased survival, tumor regression, or subjective changes. A particular chemotherapy regimen may be capable of evoking a response in one, two, or all three of these areas. Increased length of survival is a presumed goal of chemotherapy in most cases. Sometimes, however, palliation or remission of a tumor is possible, but survival is not improved. Complete remission means that all signs of a tumor mass are eradicated for at least two measurement periods four weeks apart; partial remission indicates that a decrease of 50 percent or more is observable in the total tumor area with no new lesions appearing for at least four weeks. Stable disease denotes a decrease of less than 50 percent to an increase of less than 25 percent of tumor mass, while progression indicates an increase of more than 25 percent of tumor area or the appearance of new lesions. A subjective response to a drug regimen is considered successful if a substantial improvement in well-being is reported by the patient. Generally, a patient must go through a period during active treatment when he or she feels substantially worse than before the drugs were administered. Patients are informed of this, and the vast majority choose to undergo treatment for the ultimate improvement it attempts to accomplish.

Investigational Chemotherapy

The development of any new drug to be used against cancer takes a long time and is carefully monitored. The source of new drugs varies widely, including analogs of existing antineoplastic agents, incidental discoveries, and drugs developed to respond to specific cancer cell properties. Most testing of investigational drugs is done under the auspices of the National Cancer Institute (NCI) Investigational Cancer Program. Some 15,000 new compounds are considered for testing by the NCI each year; only a very few will prove sufficiently useful for development for human trials, however (Vincent 1985). In preclinical testing, an experimental drug is first screened in animal models and in vitro tumor cell cultures for potential usefulness. If it shows appropriate biological activity, the drug enters toxicology trials. These are large animal studies in which the highest nontoxic dose, lowest toxic dose, and maximally tolerated dose are established. Once this step is completed, the drug may enter Phase I clinical trials.

PHASE I TRIALS

Phase I trials identify the possible toxic effects in patients and determine doses that may be considered safe and those that are toxic in humans. Patients with cancer of any type are potential candidates for participation in Phase I trials. Those admitted to a testing program must have a cancer for which there is no reasonable proven therapy, adequate general health and functioning, and have good metabolic function so that they can clear the drug properly.

Informed consent is a critical element for participation in Phase I trials. Patients are informed of the difficulties with present treatment alternatives for their type of cancer as well as the status of the drug being investigated. The NCI monitors patient consent practices nationally. The nurse working with a Phase I drug should assure that the patient is not confused about the potential benefits of participation, as Phase I trials are preliminary and without proven benefit to humans. If the nurse feels that the patient is misinformed, the patient should be referred back to the physician investigator for further information. Phase I trials usually involve 15 to 30 patients. Initially, some patients are started on very low doses of the drug, then successive groups of patients are given successively higher doses. Once appropriate doses and toxicities are known, the next step in drug development is taken.

PHASE II TRIALS

In Phase II trials, the specific cancers for which the drug shows maximum benefit are established. Patient selection is based on cancer type, and the cancer must be histologically confirmed and measurable. The usual cancer types that are tested are those for which there are few useful present chemotherapeutic agents available. Melanomas, lymphomas, and cancers of the breast, lung, and colon are types of malignancies commonly considered applicable for Phase II trials. A 20 percent response rate is the lowest rate allowing the drug to be used in Phase III trials. Nurses should maintain a realistic, calm attitude during investigational treatments, as patients may easily become unrealistically optimistic about their treatments when initial response is seen, only to be badly disappointed with subsequent failures. Emotional problems are common among patients who experience tumor regrowth. Nurses should share in a patient's pleasure with optimistic findings, but be careful to reinforce the experimental nature of the therapy. A broad perspective is needed to ensure that nurses working with investigational drugs are emotionally able to support patients when they need it, as well as to maintain emotional health for themselves.

PHASE III TRIALS

Phase III trials involve the randomization of patients in experiments comparing the investigational drug to standard therapy in separate arms of a trial. Clients entering Phase III trials are usually newly diagnosed and have received no prior therapy with chemotherapeutic agents or radiation. These patients are particularly vulnerable to unrealistic expectations or confusion about the benefits of investigational drugs. They need to be particularly clear on the fact that choosing not to participate in a clinical trial will in no way reflect adversely on their care and treatment. Being in the trial does not assure that they will receive the experimental drug, as they are randomly selected for an arm of the trial after they have agreed to participate. Patients should also clearly understand that they can withdraw at any time without penalty.

Another part of Phase III trials involves the use of various protocols, such new combinations of drugs including an investigational drug, new methods of administration, or new schedules of administration. Usually the patient is responsible for any costs of treatment, side effects, and extra laboratory costs associated with treatment involving an investigational drug. If a drug company is sponsoring a particular protocol, some laboratory costs may be absorbed by the company.

Once a drug has proved its effectiveness and acceptable levels of toxicity, and has completed Phase III trials, it is considered for approval by the Food and Drug Administration (FDA) for general use. It usually takes ten to twelve years from Phase I trial initiation to FDA approval of an investigational drug. The cost is counted in the millions of dollars for each drug.

Nurses play a major role in the administration of protocols, as they are expected to report immediately to the primary investigator any adverse or unusual effects observed as well as life-threatening toxicities. Nurses should report any information they have about local reactions, irritation to veins, tissue damage, and other problems encountered during drug administration for other nurses to use. The agency sponsoring the protocol should be informed about these observations, as should the professional journals, particularly *Oncology Nursing Forum* or *Cancer Nursing*. Nurses should report adverse drug reactions seen with newer antineoplastic agents to the Food and Drug Administration through its voluntary reporting system. Reporting forms may be obtained through Food and Drug Administration, Center for Drugs and Biologics, Division of Drugs and Biological Products Experience (HFN–730), 5600 Fishers Lane, Rockville, MD 20857; phone number: (301)443-5480. In dealing with patients involved in clinical trials, the nurse needs to communicate honestly and listen closely to what the patient is saying about effects both physical and emotional.

Classification of Antineoplastic Drugs

Chemotherapeutic agents are customarily divided into several classes: the alkylating agents, antimetabolites, hormonal agents, natural products, and a miscellaneous category. Within each class are various types of agents, grouped according to their mechanism of action, biochemical structure, or a physiologic action. The customary categorization of agents is somewhat arbitrary; some of the drugs could fit into two or more categories. The categorization of drugs is useful in helping physicians choose combinations that have the highest probability of success (see Table 3.1).

ALKYLATING AGENTS

These drugs act by direct attack on body compounds including DNA, enzymes, and many molecules of low molecular weight. Usually they form a covalent bond with a portion of the cell with critical physiologic importance, rendering it unavailable for normal metabolic reactions. Because the alkylating agents interact with preformed molecules, they are not phase specific, and at least some are not cell cycle specific. Their effectiveness often depends on direct toxicity, and in turn upon dose level; hence larger, more toxic doses are often more effective than small doses.

Each type of alkylating agent acts in a slightly different way, although inhibition of appropriate DNA replication leading to cell mutation or death is a common characteristic. The nitrosoureas are unique in the class with respect to being non-cross-resistant with other alkylating agents.

ANTIMETABOLITES

The antimetabolites act by interfering with metabolic pathways of dividing cells, usually with DNA synthesis. Commonly, they are structural analogs of precursor molecules or cofactors and interfere with biosynthetic enzymes or become incorporated into abnormal and nonfunctional products lethal to the cell. Because target cells are vulnerable proportionate to DNA synthesis, these agents are cycle sensitive. Since these agents require activation by specific enzymes within the cells, increasing the dose of the antineoplastic agent will not be effective if the enzyme is absent. Therefore, if the drug does not show a response, increasing the dose will not necessarily increase the effect.

The only folic acid analog in general use today is methotrexate, which inhibits the enzyme dihydrofolate reductase, which is necessary for the production of thymidylic acid. Pyridine analogs directly interfere with DNA and RNA synthesis. Purine analogs are thought to interfere with DNA and RNA synthesis as well, although their site of action is less well understood than that of the pyridine analogs.

Table 3.1   Clinically Useful Chemotherapeutic Agents

Class	Type	Examples
Alkylating agents	Nitrogen mustard-derivatives	chlorambucil, cyclophosphamide, mechlorethamine (Nitrogen mustard), mel phalan
	Ethylenimine-derivatives	triethylene thiophosphoramide (thiotepa, Thiotepa)
	Alkyl sulfonate	busulfan
	Nitrosourea	carmustine, lomustine, streptozocin
	Triazine	dacarbazine
	Metal salts	cisplatin
Antimetabolite	Folic acid analog	methotrexate
	Pyrimidine analog	cytarabine, fluorouracil
	Purine analog	mercaptopurine, thioguanine
Hormone products	Androgens	
	Corticosteroids	
	Estrogens	
	Progestins	
	Estrogen antagonist	tamoxifen
Natural products	Mitotic inhibitor	vinblastine, vincristine
	Podophyllum-derivative	etoposide
	Antibiotics	bleomycin, dactinomycin, daunorubicin, doxorubicin, mithramycin, mitomycin
	Enzyme	asparaginase
Miscellaneous agents	Urea-displacement	hydroxyurea
	Methyl hydrazine-derivative	procarbazine
	Steroid suppresser	aminoglute thimide
	Melamine-displacement	hexamethylmelamine

NATURAL PRODUCTS

These agents are grouped together because they are derived from natural sources, not because of their mechanism of action. A class of mitotic inhibitors is derived from the periwinkle plant. Since these compounds act by arresting mitosis, they are cycle-specific agents. Etoposide, an investigational drug derived from podophyllum, obtained from the root of the mayapple plant, arrests cells during the G2 phase. The antitumor antibiotics are agents produced by the Streptomyces species of soil fungus. They are far too toxic to be useful in treating bacterial infections, but their cytotoxic characteristic makes them particularly useful in cancer treatment. They all act to disrupt the function and synthesis of nucleic acids. The enzyme agent asparaginase interferes with the metabolic hydrolysis of asparagine, causing cell death.

HORMONES AND HORMONE ANTAGONISTS

Hormones act against tumors in pharmacologic doses that are 10 to 100 times physiologic replacement doses, and therefore do not function in a traditional fashion. A common characteristic of these agents is that they are effective against cancer cells that have retained some sensitivity to hormonal control of growth. An exception to this mechanism is the effect of corticosteroids on the leukemias and lymphomas, in which the steroids are directly cytotoxic to abnormal lymphoid cells with high numbers of glucocorticoid receptors.

Androgens are thought to exert their effect by altering pituitary function or by direct cytotoxic effects. Corticosteroids cause lysis of susceptible cells directly. Estrogens act through the hypothalamus to suppress testosterone production in males and also alter breast tissue response to prolactin. Progestins seem to promote differentiation of cancer cells directly. Estrogen antagonists displace estrogen on binding sites on cancer cell membranes.

MISCELLANEOUS AGENTS

Agents within the miscellaneous class act in unique ways. Hydroxyurea, procarbazine, and hexamethylmelamine, in particular, are frequently used miscellaneous agents (see Table 3.1).

Over the last thirty years, some thirty-eight such drugs have cleared all of the preclinical tests and have been made available for standard clinical use. These drugs are widely used in the United States today, either as standard therapy or in large investigational trials. A dozen or so more are at preliminary stages of investigation at comprehensive cancer centers around the country. Nurses using drugs—in any category—with which they are unfamiliar need to read available literature and observe the patient carefully for unusual or unfamiliar reactions.

Handling Chemotherapeutic Agents

Presently, there is concern about the safety of nurses who routinely admix or administer antineoplastic agents. The concern stems from the fact that many of these agents are not only toxic, but are also potent mutagens or carcinogens. Although there is laboratory evidence of increased cancer risk to animals exposed to these agents, as well as a documented increased cancer risk to patients actually receiving them, the long-term effects to health providers exposed to low levels over long time periods are still unknown. Exposure is generally in the form of direct skin contact or microdroplets of drug aerosolized during preparation.

As of 1985, the occupational risk of handling chemotherapeutic agents had not been quantified. Studies of the dangers, employing urine mutagenicity assays, chromosomal aberration studies, and blood analyses, have produced results on each side of the issue (mutagenicity or carcinogenicity of various agents is shown in Fig. 3.3). Until safety can be established, a conservative approach is warranted. Studies have shown that the urine of patients who are receiving chemotherapeutic agents of known mutagenicity is itself mutagenic (Venitt et al. 1984). This may pose a heretofore unrecognized or unappreciated hazard. When preparing these agents, complete security is not achieved by horizontal laminar-flow hoods. At M. D. Anderson Hospital, drug handler exposure occurred under the hoods, but not when Class II biological safety cabinets were employed (Nguyen et al. 1982). Type A cabinets are considered the minimal requirement. It has been demonstrated that direct skin exposure to antineoplastic agents is a risk in many roles nurses take in cancer care. The amount of this exposure varies depending on many factors and is difficult to quantify.

The best precautions nurses can take at this time include wearing latex gloves (polyvinyl chloride gloves are permeable to some antineoplastic agents) when handling the mutagenic or carcinogenic agents, minimizing direct skin contact when exposed to patient excreta, and admixing agents only when adequate protective equipment is available. Hydrophobic filters should be used with all vials and Luer-lock fittings utilized with administration equipment. Care should also be given to disposing of IV infusion equipment, syringes, and containers employed in the delivery of chemotherapeutic agents. These items should be considered biohazardous waste. Work areas

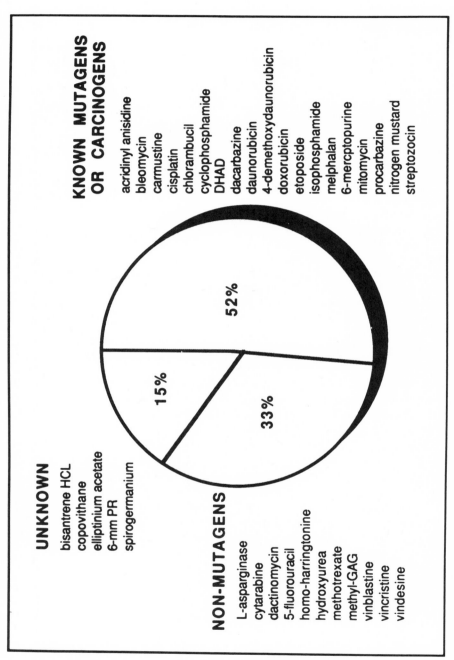

UNKNOWN

bisantrene HCL
copovithane
elliptinium acetate
6-mm PR
spirogermanium

**KNOWN MUTAGENS
OR CARCINOGENS**

acridinyl anisidine
bleomycin
carmustine
cisplatin
chlorambucil
cyclophosphamide
DHAD
dacarbazine
daunorubicin
4-demethoxydaunorubicin
doxorubicin
etoposide
isophosphamide
melphalan
6-mercptopurine
mitomycin
procarbazine
nitrogen mustard
streptozocin

NON-MUTAGENS

L-asparginase
cytarabine
dactinomycin
5-fluorouracil
homo-harringtonine
hydroxyurea
methotrexate
methyl-GAG
vinblastine
vincristine
vindesine

15%

33%

52%

Figure 3.3   Mutagenicity or Carcinogenicity of Antineoplastic Agents
Data derived from Cloak 1985; Barry 1985

for the preparation of antineoplastic agents should be washed after each preparation episode with soap and water or 70 percent alcohol, and allowed to dry before their next use. Of course, food or personal items should not be placed near the workspace. Handwashing is required after removing gloves at the finish of the procedure involving chemotherapeutic agents. Gloves are not a substitute for handwashing. If overt contamination of gloves occurs, they should be promptly removed, and hands washed well. If personnel must handle chemotherapeutic agents for long periods of time, or if contamination of gloves is likely, it is recommended that they wear two pairs of gloves.

Protocols should be established for all routine chores associated with antineoplastic agents. The National Institutes of Health Public Health Service publishes a guide for safe handling of these drugs. Other guidelines have also been published by various organizations. The national Study Commission of Cytotoxic Exposure has published a guide on all aspects of handling these cytotoxic agents. Information on their guidelines is available through Dr. Louis P. Jeffrey at Rhode Island Hospital in Providence, RI 02902. Nurses handling antineoplastic agents or caring for these patients should have guidelines available and be well acquainted with them.

Administration Principles

In order to handle antineoplastic agents appropriately, the nurse must have a basic knowledge of the routes of administration and nature of the most widely used agents. The most common routes employed are IV, IVPB, IM, Sub-cu, PO, IT (intrathecal), IP (intraperitoneal), intra-arterial, or via VADs (vascular access devices). Most of these are routes with which the general nurse is well acquainted, but others are most often seen in cancer care and will be among those discussed individually in this book in Chapter 8.

Antineoplastic agents have been divided into three categories according to their chemical effects on body tissues. They may be considered vesicants, irritants, or nonvesicants (see Figure 3.4).

A vesicant is a strong sclerosing agent. This group of chemotherapuetic agents has an acidic pH level and can cause cellular damage and destruction when even minute quantities come in contact with body tissues. The mechanism through which these agents achieve tissue destruction is not fully understood. Doxorubicin (Adriamycin) is a vesicant that can remain in tissues for many weeks and form a complex with cellular deoxyribonucleic acid (DNA). It is thought that this binding property enables doxorubicin to enter healthy cells

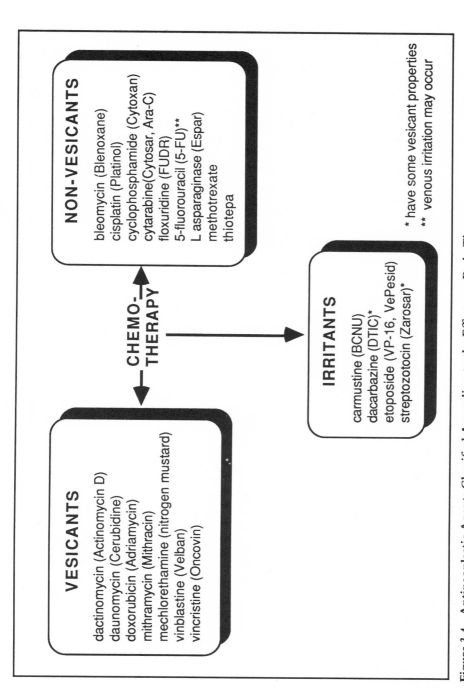

Figure 3.4 Antineoplastic Agents Classified According to the Effects on Body Tissues

and to inhibit wound healing (Laughlin et al. 1979). Its mode of action is the best understood of the vesicants. How much damage a vesicant does to tissue is directly related to the amount of drug absorbed and the site of the infiltration. Thus factors such as drug concentration and length of exposure have a large effect on the outcome of inadvertent infiltration of a vesicant into body tissues. The condition of a drug or fluid inadvertently infiltrating into the subcutaneous tissues surrounding an infusion site is referred to as "extravasation." By virtue of popular usage, when common intravenously administered drugs seep into tissues around the infusion vein, the accident is referred to as "infiltration." The term "extravasation" is generally reserved for the occurrence of infiltration by a vesicant or irritant, but this is an arbitrary use of the term. Extravasation has come to denote a condition involving potential severe tissue destruction. The damage from vesicants can lead to wounds that persist for months or years. Vesicant wounds frequently appear as severe inflammation followed in about one or two weeks by ulcers that are deep and persistent. Sometimes the wound from a vesicant must be surgically excised in order to close healthy tissue. Vesicants can cause necrosis severe enough to require amputation of a hand or limb as a life-saving measure. The result of extravasation by a vesicant can be months of surgical tissue debridement, resection, and grafting. The patient may experience pain, incapacitation, and possibly a threat to life due to gangrene or sepsis.

Irritants produce extravasation, much as their name implies, causing local inflammation and pain. The damage is generally temporary and the compromised tissue heals well over a period of days or weeks. There are differences in the way individuals may react to these drugs, however, and small ulcerations may occur. The severity of the tissue reaction depends on the drug concentration and site of damage. Patients being infused with irritants need careful nursing.

Nonvesicants do not cause tissue damage by virtue of their chemical properties. Should they infiltrate, inflammation results due to tissue compression and local disruption, and this reaction should clear in a few days. Idiosyncratic differences in response to these drugs exist, however, and some individuals may experience reactions that are more severe.

Vesicants may be administered by slow push through a well-established intravenous line, by sidearm technique, or preferably through a central VAD or an intra-arterial catheter. When the route is through a peripheral vein, care must be taken to ensure that the chosen vein has been cleanly entered, and the puncture site should not be at the antecubital fossa, over joint spaces, tendons, or neurovascular bundles. If extravasation should occur, a loss of function in the involved arm will occur if these sites are used. The entire venous network associated with the chosen vein should be evaluated, as ulceration can occur at a distal, recently discontinued puncture site, which results in minute leaks of drug into surrounding tissue.

The nurse should remain with the patient throughout the infusion of a vesicant, checking for good blood return after every 5 ml of drug is administered for adequate patency. Should swelling occur or the patient complain of pain or a stinging sensation, the infusion should be stopped at once and extravasation procedures instituted. The most common drugs given slow IV push are the vinca alkaloids, nitrogen mustard, mitomycin-C, doxorubicin, and dactinomycin, which are all small volume vesicants. Another method used for delivering small volume vesicants peripherally is the sidearm technique. This method involves the administration of drug by needle and syringe through a side port of a flowing IV line. Usually a solution of 5 percent dextrose in water or a normal saline solution is used for the running IV line. The rationale for this technique is that it dilutes the vesicant, and if extravasation should occur, it would involve a less concentrated amount of drug and so have a less intense effect.

Whenever available or if a volume larger than 20 cc of a vesicant needs to be delivered, a vascular access device (for example, Hickman right atrial catheter or an implanted Infuse-a-Port line) should be used. Occasionally, an intra-arterial line may be employed for regional drug delivery. These latter lines are often checked radiographically prior to drug administration. These methods all enable safe administration of the highly toxic vesicants. Because the drug enters the body circulation through a catheter tip distal to the point of blood vessel entry, extravasation is highly unlikely. These methods also utilize catheters that are well established in large blood vessels. Therefore, the chance of extravasation is small indeed.

Irritants are sometimes given in volumes too large for the practical use of the IV push technique. Slow, continuous infusion with mini-bags is then used as the mode of delivery. Still, the patient should be continuously monitored for signs of extravasation throughout the administration interval. With the use of both vesicants and irritants, the nurse needs to inform patients of their role in immediately reporting signs of extravasation.

Unfortunately, it has been documented that with several agents, 5–FU (a nonvesicant) and Mutamycin (a vesicant), delayed tissue damage can occur even if no evidence of extravasation occurs at the time of drug administration (Teta and O'Connor 1984; Wood and Ellerhorst-Ryan 1984). Any part of the locally associated venous network of the site used can be involved. Reactions have been seen from ten days to six months after drug administration. Even with the best delivery technique, the powerful vesicants and irritants can cause misery for the patient they are supposed to help. Even nonvesicants can cause problems in susceptible individuals.

Nonvesicants can safely be administered via peripheral lines. However, as noted above, 5–Fu in particular is showing up in the literature as responsible for tissue damage in spite of good administration technique. Nurses administering nonvesicants should use care in venipuncture and periodically monitor the site during infusions.

Extravasation Procedures

Different health care agencies have developed various extravasation protocols that successfully control extensive damage from vesicants. All work well as long as they are instituted at even the slightest suspicion of extravasation. The speed with which the protocol is begun is of utmost importance to the eventual success of the regimen. Therefore, the nurse administering these drugs should understand fully the steps of the procedures approved for extravasation at the agency involved and have ready access to necessary items.

Extravasation may be recognized immediately, but is more often recognized between one and four hours after drug administration. A few patients will not have signs and symptoms of extravasation until twenty-four to forty-eight hours after drug infusion. In any of these cases, extravasation protocols should be employed. Chemical cellulitis is progressive and the sooner it is halted, the less the ultimate tissue damage. Pain may be short-lived, so patients and nurses should not assume that if no pain is involved, no damage is occurring.

Today, there is research to indicate that conservative treatment of extravasation with prompt removal of the needle and line, ice applications, and close observation is the best protocol (Larson 1985). The following are several alternatives of management procedures that have worked well in various agencies and can be considered as general guides to appropriate care of extravasations.

- Stop the infusion quickly.
- Remove the needle and tubing, or remove the tubing and aspirate any drug in the needle and accessible tissue with a syringe.
- Inject prescribed antidotal medications. Sodium thiosulfate is a specific antidote for nitrogen mustard, but its use may cause some local toxicity. The antidote is a combination of 4 ml of 10 percent USP sodium thiosulfate and 6 ml of sterile

water. Hyaluronidase is considered antidotal for the plant alkyloids. The antidote is prepared by adding 1–2 ml of 0.89 percent saline to each 300 USP units of hyaluronidase. Use of the glucocorticoids is contraindicated with the vinca alkaloids, as it may increase symptoms of extravasation. Antidotes for doxorubicin that have been used include injected hydrocortisone, 50–100 mg; dexamathasone, 2–4 mg; and sodium bicarbonate, 1–3 mEq. Dimethyl sulfoxide (DMSO) and vitamin E have been shown to be minimally effective separately, but very effective in reducing ulcer size in extravasation in some trials. Other trials have shown no benefit to the treatment. Propranolol has recently been shown to be effective against low-dose doxorubicin extravasation in animal models. Clinicians disagree on the benefits of administering specific antidotes to the various drugs, and recently their use has begun to decrease in favor of conservative treatment.

• Apply a topical medication. The agent most commonly used is 1 percent hydrocortisone cream rubbed gently into the skin. Some agencies have reported success with dimethyl sulfoxide (DMSO) applied topically, while others have observed no benefits from DMSO applications or injections.

• Apply a dressing. Either a sterile gauze pad or plastic dressing can be used. The plastic dressing allows better penetration of topical ointments and easy observation of the site. Clinicians differ as to which procedure is preferable.

• Elevate and immobilize the affected site. For the first twenty-four hours particularly, the extremity should be elevated above heart level. Otherwise, if the patient is up and about, a sling may be useful to immobilize the arm and reduce dependent edema.

• Apply ice or heat treatments. Frequently, ice is applied for twenty minute periods four times daily beginning immediately after the initial site care. Alternatively, ice may be applied continuously for the first twenty-four hours, then on an intermittent schedule. Ice treatments are felt to minimize cellular damage by decreasing the absorption of the drug into subcutaneous tissues. Cold is also thought to decrease vesicant agents' ability to disrupt cells and decrease the inflammatory response of white blood cells. Some clinicians feel that continued intermittent ice treatments are most beneficial over the next three days (Stapczynski 1984). Although some cellulitis may occur as a consequence of this therapy, more harmful full-thickness skin loss is avoided.

Others feel that the more standard approach of heat applications after a twenty-four-hour initial cold treatment for tissue injury is best. Reabsorption of remaining drug and promotion of healing through increased migration of white blood cells and removal of cellular debris is the mechanism of action of heat. Another viewpoint is that immediate heat applications speed the dispersion of antidotes in the affected site and are thus the preferred method of treatment throughout the course of the injury.

A specific contraindication for the use of cold is with extravasation of the vinca alkaloids, and animal models suggest it may be harmful when nitrogen mustard is extravasated. In these two situations, heat treatments initially should be used.

• Document the extravasation event and treatment precisely.

Toxicity of Chemotherapeutic Agents

A major characteristic of chemotherapuetic agents is the severity and frequency of side effects seen at therapeutic doses. Toxicity is dependent on the specific agent, dose, schedule of administration, and route of administration. In addition, patients enter chemotherapy with individual debilities and idiosyncracies that may predispose them to toxic reactions.

Some toxicities are relatively common among the various antineoplastic agents. Nausea and vomiting are seen to some degree with the majority of these drugs. Other common toxic reactions stem from the action of the drugs on the rapidly dividing cells of the bone marrow and epithelium. Myelosuppression with leukopenia, thrombocytopenia, and anemia is common as are mucous membrane ulcerations, and alopecia.

Other toxicities are less common and specific to various agents or classes of drugs. Important examples of selective toxicities include:

• vinca alkaloids: neurotoxicity
• cyclophosphamide: hemorrhagic cystitis
• AMSA, daunorubicin, doxorubicin: cardiomyopathy
• bleomycin, busulfan, BCNU, chorambucil, cyclophosphamide, mitomycin, methotrexate, melphalan, 6–mercaptopurine, procarbazine, VM–26, zinsostatin: pulmonary fibrosis and pneumonitis
• asparaginase, cisplatin: anaphylaxis
• cisplatin: irreversible nephrotoxicity

• methotrexate, 5–FU, vinblastine, doxorubicin, actinomycin-D, bleomycin: photosensitivity

Future Directions of Chemotherapy

Four areas of research are currently underway in the field of oncology drug therapy that hold the promise of improvements in patient response to this modality. High–dose chemotherapy that is capable of high cell kill ratios is becoming more available because of selective rescue techniques such as the use of leucovorin after high-dose methotrexate, improved support mechanisms such as autologous marrow transplantation, and early use of antibiotics in patients at high risk for infections.

Another research area today is the use of regional chemotherapy. Although very high concentrations of drug can be delivered to selective body areas by this technique, a disadvantage is that it is less effective against any extraregional metastasis. The two most widely used methods of employing regional chemotherapy today are intraperitoneal and intrahepatic arterial routes.

Biochemical modulation is a third area of drug research. Combinations of drugs are used to increase their sum effect over that possible with their individual use. Certain drugs can enhance the biochemical activity of others, by directly increasing activity, inhibiting degradation, or modulating the tumor cell to increase the effectiveness of the other agents. Determining what specific combinations and sequencing are necessary to optimize chemotherapy's ultimate effect is the thrust of today's research in this area.

Finally, research in the area of drug resistance is of particular prominence. One theory of how drug resistance occurs is that the tumor cell is able to amplify the production of target proteins, thus escaping cytotoxicity. Efforts are underway to overcome this problem. Another interesting area of research is in the use of calcium channel blockers, which have beeen shown in animal models to overcome drug resistance. Verapamil and nifedipine are two such drugs currently being evaluated for their effectiveness in cancer chemotherapy (Skeel 1982).

Principles of Radiation Therapy

Ionizing radiation passes through matter, disrupting or damaging the atoms with which it comes in contact. Resultant cellular disruption occurs in three ways: an immediate cellular effect, which is described as damage to the DNA-replicating ability of cells and cell membrane changes; a chromosomal effect, wherein mutations, translocations, and breaks occur in the cell chromosomes; and a delayed effect, which is a factor of late disrupted mitosis of a cell that appears undamaged at the time of the irradiation. Ionizing radiation can be either electromagnetic (high energy level X-rays and gamma rays) or particulate (alpha particles, beta particles, and neutrons).

Radioactive Substances

The emission of highly energetic nuclear particles (alpha or beta) or electromagnetic (gamma ray) radiation is an attempt by an atom to gain stability. The rate of progress toward stability, which is distinctive for each radioactive substance, is measured as a half-life. The half-life of a radioactive element is the time required for it to lose 50 percent of its activity by decay. Radioactive elements are used in brachytherapy.

Electromagnetic Radiation

High energy electromagnetic emissions (X-rays and gamma rays) are described as photons—discrete bundles (quanta) of energy. Their radiation is delivered in beams with the same characteristics as light. Although their origins are different, they share the same ionizing properties, which lead to cellular disruptions.

Particulate Radiation

Atomic particles that are capable of ionization are alpha and beta particles, neutrons, protons, pi-mesons, and deuterons. They differ from electromagnetic ionizing radiation as they possess mass and can carry an electrical charge, either negative or positive. Alpha and beta particles are easily blocked; paper will impede alpha particles, and aluminum or plastic stops beta emissions. Protons, pi-mesons, and deuterons are produced in generators and cyclotrons. Neutrons, which act by disrupting atomic nuclei and releasing protons, are produced from cyclotrons and nuclear reactors.

Linear Energy Transfer

Different types of radiation vary in their rate of loss of energy along a track. This is termed linear energy transfer (LET). Radiations capable of high LET include alpha particles, neutrons, and pi-mesons. These high-LET particles are theoretically more efficient irradiators of tumors, as they can affect cells regardless of their phase in the cell cycle, impose greater damage to hypoxic cells, decrease cell repair abilities, and all but neutrons can direct energy very specifically (Richter et al. 1984). High-LET particle irradiation is currently being tested against conventional radiation and low-LET irradiation in several cancer centers. Although it has many theoretical advantages, clinical advantages to this type of radiation therapy are not always clear (ibid.). Neutron high-LET treatment facilities are currently available in Cleveland, Batavia (near Chicago), Los Angeles, Chicago, Philadelphia, Houston, and Seattle. Heavy-charged particle high-LET treatments are available in Berkeley, California.

Energy Measures

The term "rad" is used to measure the amount of energy absorbed by the tissue irradiated. One rad equals 100 ergs of energy absorbed per gram of tissue.

Radiation Oncology

The dose of radiation that can be delivered to any tumor is limited by the radiation tolerance of the normal tissues adjacent to the tumor. Injury to some normal organs or tissues may result in fatality or unacceptable morbidity. Particularly vulnerable structures are the liver, lung, brain, spinal cord, heart, kidneys, intestines, and bone marrow. Whenever feasible, shielding and radiation field construction is planned to reduce the dose to limiting normal tissues. One means employed to increase the amount of radiation that can be delivered to a tumor is by using multiple doses (or fractions) of radiation to accumulate to the total dose desired.

Four important biologic processes (called the four Rs of radiation therapy) have been shown to be influenced by fractionation: repair of sublethal radiation damage, repopulation of cells, reassortment of cells in the cell cycle, and reoxygenation of hypoxic cells (Levene and Harris 1982). The influence of fractionation on these processes is a complex relationship that varies with the tumor type and location. It is presumed that normal cells have a greater and faster capacity to repair sublethal damage than do tumor cells, so fractionation theoretically tends to favor normal cells over tumor cells. As a very general rule, best results are achieved with radiation doses of 180–200 rads given five times per week (ibid.). If a sufficient total dose of radiation is not delivered to a tumor, radioresistance can develop from a previously sensitive cancer. A radiation dose is considered lethal to a tumor type if it achieves 95 percent tumor control. With doses that achieve less than a 95 percent control rate, tumor cells that survive are more likely to produce resistant cell phenotypes, either through characteristic mutations or through radiation-induced mutations.

Radioresponsiveness

Tumors are characterized as either radiosensitive or radioresistant. Malignant tumors tend to possess the same degree of radioresponsiveness as the tissue from which they originate. Radiosensitivity is also a factor of the mitotic potential of target cells and the oxygen component of the tumor environment. Except in the case of high-LET radiation, a hypoxic environment requires two to three times greater radiation doses to achieve a biological effect than a well-oxygenated environment. Cells that divide frequently are more radiosensitive than slowly replicating cells, as the DNA-replicating damage that radiation causes affects them more immediately, so repair is less likely to be effective.

Megavoltage Radiation

Today, megavoltage (meV) equipment is replacing kilovoltage (keV) equipment for most cancer treatments in radiation oncology. Megavoltage equipment delivers the maximum radiation dosage well below the skin surface with a sharper focus than that possible with the older, lower energy equipment. Because meV equipment does not result in as much energy absorption by bone as does keV equipment, it can deliver a cancericidal dose in the vicinity of bone without causing bone damage.

Interactions with Other Treatment Modalities

Radiation is often complementary in its effect with surgery. While surgery is effective at removing macroscopic tumor, radiation therapy is able to destroy microscopic tumor with relatively low doses. When the two are used together, the choice between preoperative and postoperative radiation is not clear-cut and remains a matter of controversy.

Chemotherapy and radiation therapy can sometimes interact to the disadvantage of normal tissues. For example, both can cause bone marrow suppression, which is usually the limiting factor in the use of these modalities together. Mucositis and dysuria are both potentiated by the use of these modalities on the same tissues. It has also been observed that leukemia is more likely to occur in Hodgkin's disease patients treated with both chemotherapy and radiation therapy than if either modality is used alone. A recall phenomenon in previously radiated tissues is observed when some drugs are given as late as a year after exposure to radiation.

Radiation therapy is an integral part of the multidisciplinary treatment of cancer. Two aspects of radiation oncology that are currently being widely studied for improvements in patient response are high-LET equipment and interactions among treatment modalities.

External Beam Radiation Therapy

Most radiation to cancer patients is delivered by external beam therapy. Clinical skills required in managing these patients pertain to the side effects of radiation therapy in general and the exposure field. External beam irradiation does not render the patient radioactive, nor require restrictions on patient activity following treatments. One general precaution nurses need to take with these patients is to ensure that ink landmarks are not washed off by staff, the patient, or family members between radiation treatments.

Internal Radiation Treatments (Brachytherapy)

The administration of radiation via a source placed in proximity to the tumor is referred to as brachytherapy. Brachytherapy includes the use of permanent or temporary implants or systemic administration of a radioactive substance. Managing the patient undergoing brachytherapy focuses on two goals: patient comfort and safety.

INTRACAVITARY IMPLANTS

The most frequent use of intracavitary implants is for treatment of uterine and vaginal cancer. Safety precautions include the prevention of dislodgment of the implant and minimizing staff exposure to the radiation. Once the implant is removed, the patient is no longer radioactive.

The placement of uterine and vaginal implants requires that the patient remain on bedrest for three to four days. During this time, activity should be minimized. Generally, the patient may sit at a 45° angle and roll from side to side. A urinary in-dwelling catheter is inserted to help minimize patient movement. The patient receives an enema prior to placement of the radioactive source and is placed on a low residue diet to minimize bowel movements, which could cause displacement of the inplant. This low residue diet excludes bran products, raw fruit and vegetables, nuts, seed-containing foods and hot spices.

After the completion of therapy and removal of the implant by a technician from the radiation department, the patient with uterine or vaginal cancer will receive a Betadine douche and, once steady on her feet, go home.

Because radiation can cause tissue shrinkage over time, a woman who has had a vaginal implant will need to dilate her vagina regularly to ensure that it remains pliable for future examinations and sexual activity. Dilation can be accomplished by sexual activity or by use of a plastic dilator. After a post-radiation rest period of about three weeks, twice weekly dilation of the vagina should be undertaken. If the woman uses a dilator, she should employ water-soluble lubricants on the appliance surface and insert the dilator as far as possible without experiencing pain, remove it, and repeat this withdrawal and insertion ten times. The easiest position for accomplishing this exercise is dorsal recumbent with legs bent comfortably at the knees. After each use of the dilator, it should be washed in soap and water. Dilation of the vagina on a regular schedule should be continued for at least a year to preclude contraction with fibrosis.

INTERSTITIAL RADIATION IMPLANTS

This modality is most often used in the treatment of breast cancer, but is also employed for head and neck cancers and prostate cancer as well. It is becoming more common as the popularity of the lumpectomy procedure increases in breast cancer treatment. Combined with the minimal surgery, and sometimes external beam radiation, interstitial irradiation preserves the cosmetic appearance of the breast while decreasing the potential for local recurrence of disease. Safety precautions include checking for loose seeds or needles that may have become dislodged and minimizing staff exposure to the radiation. When working with these patients, care must be taken with linen to check for loose implants. The patient may not be aware of the loss of these objects. Nurses have been known to walk on loose radioactive seeds in a room without being aware of their initial source!

Interstitial implant treatment generally lasts for forty-eight hours and delivers 2,000 rad to the underlying tumor. Patient activity is not greatly limited during the duration of treatment, but the patient is confined to a private room. At the completion of therapy, the implants are removed and the patient is no longer radioactive.

SYSTEMIC RADIATION TREATMENT

Radioactive substances may be administered systemically via an intravenous or oral route. A common use of this modality is for thyroid cancer, and involves the ingestion of I–131 (radioactive iodine). When this treatment is employed, the patient's body secretions—urine, stool, emesis, sweat, mucus, tears, and saliva—are contaminated. To avoid the spread of radioactive contaminants, disposable food trays are employed for the hospitalized patient. Nurses should take care to wash skin or items which may be contaminated by the patient's secretions.

The patient should avoid tub bathing and employ three to four flushes after each use of the toilet to dilute and remove radioactive material. The half-life of I–131 is 8.05 days, so these precautions are usually employed for one week. Once the I–131 has decayed, the patient is no longer radioactive.

INTERNAL RADIATION INSTILLATIONS

Radiation is frequently used for malignant effusions; both pericardial or pleural effusions may be treated. This mode of treatment is not selected if the patient presents with an acute condition; for example, if severe dyspnea is present. However, symptoms such as cough, dyspnea, and pleuritic chest pain can be treated by a sclerosing agent such as P–32 in the same way chemical sclerosing agents such as nitrogen mustard or tetracycline are used. Since the pleural drainage will be contaminated, special precautions need to be taken for its disposal. The nurse needs to assure that the fluid is drained in a manner without spills and that all associated materials are appropriately handled.

BOUGIE IMPLANTS

A radium bougie implant is sometimes used to deliver radiation close to the tumor. In the case of esophageal cancer, where this treatment may be useful, a radioactive source is placed in a nasogastric tube. It is positioned so that after the tube is passed, the radioactive source is next to the cancer, where it stays until treatment is over, usually within forty-eight hours.

GENERAL PRECAUTIONS WITH BRACHYTHERAPY

The nurse working with patients receiving brachytherapy should understand the principles of distance, time, and shielding as they relate to radiation. The closer and longer the exposure, the higher the risk of radiation exposure. The intensity of the radiation decreases in proportion to the distance from the radioactive source.

To keep staff and visitors at a reasonable distance from the radioactive source, the patient is given a private room with the bed placed at the end farthest from the door. As a wooden or plastic door will not stop gamma radiation, there is no need to close the door to the room. However, signs need to be prominently placed warning people to restrict unnecessary exposure. These precautions include standing at the door of the room or no closer than about six feet from the patient unless closer care is needed. The time spent in the room should be minimal. Generally, a restriction of fifteen minutes per day within the patient room is maintained for both staff and visitors.

The actual amount of radiation exposure received by staff and visitors is a product of the length of exposure and distance from the source. Badges are required for nurses who work with patients receiving brachytherapy. These badges simply record exposure and, of course, offer no protection. To be most informative, they should be worn at a level of the body that receives maximum exposure, such as the waist or abdomen. Individuals should be exposed to no more than 500 millirems of radiation per year. The maximum allowable dose to personnel is 5 rems of exposure for the whole body. Because of the danger of radiation to a fetus, pregnant visitors or staff are not allowed in the patient room. Visitors under age eighteen are also restricted from entering the patient's room to avoid hazards to growth and development. Women of child-bearing age are routinely excluded from pelvic radiation except during the ten day period immediately following the menstrual period in order to avoid radiating a ovum that could be fertilized.

Shielding of the body is applicable with alpha, beta and "soft" gamma radiation, but will not stop higher-energy "hard" gamma radiation. A lead apron is useful in some situations, but not in others. Direct contamination of the skin with radioactive material during patient care can be avoided by wearing gloves. Should a radioactive implant become dislodged, it must be picked up with special long-handled tongs and dropped into a lead container.

Alpha radiation is stopped by the skin and when given internally poses no risk except by direct contamination. Beta radiation is generally stopped by tissue; aluminum and lucite are often employed to shield workers against this type of radiation. Lead of varying thicknesses is needed to protect against gamma radiation; the width needed depends on the energy level of the source.

General Radiation Side Effects

Many of the side effects associated with radiation are also seen with chemotherapy treatments. They include bone marrow suppression, stomatitis, anorexia, alopecia, diarrhea, nausea and vomiting, and infection. Such side effects as well as those specifically related to radiotherapy will be discussed in detail in Chapter 4.

Most side effects of radiation therapy occur at the irradiated site. Therefore, by recognizing the most likely side effects associated with various body parts, the nurse will be able to guide assessments appropriately and instruct the patient.

SKIN REACTIONS

In the past, the dosage of radiation that could be delivered was limited to that tolerated by the skin, as severe radiodermatitis would otherwise occur. Today, megavoltage equipment can deliver most of the radiation below the level of the skin closer to the tumor site. Although skin reactions have decreased in recent years, care of radiated skin remains a priority in oncology nursing. As a rapidly renewing body part, the skin is especially sensitive to radiation effects, and some treatments require high skin dosages.

Today, the term "radiodermatitis" is fading from the literature and "radiation skin reaction" is taking its place to reflect changes in the degree of impairment now primarily seen. Long-term sequelae of radiotherapy have been largely eliminated with the advent of megavoltage equipment, but patients treated with lower energy photon or electron beam radiation may experience erythema, dry desquamation, or moist desquamation. These conditions may be described as follows (Hilderley 1983):

erythema: pink, bright, brisk, deep, dusky
dry desquamation: scaly, flaking, slight, itchy, moderate
moist desquamation: mild, moderate, severe, painful, weeping, sloughing

Nowadays, it is best to describe skin reactions to radiation by their character, not by "stages" or as "burns." Areas most at risk for a reaction are skin folds, the axillae, groin, perineum, and gluteal folds. Treatment of skin impairment is not standardized. Erythema or dry desquamation may be appropriately treated with minimal washing and careful handling. Areas of moist desquamation should be gently cleansed with saline or plain water. It is now understood that healing is promoted in a clean, moist environment, and this has begun to change the goals of therapy for moist desquamation. Instead of seeking to dry out the areas as quickly as possible, polyethylene film dressings are being used successfully. Vigilon brand dressings are another type of dressing used. With the wound-side film layer removed and a protective dressing applied over the Vigilon, a therapeutic environment is created that promotes healing.

Radiation skin reactions can be evoked or "recalled" with adminis-tration of certain chemotherapeutic agents, particularly Adriamycin and actinomycin-D. Methotrexate, bleomycin, cyclophosphamide, 5–fluorouracil, hydroxyurea, vincristine, and vinblastine are also known to cause radiation recall. Treatment of these recalled reactions is the same as for initially seen radiation skin reactions.

Epilation, or hair loss, can occur to areas within the radiation field. If between 1,500 and 3,000 rad are delivered, temporary hair loss may result. With radiation doses above 4,500 rad, permanent, complete hair loss occurs. At two to three weeks after the start of radiation therapy, hair may begin to fall out; regrowth begins after two or three months, and often the new hair is of a different color or texture. When scalp hair is lost, psychological distress usually results. It is sometimes not appreciated by care givers that even though a life-threatening disease is being treated, the stigmatizing effects of ther-apy can be of greatest concern to patients. Hair loss is often reported as the worst part of their therapy (Yasko 1983).

LYMPH NODE REACTIONS

Direct radiation of lymph nodes may cause fibrosis, which can occlude the lymph system and contribute to distal edema or infec-tion. While avoidance of such unfortunate conditions may not be possible, the nurse needs to assess extremities that are involved in a radiation field for these side effects. Teaching about care of the limb to avoid infection and minimize edema needs to be done early. Eleva-tion of the affected limb when recumbent, loose clothing over the associated area, and trauma avoidance are key points to cover.

ORAL SIDE EFFECTS

The oral side effects from radiation include stomatitis, muco-sitis, esophagitis, taste alterations, saliva production decreases leading to xerostomia, and trismus. Stomatitis, mucositis and esophagitis, which are also seen with chemotherapy patients, are covered in Chapter 4. Taste alterations that occur secondary to radiation therapy are a result of direct damage to taste buds of the tongue and are not the same as the taste alterations associated with cachexia. The de-crease in saliva production that may occur, particularly if the parotid glands are irradiated, also contributes to an altered taste sensation. These alterations to taste can be subtle or severe and may persist for the patient's lifetime, or if transitory, for as long as a year after therapy. Experimentation is the only way to find what foods the patient can enjoy, although the nurse needs to stress balance and adequacy of the diet. In the presence of xerostomia, the patient needs to lubricate the oral mucosa by frequently drinking fluids or by using commercially prepared artificial saliva, which is a prescription item. Sucking on items that stimulate saliva production, such as sugarless candy, may be helpful. Dental caries are more frequent in the patient with xerostomia. This problem can be ameliorated by the use of fluoride gel in a mouth mold daily, particularly during the period of radiation therapy. In addition, it may be helpful to avoid items that irritate mucous membranes, such as tobacco, alcohol, hot spices, or very hot or very cold foods. Dentures should fit well and snugly to avoid trapping food particles under them, which will irritate the oral lining.

In order to control or prevent oral side effects of radiation therapy, the patient needs to be consistent in applying good oral hygiene. During times when acute symptoms are present, oral care is necessary every two hours. Unfortunately, the epidemiology of oral cancer tells us that many of the patients afflicted with oral cancer have had poor oral hygiene for many years, and they will require patient, persevering guidance in developing new habits.

Trismus is a late effect that may occur subsequent to direct radiation therapy. It is characterized by contraction and fibrosis of the masticating muscles around the mouth, resulting in inability to open the mouth more than part way. The condition can be largely avoided if the mouth is routinely and consistently expanded or appliances are used to control distortions from defects associated with the surgery that is done on oral cancers. The social and psychological implications of the resulting communication impairment should be considered by the nurse caring for the patient with trismus. Approaches to managing side effects involving the gastrointestinal tract are treated in Table 3.2.

PULMONARY SIDE EFFECTS

Initial reactions seen from radiation to the lungs are a mild dyspnea and nonproductive cough. Between two and three months after therapy, radiation pneumonitis can occur, varying from asymptomatic radiographically seen lung changes to severe fibrosis. The fibrosis may be severe enough to compromise excursion and increases the patient's risk of pneumonia. Bleomycin administration compounds the risk for pulmonary fibrosis. Steroids may be helpful in reducing symptoms of early pneumonitis. If damage to the lungs does not reverse itself, the patient may be subject to a restricted lifestyle on a permanent basis and will need to be cautious about exposure to upper respiratory infections.

Table 3.2   Nursing Interventions and Dietary Guidelines for Side Effects Connected with Nutritional Problems

Problem	Cause	Nursing interventions/dietary guidelines
Mucositis, esophagitis	Radiation, chemotherapy	Pretreatment dental exam. Written and oral instructions for oral hygiene. Soft toothbrush and fluoridated toothpaste. Dental floss and daily fluoride treatments. Anesthetic mouthwashes or lozenges before meals and prn. Soft, moist foods: eggs, macaroni and cheese, chicken, soft fish, cheesecake, custards, puddings, ricotta cheese, yogurt, cooked cereal, rice, noodles, canned pears, peaches, apricots, applesauce, bananas, well-cooked soft fruits and vegetables. Food chopped into small pieces or mixed with gravy, sauces, or butter. Firm foods soaked in liquids to soften. Use of herbs rather than spices or peppers. Avoidance of coarse, crisp, crunchy, spicy, or hot foods; extremes in temperature; citrus or raw fruits; caffeine; alcohol; and tobacco.
Salivary changes	Radiation	Oral irrigations with pulsating water jet device and hydrogen peroxide and normal saline. Artificial saliva. Increased air humidity. Moist foods; stews; casseroles; simmered foods; pureed or blended foods mixed with milk, cream, or butter; clear soups with chopped cheese, meat, vegetables, beans, or noodles. Use of tart foods to stimulate saliva: lemon juice, lemonade, tea with lemon. Use of sauces, gravies, yogurt, sour cream, and salad dressings over foods to moisten. Avoidance of meat, bread products, and soft fish.
Inability to manipulate or control food	Resection of tongue, larynx, or mandible	Exercises to avoid aspiration. Referral to speech therapist and prosthetist. Firm, slippery foods: pasta, soft fruits, puddings, cheeses, hot dogs, hamburger, scrambled eggs, canned fruits, ground foods, foods with sauces or gravies, and bananas. Stimulation of visual, olfactory, and tactile awareness with colorful, aromatic, spicy, and strong-flavored foods. Avoidance of dairy and citrus foods.
Trismus	Radiation	Finely chopped, soft, or semiliquid foods. Exercises to relive spasm with tongue blades or mechanical devices to stretch the occlusion.

Table 3.2   Continued

Problem	Cause	Nursing interventions/dietary guidelines
Dysphagia	Tumor or radiation	Soft, semiliquid, or liquid foods as needed. Increased calories: extra butter, sugar, honey, marshmallows, whipped cream. Mayonnaise instead of salad dressings. Use of sour cream, yogurt, sauces, gravies, and cream as garnish for blended foods. Increased protein by addition of dry milk powder, cream, cheese, ground meat, or fish to soups, casseroles, eggs, or vegetables. Addition of eggs to milkshakes, puddings. Cream, bean, or meat soups instead of broths.
Early satiety	Gastrectomy or tumor	Small, frequent meals. Slow chewing. Choice of only high-calorie, high-protein foods. Avoidance of greasy foods, rich sauces, butter, liquids drunk with meals.
Dumping syndrome	Astrectomy	Low-carbohydrate, high-protein, high-fat diet. Fluids between meals only. After-meal rest periods of 30 to 60 minutes. Anticholinergic drugs before meals.
Diarrhea	Small bowel resection or radiation	Small, frequent meals. Choice of refined-grain breads, pasta, crackers; cream of wheat, white rice, tapioca, bananas, cheese, fish, chicken, cooked vegetables, boiled milk, applesauce, juice, and tea. Avoidance of whole-grain bread products, fruits or vegetables with skins and seeds intact, gas-forming foods (broccoli, onions, garlic), chewing gum, citrus fruits and juices, and pork. Defined formula diet as needed. Antispasmodics, antiemetics, anticholinergics, and antidiarrheal agents as needed.
Constipation	Drug therapy	One liter or more of fluid per day. Choice of whole-grain bread products, bran products, nuts, coconut, corn, popcorn, raw fruits and vegetables with skins and seeds intact, raisins, prunes and prune juice, dates, hot lemonade. Avoidance of cheese, refined bread products, rich pastries. Use of stool softeners and laxatives as needed.

Source: A. J. Kempen, in *Nursing Care of the Cancer Patient with Nutritional Problems.* Report of the Ross Oncology Nursing Round-Table. (Columbus, Ohio: Ross Laboratories, 1981), 59.

CARDIAC SIDE EFFECTS

If the heart is in the radiation field, acute transient pericarditis can occur. Even months or years following treatment, pericarditis, myocarditis, or cardiac tamponade can develop as a consequence of the radiation therapy. Assessments of patients with a relevant history need to include particular attention to signs or symptoms of cardiac inpairment such as chest pain, tachycardia, a narrowing pulse pressure or shortness of breath with normal activity.

URINARY SIDE EFFECTS

If the bladder is included in an external beam radiation field or if internal radiation sources are proximal to the bladder, cystitis can develop. Burning, frequency, urgency, and hematuria are signs of developing radiation cystitis of which the nurse should be aware. Increasing fluids to 3,000 cc over the course of a day, and avoiding bladder irritants such as coffee, tea, alcohol, hot spices, and tobacco may help reduce symptoms.

Radiation nephritis can occur if the kidneys are exposed to radiation doses beyond 2,300 rad over four to five weeks (Yasko 1983). Within a year's time renal hypertension and renal failure can develop, as well. Ureteral obstruction subsequent to abdominal radiation is another potential side effect of radiation therapy.

Immunology and Biological Response Modifiers

The central concept of contemporary tumor immunology is that tumors possess antigens distinct from those of normal cells that may permit the host to recognize the tumor as foreign. Biological response modifiers (BRM) act to alter the patient's biological response to tumor cells in a therapeutic manner. Generally they are categorized into two groups: (1) modulating agents, which are compounds that stimulate the patient's resistence to tumor growth or metastasis, and (2) biologicals, which are cells or cell products that act directly against tumor cells. Some substances are active in both categories. The first group largely includes immunomodulators, which suppress, inhibit, or increase various immunologic mechanisms. The second group acts by cytotoxic effects or as an inhibitor of tumor growth or metastasis directly.

Classic immunotherapy is a part of BRM therapy, categorized in the first group described above. The biologics that are under current review or are currently in clinical trials are interferon, thymic factors, monoclonal antibodies, and several cytokines. Some agents, such as interferon, act as either immunomodulators or biologics, depending on the dose. It is probable that although not widely used today, some of these therapeutic agents will be standard therapy by the late 1980s (Suppers and McClamrock 1985).

Lymphokines and Cytokines

The term lymphokine refers to the soluble cell products of lymphocytes; cytokines are the soluble products of cells in general. Interferon is a cytokine as it can be produced by any body cell. There are over one hundred lymphokines and cytokines that can be described at the present time; many more may exist. The use of the biologicals is not restricted to cancer therapy; in fact, many will probably prove useful for autoimmune, inflammatory, and infectious disorders.

Some agents that are being vigorously studied at the present time include interleukin–1 (IL–1), interleukin–2 (IL–2) (also known as T-cell growth factor), colony-stimulating factor, macrophage activating factor (MAF), tumor necrosis factor, and leukoregulin. IL–2 is receiving a lot of attention recently as it has shown some activity in Acquired Immune Deficiency Syndrome (AIDS). Patients with this disorder have a selective defect in T-helper cells. There have been encouraging results so far with the limited supplies of the compound tested. Another use of interleukins being studied is the administration of these substances as an adjunct to chemotherapy to hasten recovery of the immune system.

Interferon

The interferons (IFN) are proteins that regulate cell function, slow cell proliferation, and inhibit virus replication. Interferons slow proliferation of cells by prolonging all phases of the mitotic cycle. With removal of the IFN, normal growth resumes within twenty-four to seventy-two hours. Interferons are thought to act against virus-caused disease by stimulating uninfected cells to change their cell membrane, preventing viral penetration. Interferon acts against viral oncogenes by this mechanism, but some other mechanism is responsible for their observed efficacy against differently induced cancers. Interferons from various cell lines exhibit dissimilar pharmacokinetics, thus complicating clinical trials. They have been shown to be active in human breast cancer, malignant lymphoma, multiple myeloma, acute and chronic leukemia, melanoma, Kaposi's sarcoma, renal cancer, bladder carcinoma, gliomas, and nasopharyngeal cancer. Discovered in 1957, they are currently being evaluated in clinical trials around the world. IFN-alpha is the best understood type of interferon being used today. IFN-beta and IFN-gamma are the two other main forms of interferon that have been identified, and they are presently undergoing earlier steps in the evaluation process than IFN-alpha.

There is confusion in the literature concerning the nomenclature for the various interferons. An international group sponsored by the National Institutes of Health and the World Health Organization recently has made recommendations, which are being generally adopted. Interferon should be abbreviated as INF. Each interferon should be identified by the animal of origin, antigenic specificities, and cell line origin. For example, human interferon from leucocyte cells would be abbreviated as HuIFN-alpha(Le).

IFN-alpha therapy has resulted in both complete and partial regressions of tumors in patients with disseminated or metastatic disease, perhaps by its ability to support T-cell proliferation (Oldham et al. 1984). Response has been dramatic and rapid; although only small numbers of patients have received IFN-alpha therapy to date, a significant number have moved from a life-threatening condition to a virtually normal state within six to eight weeks (Quesada et al. 1985). Most IFN studies are still in Phase I and Phase II of development, so all results are preliminary and limited. The nurse caring for patients undergoing IFN-alpha treatment can expect to observe transient fever of between thirty-eight to forty degrees Centigrade during the first few days of therapy. A drop in the leucocyte count to between 2,000 and 4,000/cu mm is common, but quickly reverses when therapy is stopped. With high doses, anorexia and fatigue are often dose-limiting. Diarrhea may be a problem. Opportunistic herpes infections sometimes develop during therapy. SGOT values are commonly elevated and if high values persist, the interferon therapy sometimes has to be discontinued. A commonly used schedule of administration of IFN-alpha is a daily intramuscular injection of 3–9 x 10–6th power units for twenty-eight days. The most effective route, dose, and schedule are not yet known, and the nurse may see a variety of other regimens used.

IFN-gamma may act as an interleukin (endogenous pyrogen). Although trials of this interferon class are new, it may prove to be the most powerful and diverse immunomodulator of the three interferon forms currently being used clinically. There is some evidence that IFN-gamma may be responsible for some of the biological activity ascribed to other lymphokines and cytokines (Zlotnik 1983). Toxicities seen with IFN-gamma use are similar to those described for IFN-alpha. In addition, dose-limiting hypotension has occasionally been seen in these patients.

Monoclonal Antibodies

In the late 1970s, Kohler and Milstein developed a method of producing pure monoclonal antibodies (MAB) from the cloned cells of mice. This breakthrough allowed scientists to develop specific antibodies to antigens of interest. It has been found in some clinical trials that MAB therapy has an immediate, but transient, antitumor effect. One problem encountered has been the antigenic modulation of tumor cells and the heterogeneity of tumor cell colonies. The development of a pure antitumor cell antibody may be effective only against a proportion of the total number of cancer cells, and then only for a limited period of time. Another means of dealing with the problem of a subpopulation of primary tumor cells with a predefined metastatic potential is the development of MABs to metastasized tumor cells. In order to be most effective in prolonging patient survival, however, it is preferable that therapy be used as soon as possible, particularly prior to detectable metastasis, if possible. Cocktails of mixtures of MAB may be required for clinical effectiveness in this instance. If MABs are used to carry drugs, toxins, or radioisotopes to cancer cells specifically, the problem of tumor cell modulation and diversity may be largely irrelevant. This use of MAB is being vigorously investigated.

Relatively low toxicities are associated with the administration of MABs. Mild fever, mild nausea, anorexia, chills, and headache are seen in some patients, along with urticaria.

Classic Immunotherapy

It has been clearly shown in the past that tumor cells carry on their surfaces specific antigens that can be recognized by the host as foreign. These surface antigens appear as a probable result of cellular or viral oncogenic modulations of normal cell products. Two types of immunological responses are seen in the human host to counter this threat of foreign cancer cells. The humoral immune response is one in which the body produces antibody immunoglobulin specific to the foreign antigens. This humoral immune response originates with antigen binding cells, which are lymphocytes termed B cells, that develop with a capacity to bind cells with foreign antigens that may be introduced into the host. These lymphocytes then produce antibodies specific for the antigens they have bound. This is the mechanism of the body's humoral response mediated by immunoglobulins. B cells originate in the bone marrow, and are specific for a particular form of antibody immunoglobulin (five forms). When B cells are stimulated by foreign antigen, they undergo transformation into what are termed "plasma cells." It is plasma cells that actually produce specific immunoglobulins in the body.

The cell–mediated immune response of the body is generally effected through T-cells. The thymus of the body produces T-cells, a type of lymphocyte, which reside in the spleen and lymph nodes and circulate in peripheral blood. When T-cells are stimulated by a foregin antigen, they proliferate as activated, or "effector," lymphocytes, causing a cell–mediated immune response. Graft-versus-host disease, delayed hypersensitivity, and resistance to microbial infections are examples of T-cell mediated immune responses. T-cells also function as "helper" cells, which assist the body in the production of immunoglobulin, or as "suppressor" cells to inhibit the immune response.

Macrophages are nonspecific mediators of the immune response. Macrophages develop from bone marrow monocytes and circulate for several months. They serve to regulate the B cell response, actively participate in antibody–antigen reactions, and phagocytose foreign cells, releasing many antigens for immunological response from other cells.

Since tumor cells possess distinct surface antigens that should be recognized by the body as foreign and thereafter eliminated by an immune response, yet cancers do develop, so either the tumor cells can mask their foreign nature or the immune system is defective in eliminating them. Theories that are being studied to explain the phenomenom of cancer growth include the consideration that the cancer cell antigen was present in early life so that B cells did not develop receptors for it as foreign; that tumor growth exceeds the capacity of the immune response; that tumor cells that survive have modulated their surface antigens so that only a minimal immune response is induced; and that blocking immune factors may enhance tumor growth through some unknown pathway.

Hyperthermia

Perhaps the best known historical investigator in the use of hyperthermia in the treatment of cancer is W. B. Coley, who in the early 1900s had some success with the use of hyperthermia caused by fever from the bacterial infections he induced in cancer patients. Fever is important as a natural defense against bacterial, viral, and parasitic infections, and is now considered to have a role in cancer treatment. In the early part of the century, advances in surgical techniques, radiation therapy, and then chemotherapeutic drug therapy led to a general decrease in interest in systemic fever in cancer treatment. In the 1960s this interest was rekindled when Cavaliere et al. (1967) demonstrated that cancer cells were more sensitive to heat than normal cells, and that regional hyperthermia was effective in treating some cancers. Today it is cautiously suggested that hyperthermia either alone or in combination with other treatment modalities is responsible for a 25–50 percent response rate in various cancers.

Today, it has been demonstrated that there is a synergistic effect between temperatures of 41 to 42 degrees C. and radiation therapy and some drug therapy. Efficacy of hyperthermia is increased at temperatures of 43 to 45 degrees C., but humans can only tolerate these high temperatures in regional therapy rather than whole body treatment. Whole body hyperthermia at 41–42 degrees C. has been clearly shown to be safe, reliable, and effective in increasing the effects of other cancer treatment modalities.

There are three basic methods of evoking systemic fever. The first is by administration of exogenous agents such as bacteria or chemicals that cause fever. It is difficult to control the degree of temperature elevation produced by this method, however, so it is not being tested clinically to any great extent. Secondly, temperature can be elevated by increasing the amount of heat in contact with the skin. The most frequently employed methods for skin surface heating are immersion of the patient in a heated water tank or water-filled space suit; placement in a heated enclosure; or immersion in hot parafin wax. The third method available is through use of a blood warmer that works via a femoral arteriovenous shunt. Regional and local hypertherapy may be induced by concentrated energy from interstitial implants and focused ultrasound as well as microwave, capacitive, and inductive forms of electromagnetic applications (Storm and Morton 1983).

The mechanism of heat destruction of tumor cells remains poorly understood. Several investigators have found that a major factor in cell killing at about 42 degrees C. is the irreversible damage to cancer cell respiration. The upper threshold of applied heat for humans is 45 degrees C., a temperature above which unbearable pain and generalized cell destruction occur. At temperatures above 45 degrees C., normal tissues as well as cancerous ones begin to die from protein denaturation. Because the blood flow in tumors is usually less well regulated than in normal tissue, tumors tend to retain applied heat while normal tissues are more readily cooled. Thus, selective tumor heating can be quite effective. Some investigators believe that hyperthermia stimulates the immune system, perhaps by releasing tumor cell products that increase lymphocyte activity. Studies have shown that fewer distant metastatic sites develop in those treated with local hyperthermia, lending credence to the immune response theory.

Whole body hyperthermia is currently being used at cancer centers around the country. Various methods of heat production are used; usually with the patient under general anesthesia with mechanically controlled breathing or under heavy sedation during the treatment. This induced sedation is used because the induction and treatment process takes about four hours. Whole body hyperthermia can have significant toxicity. Heating the body by the skin surface causes profound cardiovascular stress. Blood pressure falls, and heart rate increases concomitant to temperature elevation. No cardiac damage has been documented by the hyperthermic treatment, but the patient remains in a high cardiac output state throughout the procedure. Patients also lose large amounts of fluid in sweat with all methods of inducing whole body hyperthermia, which is controlled through intravenous infusions at rates of 500 to 1,000 cc per hour. Serum creatine phosphokinase (CPK) values are usually elevated at twenty-four hours post-treatment, and there may be a decrease in creatinine clearance during the procedure, which quickly reverses once treatment is stopped. Hypophosphatemia occurs during whole body hyperthermia by unknown mechanisms. When the skin surface heating method is used, nausea and vomiting have been shown to occur in 50 percent of patients during the first twelve hours after therapy. About 40 percent of patients develop diarrhea. It is interesting that 20 percent of patients experience posthyperthermia fevers as high as 41 degrees C. beginning six to twenty-four hours after cooling (Bull 1982). All investigators of whole body hyperthermia have reported instances of reversible peripheral neuropathy. There appear to be fewer toxicities associated with the blood warming technique of heat production. Cardiac output may be elevated, but pulmonary artery wedge pressures are usually little affected by the hyperthermia. Urine phosphate levels may be elevated during treatment, but return to normal with body cooling. Organ and tumor vascular response to the hyperthermia produced by skin surface heating and blood warming need to be compared further before one or the other is determined to be preferable for treating cancer. Furthermore, there is still no firm information to suggest with what frequency the hyperthermia should be given, the optimum duration of therapy, and what types of tumors respond best to this modality.

Clinical trials to date have studied the combination of whole body hyperthermia and chemotherapy administration used concomitantly; future studies must be undertaken to determine the importance, if any, of sequencing on the tumorcidal effects of the combination. Hyperthermia has been used clinically immediately after radiation therapy, with remarkable regressions achieved. Dose and fraction (interval) schedules need to be more fully understood so that optimum use of the combined modalities can be achieved. Because the core of a tumor is in a hypoxic state and hypoxic cells are more heat sensitive than well-oxygenated tissue, hyperthermia therapy combines well with radiotherapy, as hypoxic cells are less radiosensitive than oxygenated ones. Thus the two modalities complement each other to provide increased efficacy to that seen by use of the methods used singly.

Today, most local tumor heating is done with electromagnetic (EM) coupling or ultrasound. The three commonly used forms of EM coupling are all relatively easy to use. A capacitive system utilizes electrode paddles to create an electrical circuit across the skin surface between two electrodes. Fat necrosis and severe skin reactions can result from high temperatures created by the electrical circuit, limiting its effectiveness. Inductive heating is accomplished by means of placing the body part within a magnetic field created by one or more pancake coil electrodes. Deep penetration is made possible by arranging the coils circumferentially around the body part. Microwaves are the third type of EM heating system used. Because the frequency of the waves can be easily manipulated for good localization of energy, the microwave system offers the advantages of deep penetration and area specificity. Ultrasound heating can penetrate very deeply into the body except in areas where air or bone need to be passed, such as the lungs. Ultrasound does not pass through air and is reflected by bone, so treatment of the lungs, bowels, or tumors beneath large bones is not useful with ultrasound techniques (Moore 1984b).

One major difficulty encountered in hyperthermia treatment is that of thermal resistance. It appears that cells can adapt to the application of heat over short or long periods of time. Cell repair seems to take place between thermal treatments, as it does in the case of radiotherapy. As research provides answers to the questions of how to overcome resistance and what schedules and doses are optimal, hyperthermia is expected to become an integral part of cancer treatment.

4

Commonalities in Clinical Cancer Care

Some problems associated with cancer are common to many different forms of the disease. While elsewhere some specific problems associated with major cancer sites are described, this chapter will portray those problems and commonalitites in cancer care that may be evidenced in patients having cancer of various sites of origin or metastasis.

Management of Signs of the Cancer Process

Paraneoplasia

The concept of paraneoplastic (PN) syndrome, which has only been recognized since 1962, refers to conditions that arise from metabolic effects of cancer on tissues remote from the tumor, and that may resemble primary endocrine, hematologic, or neuromuscular disorders. There is evidence that malignant tumors may produce large numbers of different substances, most of which may be clinically inactive. It is now thought that cancer cells produce active and inactive peptides which are responsible for many of the syndromes seen. These syndromes are not unusual; it is thought that as many as 50 percent of patients with a malignancy will be affected by PN at some time in their illness. The nature of the underlying malignancy is a factor in the expression of PN. For example, small cell cancers of the lung are often associated with them, while colorectal cancers rarely involve their appearance. PN most frequently is seen when disease is advanced and metastasis present, although it may appear at any stage and is occasionally seen years or months before any other signs of cancer develop.

Tumor cells arising from tissues that normally produce hormones may secrete these polypeptides far in excess of normal body amounts, giving rise to clinical syndromes. This is referred to as "eutopic" substance production and secretion. In addition, tumor cells arising from tissues that do not normally elaborate a particular hormone

106

may secrete it. This, in contrast with the normal hormone produced by tumor cells of relevant origin, is called "ectopic." Ectopic synthesis and secretion of hormonal substances, almost always polypeptides, is now found to be a frequent clinical phenomenon. The hormones produced by tumor cells are identical or very similar to normal body polypeptide hormones. Even among normal human hormones there is heterogeneity, so differentiating hormones of tumor origin from those of normal tissue origin is not yet possible.

Treatment of a paraneoplastic syndrome is generally accomplished by eliminating the tumor, which stops the hormone production, or when that is not possible, by controlling the symptoms themselves to contribute to a better sense of well-being in the patient. Ectopic hormones serve to some extent as indicators of the presence of a tumor, and are used to indicate tumor regression or advance. Radioimmunoassays for human chorionic gonadotropin are used in the management of gestational choriocarcinoma and testicular cancer, while levels of oncofetal proteins, carcinoembryonic antigen, and alpha-fetoprotein help monitor disease progression. It is always a possibility that what is thought to be PN is actually a sign of infection, nutritional deficiencies or drug toxicity that can be treated directly. Differentiation of PN from other similar clinical presentations involves the testing of hormone levels in various tissues at varying times after tumor manipulation.

SECRETION OF INAPPROPRIATE ANTIDIURETIC HORMONE (SIADH)

Endocrine paraneoplastic syndromes are very common and well characterized. Nearly every polypeptide hormone normally secreted by normal endocrine tissue has been shown to be produced ectopically by various tumors of nonendocrine origin. One of the most frequently encountered endocrine paraneoplastic syndromes seen is ectopically produced antidiuretic hormone (ADH) secretion, leading to water intoxication. It is generally seen in small cell lung cancer patients, as many as 10 percent of whom show clinical signs of the syndrome at some point in their disease and about 70 percent demonstrate abnormal water metabolism when tested. A variety of other tumors have been associated with SIADH to a lesser extent. SIADH may also be caused by certain other classes of drugs (Oncovin, Velban, and Cytoxan) and a number of other classes of drugs, as well as by a paraneoplastic mechanism. Paraneoplasia of ADH is characterized by very dilute urine, absence of volume depletion, and sustained renal excretion of sodium in the face of normal renal function. Hyponatremia results. In its mild form this is associated with weakness and lethargy; if sodium falls below ll5 mEq/L, coma and seizures may result. The basic pathophysiology of excess ADH production is inordinate retention of free water. In its mild form, it can be treated by restricting water to 500 ml to one liter per day, although the chronic nature of SIADH makes this treatment impractical over extended time periods. With severe symptoms, slow and careful saline infusions and furosemide (Lasix) administration are given to treat volume overload. There are drugs available that induce a mild nephrogenic diabetes insipidus, which counteracts the ADH effects. Demeclocycline, which acts by this mechanism, given along with moderate water restrictions has been found highly successful. Lithium treatment has been largely replaced by demeclocycline, as lithium is more toxic and inferior in its effect.

HYPERCALCEMIA

Hypercalcemia is a relatively common finding in patients with cancer, and cancer is the most common cause of hypercalcemia in hospitalized patients. Between 10 and 25 percent of breast cancer patients have associated hypercalcemia during the course of their illness. This phenomena may be the direct result of bony metastasis with rapid turnover of bone or may be a true paraneoplastic effect. With other cancer types, including lung (particularly the squamous cell type), head and neck, kidney, ovary, cervix, pancreas and hepatomas, hypercalcemia is usually seen without evidence of bony metastasis. A hyperparathyroidism is produced by the tumor cells, with a few uncharacteristic aspects. Bicarbonate levels are elevated, resulting in metabolic alkalosis rather than the metabolic acidosis seen in primary hyperparathyroidism. In addition, the clinical course is much more rapid than with the primary condition. It has been recently found that there are additional paraneoplastic mechanisms of hypercalcemia. Ectopic prostaglandins and other substances have been implicated in hypercalcemia associated with various cancers such as renal cell carcinoma and lymphomas.

Hypercalcemia often causes symptoms that may be the patient's primary problem. Polyuria and nocturia occur in the early stages; and anorexia, nausea, constipation, muscle weakness, and fatigue are commonly experienced. As hypercalcemia becomes severe, dehydration, azotemia, mental obtundation, coma, and cardiovascular collapse may occur. Hypokalemia and elevated levels of BUN and creatinine may be associated with the hypercalcemia. Treatment is by resection of the tumor, or, when that is not possible, by controlling the symptoms and observing for prevention of life-threatening, severe hypercalcemia.

Mild to moderate hypercalcemia is associated with serum calcium levels of 12 to 13 mg/100 ml. Generally the patient is asymptomatic or only shows mild symptoms with calcium at this level, and adequate hydration is generally considered sufficient treatment. If hypercalcemia becomes more severe, saline diuresis, glucocorticoid administration, calcitonin infusions, oral phosphate therapy, and mithramycin or nonsteroidal anti-inflammatory agents may be used to treat this potentially lethal condition (Oncologic emergencies are more fully discussed later in this chapter.)

HYPOGLYCEMIA

Aside from hypoglycemia associated with pancreatic cancer, this condition is rarely seen except in terminal disease, when it is quite common as a paraneoplastic phenomena. Confusion, lethargy, irritability, and coma are presenting symptoms with plasma glucose levels of from 45–50 mg/100 ml. Palliation is difficult because specific agents are not available. Sometimes removal of the tumor yields relief even when metastasis is present. Diet control is the primary form of therapy. Frequent feedings, even through the night, may be required to prevent hypoglycemic attacks. With difficult cases, placement of a feeding tube for continuous feedings may be necessary. Sometimes even continuous 10–20 percent glucose infusions are required in addition to the feedings. Temporarily, glucocorticoids such as prednisone, or glucagon or human growth hormone, are helpful. Diazoxide, an agent that causes hyperglycemia, is usually ineffective in the hypoglycemia associated with malignancies.

ZOLLINGER-ELLISON SYNDROME

The Zollinger-Ellison syndrome is characterized by severe peptic ulcers of the stomach, duodenum, and jejunum in the presence of a pancreatic tumor. Diarrhea and steatorrhea (excess fat in the feces) are also commonly seen. The pancreatic tumor causes eutopic production of gastrin by islet cells. A total gastrectomy and removal of the pancreatic tumor may be utilized to control symptoms. Cimetidine or newer related drugs, such as ranitidine, are used to block hydrochloric acid secretion, and streptozotocin has been found to be helpful in some cases.

FEVER

Fever not associated with infection is commonly seen in various cancers and may be the result of tumor necrosis or be produced by pyrogens secreted by tumor cells. It is most often seen with renal cell carcinomas, lymphomas (particularly Hodgkin's disease), and with liver metastasis from gastrointestinal cancers. Nearly half of all lymphoma patients will present initially with a fever of unknown origin. It needs to be borne in mind, though, that most fevers experienced by the patient during the course of cancer are related to infections. If antibiotics are not helpful in reducing fever, symptomatic relief is found with antipyretics or nonsteriodal anti-inflammatory agents.

CACHEXIA

Cachexia is considered to be a paraneoplastic syndrome. Because it is so common in lung, gastrointestinal, lymphoma and breast cancer and is almost universal in terminal disease, it is described separately in this chapter.

ANEMIA

Anemia is commonly seen in cancer patients and is due to a variety of causes, including direct infiltration of the bone marrow, anemia associated with chronic disease, antibody-mediated hemolytic anemia, and iron deficiency. The anemia associated with chronic disease is not clearly understood, but is frequently seen in cancer patients and thought to be a paraneoplastic phenomenon.

HEMATOLOGICAL DISORDERS

Coagulation disorders in cancer patients are commonly seen and may be paraneoplastic phenomena or direct complications of the cancer itself. Thrombocytosis, with platelet counts above 400,000/cu mm, is especially common in lung cancer, Hodgkin's disease, and myeloproliferative disorders. Unexplained thrombocytosis may indicate a subclinical malignancy and present as thrombophlebitis or pulmonary embolism. Thrombocytopenia secondary to chronic subclinical disseminated intravascular coagulation (DIC) is commonly seen in cancer patients. The DIC itself may be related to tumor production of thromboplastic materials or tumor activation of fibrinolytic enzymes.

BONE AND SOFT TISSUE ABNORMALITIES

Clubbing of the fingers and toes, as well as joint inflammation and periosteal proliferation, may be seen in malignancies (particularly lung cancer) as PN. When these three conditions are associated, they are more commonly part of a neoplastic process than related to benign causes. The joints most frequently involved are the knees, ankles, elbows, wrists, and metacarpophalangeal joints. Patients complain of joint or leg pain. Salicylates or glucocorticoids may offer relief and, of course, successful resection of the tumor responsible provides prompt regression.

CENTRAL NERVOUS SYSTEM ABNORMALITIES

A syndrome of cerebellar ataxia, dysarthria, dysphagia, and sometimes dementia is a form of PN with an unknown underlying pathology. It has been most commonly associated with small cell lung cancer, ovarian carcinoma, and breast cancer. This unfortunate and dramatic syndrome causes enormous pain for the patient and family and is only poorly responsive to palliation, which is limited to tumor resection if possible.

NEUROLOGICAL ABNORMALITIES

Motor, sensory, or mixed neurologic abnormalities are commonly encountered in malignancies. Mild symmetrical sensory peripheral neuropathy is the most common of the neuropathies considered to be paraneoplastic events and is seen in terminal disease. The role of general debility and poor nutrition in these clinical syndromes needs to be elaborated and the mechanism of the PN determined before adequate control of these neuropathies can be effected.

The syndromes described above are but a few of those that are tentatively identified in relationship to cancer as paraneoplastic phenomena. As research continues and more is understood about the role of oncogenes and viruses in cancer events, the list will change. One example of the way that research is changing our understanding of cancer's effects on the body in general is the case of progressive multifocal leukoencephalopathy. This syndrome was considered to be a paraneoplastic event associated with hematologic malignancies until the 1980s, when compelling evidence was accumulated of its viral origin. A DNA virus of the popova group has been shown to be the etiologic agent in the syndrome's course. The viral infection may be a reactivated latent infection or an opportunistic infection related to immunosuppressive therapy.

The nurse should be aware that these paraneoplastic phenomena are extremely common and not always amenable to standard therapies associated with their occurrence from other causes, and may have devastating consequences. Those described above are some of the most familiar ones seen in cancer centers today.

Cancer Cachexia

Cancer cachexia is a clinical syndrome, based on metabolic dysfunction, which is seen in over half of all cancer patients and in most who are in a terminal phase. It is distinct from protein-calorie malnutrition in its pathophysiology and response to nutrition therapy. Two types of cancer cachexia are described: primary, which has an unknown cause, and secondary, which is related to decreased food intake from obstruction, anorexia, and so on. The syndrome is characterized by wasting, whether or not nutrient intake is maintained or even increased. In fact, primary cachexia does not respond to aggressive management; total parenteral nutrition (TPN) is not effective. Even if weight is gained while on TPN, it is not lean body mass, but mostly fat and water. Therefore, the early promise in the 1970s for TPN in controlling cachexia has not been realized, and its use in these cases is diminishing. TPN has been shown in many national trials to have no effect on cancer survival time after metastasis. Candidates for TPN among cancer cases include those in whom the tumor is potentially curable, or who are thought to need nutritional support during therapies. Once liver metastasis has occurred, TPN is not considered useful. However, with the advent of more clinically useful hepatic chemotherapy infusion systems such as the implanted pumps, the extremely poor prognosis heralded by liver metastasis may be modified and some of these patients found to be helped with nutritional support in potentially curable disease.

The cachexic individual is seen progressively to deteriorate physically. Sodium and water retention occurs in the syndrome, sometimes initially masking weight loss. Nausea, dysphagia, anorexia, early satiety, and altered taste sensations are also experienced to varying degrees. As the condition progresses, weakness, apathy, and emaciation occur. As standard treatment has prolonged survival time for some cancers, more cachexia is being seen, probably because other disease manifestations killed the patients before cachexia developed.

Cancer cachexia is not a result of starvation or inadequate nutritional support. Encouraging the patient to eat more will not reverse the effects of primary cachexia and may only add guilt to the patient's burdens. Sometimes helpless families and even professionals who know better will aimlessly encourage the patient to eat throughout the day. The patient may find the thought of food nauseating or be able to tolerate only very specific foods that may not be considered "best" for him or her. The main point to nursing care of the cachexic patient is to include the patient in planning nutrition and adhering to the limits the patient feels comfortable with.

The metabolism of all nutrients is altered in cancer cachexia. It has been postulated that the pathogenesis of cancer cachexia is related to the production of peptides by cancer cells that alter the normal enzyme functions of the body's cells. Consequently, the body is unable to utilize nutrients properly. Other constitutional effects may also occur. Alterations in biochemistry that occur in cancer cachexia (Kempen 1981) include:

> endocrine homeostasis
> enzyme activity
> carbohydrate metabolism
> lipid metabolism
> protein metabolism
> water content
> electrolytes and acid–base balance
> mineral concentrations
> vitamin concentration and effects
> energy metabolism

If the cachexia is not of the primary variety, but due to effects of the cancer such as obstruction or the side effects of chemotherapy, then modification of eating patterns, nutrient supplementation with tube feedings or TPN, and control of symptoms such as pain and depression can be helpful. Although cancer cachexia cannot be prevented, the nurse should be alert to signs of this syndrome and initiate measures to attempt reversal of early manifestations. Guidance should be given to patients and family members about small, frequent meals that are high in proteins the patient tolerates well. Tube feedings (see Table 4.1) or TPN should be initiated before muscle wasting is severe in potentially curable disease. This is when gains in well-being are most likely to be achieved. It is not clear what proportion of anorexia is due to symptoms such as pain or depression, but it is probably large. The nurse should always consider these associated factors in dealing with cancer cachexia. Once it is clear that cachexia is progressing, the patient and family should be taught that it is a syndrome associated with cancer that is not related to the patient's adherence or nonadherence to appropriate nutritional intake.

Skin Lesions

When tumors near the skin surface become large, they may cause fungating wounds that are necrotic, painful, and malodorous. This type of wound is most commonly seen in advanced breast cancer and can be difficult to treat.

A useful regimen for handling this type of wound is to irrigate it well with normal saline, then apply a thin layer of Silvadene (silver sulfadiazide) to the wound surface using a sterile glove, and cover

Table 4.1 Tube Feeding Routes

Indications	Advantages	Disadvantages	Precautions
Nasogastric Anorexia, lack of weight gain due to decreased intake, laryngeal or pharyngeal tumors, obstruction, or reconstruction (Some esophageal tumors, depending on obstruction)	No surgery required. Patient can feed self. Patient upright for feeding. Small, flexible, polyurethane tubes are comfortable	Irritating to nose, throat, pharynx, and larynx. Interferes with cough reflex, increasing risk of pulmonary complications. Disoriented patient may disturb tube or feeding. Tube may interrupt sutures. Possible ulceration of nares, sinusitis, skin breakdown. Reinsertion can cause wound damage. Unesthetic and socially limiting.	Elevate head of bed while feeding and for 30 minutes afterward. Vary the method of anchoring the tube to prevent pressure sores. Prolonged intubation creates the possibility of refluxed gastric acid and distal esophagitis.
Nasointestinal All of above, plus gastric resection	All of above. Eliminates esophagitis.	All of above.	All of above except esophagitis.
Gastrostomy Total obstruction of head, neck, or esophagus	Patient can feed self. Easy to reinsert.	Requires abdominal surgery. Requires supine feeding position. Patient must open or remove clothing for feeding. Skin excoriation.	Provide skin protection with stoma adhesive, Karaya ring, zinc oxide, or aluminum paste.
Cervical esophagostomy Tumors, resection, or irradiation of nasal, oral, pharyngeal, laryngeal, or esophageal	Avoids abdominal surgery. More physiologic than gastrostomy. Patient sits during feeding. Stoma	Cannot be used after certain radiation treatments or for obstruction distal to lower esophagus.	Assess hoarseness, coughing reflex prior to first feeding to rule out damage to 10th cranial nerve.

Table 4.1 Continued

Indications	Advantages	Disadvantages	Precautions
passageways; permanent or temporary loss of swallowing; need for long-term tube feeding	concealed by clothing. Tract closes promptly after tube removed. Easy to replace if accidentally removed.	Possible carotid artery erosion. May cause stricture or esophagitis.	
Jejunostomy			
Tumor, obstruction, or resection of head, neck, or upper GI tract	Aspiration unlikely.	Requires abdominal surgery. High incidence of diarrhea and skin excoriation.	Skin care. Give low osmolarity feedings at slow rate.

Source: A. J. Kempen, in *Nursing Care of the Cancer Patient with Nutritional Problems,* 51. Report of the Ross Oncology Nursing Round-Table. (Columbus, Ohio: Ross Laboratories, 1981).

with sterile gauze. Instead of tape, the use of cling gauze around the body part is usually found to be more satisfactory. Silvadene is a soothing ointment, which decreases odor and fights infection. It is a frequently used agent in the treatment of burns. When applied as described above, it promotes ease in dressing changes as well, which is important as these wounds can be excruciatingly tender or bleed easily. Cleansing of open wounds that are healing should not be done with hydrogen peroxide as this may cause destruction of granulating tissue.

Odor may need special attention. Secondary to skin or soft tissue breakdown or infection, it can result in social as well as personal distress for the cancer patient. Just when the patient and family want to be close to each other, odor can stand between them. Room deodorants are not an adequate means of dealing with odor problems. They are progressively more effective at increasing distances from the odor source (the patient) and frequently simply result in the addition of another odor to those that continue to be present. Several alternatives are available.

The use of Silvadene alone may be effective in controlling odor. In those patients for whom it is not appropriate, an alternate solution is to use charcoal-impregnated dressings over regular wound dressings. As long as these charcoal dressings are not contaminated, they may be reused when dressings are changed. Chlorophyll tablets can be useful in odor control. They are soaked in warmed water until they dissolve, then gauze pads are soaked in the solution, wrung out and applied over regular wound dressings. This latter method may be cheaper than the use of charcoal dressings, but is less convenient. Both methods work well.

For appropriate control of infection as well as better control of odor, dressings should be changed when saturated with wound discharge rather than simply reinforced. Removing the soiled dressings from the room in closed plastic bags should be part of routine wound dressing care. Attention to the esthetics as well as the asepsis of skin wounds is required for holistic care of cancer patients. The care of radiation skin reactions is covered later in this chapter.

Stomatitis, Mucositis, Esophagitis

Stomatitis and mucositis are conditions characterized by inflammation of the oral mucosa, often accompanied by mouth sores and inflammation of oral structures. Some cancer centers around the country are reporting excellent results from using vitamin E directly on stomatitis lesions. The vitamin E can be easily used by puncturing vitamin capsules with a needle, then directly applying the contents to the sores. Pain is well controlled and healing promoted with this method of treatment. In addition, a bland diet, by not aggravating discomfort, may encourage patients to continue to eat. Oral care every two hours with half strength hydrogen peroxide and Cepacol brand mouthwash in equal parts is often used as the regimen for control of stomatitis. Topical anesthetics such as viscous Xylocaine or Orabase may be used before meals for discomfort. Topical antibiotics, such as Mycostatin, may be required as well as analgesics in severe cases.

Specific agents in frequent use for mild stomatitis and mucositis are lemon-glycerine swabs, hydrogen peroxide, Maalox, Cepacol, and milk of magnesia. Although there is a lack of general agreement, the best research seems to indicate that lemon glycerine swabs are ineffective in promoting oral hygiene except as a possible adjunctive measure to improve lubrication, and that weak hydrogen peroxide solutions are the most effective agent for oral care. Hydrogen peroxide should be used in weak solutions as it may be damaging in strong concentrations to newly granulating tissue.

Prevention of severe stomatitis should be the goal of cancer care providers. As this debilitating condition is frequently associated with chemotherapy and some radiation therapy, it should be anticipated in most of these patients. An oral care protocol for the prevention of stomatitis is only as good as the persistence with which it is applied, however. Research confirms that oral care must be given regularly at frequent interviews to be of any real benefit. Frequency of application of the protocol seems to be more important than the specific agent used, and omitting oral care for only two to six hours can cause significant loss of mucosa integrity.

Prophylactic dental cleaning and plaque removal prior to beginning chemotherapy or radiation therapy to the head and neck are recommended, as these practices tend to limit the incidence of stomatitis (Lindquist et al. 1978). Patients should be informed about the possibility of stomatitis and given an appropriate schedule of oral hygiene for prevention or amelioration of the condition. Specific routines and agents employed vary among centers across the country. Generally, however, a program of gentle brushing of the teeth after each meal and rinsing with Cepacol mouthwash can be recommended. Some nurses advocate brushing the teeth before and after meals. In addition, at the first sign of impaired integrity of the oral mucosa, a diligent program of care every two hours should be implemented. The goals of this oral care are to keep the oral mucosa and lips clean, moist, soft and intact; and to alleviate pain and discomfort should they occur.

It is not sufficient to assume that the patient will detect and begin to treat stomatitis and mucositis as they occur. The nurse should include observation of the oral mucosa for signs of stomatitis in a routine assessment.

Pain and difficulty swallowing are the initial symptoms of esophagitis. As the condition progresses, substernal pain, which may be confused with heart pain by its location and character, develops. Esophagitis is treated by minimizing trauma related to harsh-textured foods, very hot or cold food or beverages, and the use of tobacco and alcohol. Milk, milk products, and antacids may be helpful in relieving symptoms, as they coat the tender epithelium. Liquid analgesics, such as acetaminophen, are often used to provide relief, although analgesic systemic narcotics may be necessary in severe cases.

Thrombocytopenia

Thrombocytopenia is commonly seen in malignancies and may be due to a variety of causes including leukemia, enlarged spleen, bone marrow suppression, antigen–antibody reactions, disseminated intravascular coagulation (DIC), and chemotherapy or other drug use. Platelets have a very rapid cell turnover rate (between eight and ten days), and thus are particularly vulnerable to the effects of chemotherapy. Normal platelet values are 150,000–300,000/cu mm. The effects of thrombocytopenia on the patient can range from mild to life-threatening. Moderate reductions in the platelet count can result in petechiae, ecchymosis and hematomas. Although these signs may be frightening to the patient or family, they are not dangerous. As the platelet count continues to fall to around 50,000/cu mm, microscopic hematuria, epistaxis, scleral hemorrhages, and gingival bleeding may occur. Inordinately heavy menstrual periods may occur in women. If the platelet count drops below 20,000/cu mm, the danger of life-threatening hemorrhage is dramatically increased. The most common sites for hemorrhage are the gastrointestinal tract, lungs, and central nervous system. With a platelet count below 20,000/cu mm, hemorrhages can occur spontaneously or as a result of trauma. If the platelet count drops below 10,000/cu mm, platelets are usually transfused even if no symptoms are present. Other factors can influence the risk of bleeding for the patient. The presence of several causative factors, infection, increased friability of tissues, and the use of drugs such as aspirin, indomethacin, phenylbutazone and high-dose penicillin can exacerbate bleeding tendencies.

Initial symptoms of intracranial bleeding may be nonspecific and insidious. Visual disturbances, loss of motor function, pupil changes, headache, and changes in the level of consciousness may herald dangerous hemorrhage. Gastrointestinal hemorrhage may present as melena or hematemesis, or be picked up by testing of the hematocrit and hemoglobin, which show a drop without obvious cause. Pulmonary hemorrhage results in rapid dyspnea, labored, shallow respirations and rales in the affected lobe. Coughing of copious blood-streaked sputum is seen. Hemorrhage at any of these three sites can be lifethreatening.

In the case of gastrointestinal bleeding, treatment consists of passing a nasogastric tube to prevent abdominal distention, and initiating ice lavages to help control bleeding. Blood loss may be replaced with packed cells (PC), platelets transfused, or fresh frozen plasma with clotting factors administered. In the case of intracranial bleeding, treatment with a platelet transfusion must be started quickly or irreversible brain damage can result. With intrapulmonic hemorrhage, platelets also must be administered quickly. Fresh frozen plasma with clotting factors and PC are given as well. Mechanically assisted breathing with intubation and a ventilator are usually required.

Nurses caring for patients with thrombocytopenia need to assess routinely for signs of occult bleeding as well as for bleeding from obvious sources. Intramuscular injections, blood draws, and oral care need to be done carefully, with pressure applied to sites of bleeding for prolonged periods until all bleeding has stopped. Bladder catheterization if needed should be done with a small lumen catheter and the liberal use of lubricant, and with extreme care. Safety becomes of prime importance, as an accidental fall can have enormous consequences. Should epistaxis occur, the nurse should apply direct pressure to the nostrils and place the patient in a high Fowler's position. Ice to the bridge of the nose and nape of the neck will help control bleeding. If bleeding is not controlled by these measures within ten minutes, the physician should be notified so that actions can be taken such as neosynephrine-soaked gauze packing of the affected nostril. In order to minimize intracranial pressure increases in the patient at risk for bleeding within the skull, stool softeners should be used, and the Valsalva maneuver and strenuous lifting avoided. The patient should be taught to be careful about vigorous nose blowing, the use of sharp objects, and the importance of reporting any unusual symptoms. Patients are not always able to appreciate the possible relationship between a particular symptom and hemorrhage; for example, nausea may be an early symptom of gastrointestinal bleeding, although not necessarily an obvious one.

Thrombocytosis

Thrombocytosis can occur as a consequence of chronic myelogenous leukemia or as part of a paraneoplastic syndrome. Platelet pheresis is employed periodically to control this event.

Disseminated Intravascular Coagulation

Disseminated intravascular coagulation (DIC) may be caused by the release of thromboplastic substances into the blood stream of patients with tumors. These substances trigger the formation of thrombin. As a consequence, generalized intravascular clotting occurs throughout the capillaries, which in turn leads to a deficiency of platelets, fibrinogen and Factors V and VIII due to the exhaustion of the supply of these materials. Paradoxically, when the platelets and related factors are no longer present in sufficient quantities, this generalized clotting syndrome produces hemorrhage. It is the risk of dangerous hemorrhage that presents a problem in DIC.

The laboratory features of DIC are somewhat variable, depending on its severity and other underlying problems. Generally, prolonged PT, APTT, and thrombin time values are seen, as well as thrombocytopenia, reduced fibrinogen, low Factor V and VIII levels, and hemolytic anemia.

DIC is often associated with hypotension or frank shock. In addition, renal, pulmonary, and CNS hemorrhage may occur (see section on "thrombocytopenia" for a complete discussion). The definitive treatment of DIC is to address the underlying cause of the generalized clotting phenomena; unfortunately, this is quite often not possible in the case of cancer patients.

Infection and Granulocytopenia

Infection is the leading cause of morbidity and mortality in patients with cancer. Patients at particularly high risk are those with leukemia, but with aggressive therapies extending the remission period or survival for other cancers, infection is becoming a larger problem with solid tumors. Increased risk is associated with those patients on chemotherapy, radiotherapy, with granulocytopenia, undergoing immunosuppression, with compromised pulmonary or renal function associated with metastasis, or those with far advanced disease. Granulocytopenia, which is associated with leukemia, but is more often a consequence of chemotherapy or radiation therapy, occurs when bone marrow is suppressed by disease or therapy. The threat or occurence of granulocytopenia frequently dictates drug protocols rather than cancer cell kinetics because of its risk to the patient. Moreover, normal neutrophils may be more sensitive to chemotherapy than malignant neutrophils, which become resistant, so sometimes chemotherapy must be curtailed on this account.

Granulocytopenia impairs the body's major defense system against bacteria and fungal infections, and is considered to be the biggest risk factor for serious infectious complications in the cancer patient. The condition of granulocytopenia may be aggravated by certain drugs that have been shown to cause abnormal function of leukocytes that continue to circulate in the blood. The implicated drugs include corticosteroids, vinca alkaloids, asparaginase, and the opiates. Similar abnormalities in bactericidal activity of leucocytes have also been noted in patients during a three-month period following craniospinal irradiation for leukemia. Another factor that aggravates the granulocytopenic condition is the frequent presence of altered integrity of the patient's physical defense barriers, such as mucositis, indwelling catheters, and intravenous lines.

Because the inflammatory response is impaired in the granulocytopenic patient, it is sometimes difficult to differentiate life-threatening infection from a nonlethal condition when the patient becomes febrile. It is now standard practice to begin antibiotic therapy as soon as the patient becomes febrile. Third-generation cephalosporins and extended-spectrum penicillins are currently the drugs of choice in many cancer centers (Pizzo 1984).

In the last ten years, it has been recognized that fungal invasion is a concomitant major problem to bacterial infection in the granulocyto-penic patient. Antifungal therapy in some high-risk patients with amphotericin B is now a frequent adjunct to antibiotic therapy. Candida, Aspergillus, and the Phycomycetes are the major fungal organisms seen in the granulocytopenic patient (ibid.). Because fungal infections are difficult to diagnose early and difficult to treat once established, early antifungal therapy is advocated by some clinicians.

The appropriate length of therapy with antibiotics and antifungal agents remains unclear. Some centers continue these therapies until the patient's granulocyte count has recovered to greater than 500/cu mm, while others have shown good results with selected patients who were removed from these therapies after one week. Because of the possible rapid deterioration of patients with granulocytopenia, overtreatment of some patients is generally done to provide safety in treatment regimens for all the patients affected.

Although it would seem reasonable that granulocyte transfusions be included as a major component of the management of the granulo-cytopenic patient, their use has not clearly proven useful. With recent advances in the effectiveness of antibiotic agents and the addition of antifungal medications to standard treatment of febrile granulocyto-penic patients, the role of granulocyte infusion has diminished in recent years. Until the technology for collecting granulocytes for transfusion and the leukopharesis filtration process is improved, and other technical and biological problems associated with granulocyte transfusion remedied, this treatment will probably not regain the popularity it attained ten years ago (Pizzo 1984). The risks associated with granulocyte infusions are currently felt to outweigh the benefits in many instances. Pulmonary toxicity has been the most critical sign noted with the use of these transfusions. It is exacerbated by the use of amphotericin B, so use of granulocyte transfusions may compro-mise the use of antifungal therapy, which could be critical to the patient's well-being. It has also been demonstrated that granulocyte infusions can transmit pathogens, including cytomegalovirus, which can be difficult to treat.

Use of a total protective environment, including a laminar air flow room with sterile technique maintained, has proven somewhat useful to the granulocytopenic patient, although virtually all patients still required systemic antibiotics during their period of isolation. The tremendous expense, awkwardness of care, and variable patient compliance have restricted the usefulness of this treatment in the management of granulocytopenia. When careful handwashing is performed, the use of other isolation protocols has proved unnecessary. The addition of reverse isolation offered no significant benefit in preventing the acquisition of new organisms and did not reduce the incidence of infection.

Although a wide variety of treatments have been used over the past few years, today the most reasonable protocol for the granulocytopenic patient appears to be early use of antibiotics with antifungal therapy and careful aseptic technique. Other forms of treatment such as passive immunization and gastrointestinal decontamination are currently being evaluated for their potential use as adjuncts to the above management techniques.

If infection progresses to general septicemia in any cancer patient, an emergency situation exists and must be aggressively treated. In general, nursing care of even small infected skin sites should be vigorously treated, as these patients are frequently debilitated and at risk for colonization and spread of microorganisms.

Renal Dysfunction

Dysfunction of the uninary system can occur due to a deficit in the kidney's ability to regulate the volume, osmolality, pH, and electrolyte balance of the plasma, or from a disruption in the urinary transport and collection organs.

OBSTRUCTION

The ureters, bladder or urethra may become occluded or compressed, leading to dysfunction of the kidneys. This occurs from direct cancer cell invasion of the renal system from a primary renal carcinoma or from metastasis.

ABNORMAL HORMONE SECRETION

Kidney function is partly under the control of three hormones: antidiuretic hormone (ADH), parathyroid hormone, and aldosterone. ADH serum level elevations cause retention of water by the kidney distal tubules. An increase in parathyroid hormone causes an increased serum calcium level and decreased phosphate level. Aldosterone increases result in increased serum sodium levels and decreased potassium levels. All three of these hormones may be abnormally secreted as a paraneoplastic phenomenon of the cancer process, causing abnormal renal function.

RENAL PARENCHYMA DISPLACEMENT

Primary renal carcinomas as well as metastatic disease can result in the replacement of normal kidney cells by abnormal tumor cells, resulting in abnormal function. In particular, tumor cells of acute myelogenous leukemia, acute lymphatic leukemia, and Hodgkin's and non-Hodgkin's lymphoma can invade the kidney parenchyma, disrupting normal function.

RENAL VEIN THROMBOSIS

Thrombosis of the renal vein can result from impaired blood flow secondary to tumor cell agglutination or obstruction.

NEPHROTOXIC TUMOR PRODUCTS

Bence Jones protein, common in patients with multiple myeloma and sometimes seen in lymphoma patients, is a cause of renal dysfunction by its action on the renal tubule system. The amyloid fibril of amyloidosis in patients with multiple myeloma can cause destruction of the glomerulus of the kidney. Immune complexes that can occur in a variety of cancers also act to destroy kidney cells. Tumor lysis syndrome can produce quantities of nephrotoxic tumor by-products that act to obstruct and destroy the kidney parenchyma.

SIDE EFFECTS OF CHEMOTHERAPY

Prolonged administration of chemotherapeutic agents can reversibly or permanently damage the kidneys. Hypercalcemia and hyperuricemia are especially common potential causes of reversible renal failure in patients receiving chemotherapy. Both cisplatin and methotrexate affect renal function and are among the most commonly administered agents. Unfortunately, considerable kidney damage may occur before a rise in serum creatinine occurs with their use. Aspirin, sulfonamides, phenytoin, cefoxitin, and gentamicin may all decrease methotrexate clearance and increase the toxicity of this drug. Before administration of high-dose methotrexate, sodium bicarbonate is infused, and allopurinol given for one to three days prior to beginning chemotherapy. These precautions cause alkalinization of urine and decrease hyperuricemia. Dehydration in conjunction with the administration of any of the nephrotoxic drugs greatly increases their toxic effects. This is a particular problem with cisplatin, which readily produces a cystitis when concentrated in the bladder. Prehydration is routinely done with cisplatin administration to decrease kidney damage potential.

Chemotherapeutic agents associated with nephrotoxicity include the following:

cisplatin	methotrexate (high doses)
cyclophosphamide	semustine
dacarbazine	streptozocin
hydroxyurea	

SIDE EFFECTS OF RADIATION THERAPY

Fibrosis of the kidney or bladder can occur secondary to radiation exposure. Immediate reactions of renal system organs that can occur subsequent to radiation are cystitis or nephritis. Nephritis can progress to hypertension and impaired renal function months after the final radiation dose. Generally, the kidneys are shielded from radiation after receiving 2,000 rads, to protect them from a dose above their tolerance, which would lead to nephritis. With abdominal radiation, obstruction of the ureters can develop with retroperitoneal fibrosis.

RENAL FAILURE

The nurse must be observant for signs of impending renal failure. These include changes in urinary output from polyuria to oliguria, or anuria in actual failure. Malaise, fatigue, edema, pruritus, and anorexia may be seen. A metallic taste and diarrhea are often reported by renal failure patients. Fluid and electrolyte imbalances occur along with anemia, hypertension, and uremia. Laboratory tests reveal an increase in plasma creatinine and blood urea nitrogen levels. Urinalysis may reveal red blood cells, white blood cells, and casts (mucoproteins shaped like renal tubules). Renal failure affects every system of the body and has profound effects on the quality of life. Once renal impairment is present, efforts are made to reduce the burden on the kidneys. Fluids are limited to compensate for the decreased ability of the kidneys to excrete urine.

Obstructive disease may be confused with renal failure initially, since the signs and symptoms are similar. In addition to the effects mentioned above, flank pain may be present along with fever if obstruction is causing renal dysfunction.

CYSTITIS

Cystitis is recognized by the symptoms of frequency, urgency, and pain when voiding. The patient may also complain of low back pain. Urine may appear cloudy or bloody. If cystitis occurs subsequent to chemotherapy, the patient should be encouraged to increase fluid intake to at least 3,000 ml per day. Intravenous therapy may be required for the patient experiencing vomiting, stomatitis, or other conditions that tend to limit fluid intake. Coffee, tea, alcohol, hot spices, and tobacco use are irritating to the bladder lining and should be avoided. Maintenance of an acid urine pH (7.0 or lower) may help prevent infection. Ascorbic acid, 500 mg daily, is most effective in acidifying urine. Cranberry juice is not an effective means of acidifying urine since at least 3 quarts daily must be consumed for the effect. The patient should be encouraged to empty the bladder frequently to minimize the time that irritating substances are in contact with the bladder epithelium. If the cystitis is due to a bacterial infection and is not from irritating substances, some clinicians recommend allowing the bladder to become full if the patient is on antibiotic therapy, so that the lining is stretched sufficiently for the antibiotic-rich urine to come in contact with the entire epithelium.

Symptom Management

Pain

It is estimated that 60 to 80 percent of hospitalized cancer patients experience severe pain, usually in the terminal stage of disease. This aspect of cancer looms as the most significant problem associated with cancer for many patients. As it is usually associated with a deteriorating condition, it has both psychological and physiological dimensions that may have a greater impact on the cancer patient than on other types of patients experiencing pain. Fear that the pain will not be relieved can completely shatter the patient living with the chronic, increasingly intense pain of cancer. In the early stages of cancer, pain is reported by 5 to 10 percent of patients (Cleeland 1984), interfering with mood and activity. Its prevalence increases most consistently thereafter with the onset of metastasis.

Today, the use of continuously infused morphine sulfate (MS) is the hallmark of severe pain control. Because constant blood levels are maintained, more consistent relief is achieved, often with fewer side effects and lesser amounts of drug required overall. Anxiety about possible delays in getting the next dose are eliminated and the infusion rate can be easily changed to titer the drug dose. Besides continuous subcutaneous infusions of MS, newer techniques such as intermittent intrathecal or intraventricular morphine injections are also used to control pain. These methods can be employed on an outpatient basis for satisfactory pain control.

A disturbing finding concerning pain control (Randin and Snider 1984) was that almost 60 percent of nurses they studied felt that the goal of narcotic administration was to reduce pain rather than to relieve it for cancer patients. Success might be inferred, since in a parallel study, 70 percent of patients noted that their pain was reduced but not eliminated in the narcotic regimens. The authors interpreted data from the study as indicating that these nurses often perceived moderate relief of pain as an adequate goal. In light of available modalities that can relieve pain on a relatively consistent basis, settling for moderate pain for cancer patients is not appropriate.

Bones figure prominently in the incidence of cancer-associated pain, with 50 percent of patients in one series citing this area as the source of their pain (Foley 1985). Half that rate had pain associated with nerve compression or infiltration, with other sources of pain mentioned much less often. These results have been confirmed in other studies. Unfortunately, bone pain has been shown to be that which is most resistant to multimodal pain therapy.

A most interesting finding of Schittmann et al. (1983) was that patients used specific descriptions of their pain that varied with the physical site. "Throbbing" was most often used by patients with bone pain; "aching" with nerve-related pain; "sharp" with soft tissue pain; and "tender" and "burning" with treatment-related pain.

SUBJECTIVE NATURE OF PAIN

While not all patients with cancer experience pain, those who do may require concerted nursing efforts in order to find relief. The experience of pain is an entirely subjective phenomenon. A response to both physical and psychological stimuli, it is a composite affected by past experiences, expectations for the future, cultural role expectations, current circumstances, individual neurophysical characteristics, and the emotional state of the patient.

A similar physiological assault on two different people will be experienced differently and may require different levels of pain relief between the two. There is no standard amount of pain that can be considered appropriate for a specific injury. The nurse is totally dependent on the patient's report of pain and must respond to the pain as reported by each individual patient at whatever level of intensity the patient states exists. To do less is to substitute one's own expectations about what is "normal" or "appropriate" in favor of the patient's actual experience.

TIMING OF RELIEF

Due in part to the intense training given nurses about the potential ill effects of medicines in general, and narcotics in particular, there is sometimes a subconscious tendency by the nurse to limit addictive medications until a preconceived "appropriate" level of pain intensity is reached by the patient. This must be carefully guarded against. Evidence exists that pain is more satisfactorily controlled by medication when it is treated at a mild level than if it is allowed to become full-blown. Studies have repeatedly shown that the total amount of pain medication taken over time is less if pain remains under control at all times than if it is allowed to become intense before medications are administered. The lessons for treating the cancer patient are clear: prophylaxis and scheduled pain medication make sense both in terms of patient satisfaction and efficient use of medications.

CONTROL OF RELIEF MEASURES

Research has also given nurses another tool for understanding how to control pain: control over the method of pain relief and the ability to control the administration of medication increases patients' perceptions of pain relief. Utilizing this principle, the use of the patient-controlled analgesia system (PCA) is revolutionizing pain control for many surgical and cancer patients.

GATE CONTROL THEORY OF PAIN

Another piece of information will prove useful to the nurse in establishing a comprehensive pain relief program for cancer patients; that is, the gate control theory of pain. This most popular theory of how pain is experienced is premised on the notion that pain and thermal impulses travel over small-diameter, slow-conducting afferent nerve fibers to the spinal cord dorsal horns. Within the dorsal horns lies the substantia gelatinosa, an area of grey matter, which opens a theoretical gate for transmission of pain impulses to the brain once they have reached a critical threshold intensity. In contrast, large-diameter fibers, which carry cutaneous impulses, close the gate to the small-diameter fibers when stimulated. Thus, any practice which stimulates cutaneous nerve fibers will help to inhibit the conscious experience of pain. Applications of heat and cold, acupressure, and transcutaneous electric nerve stimulation utilize this theory to explain their effectiveness.

A second conception of the gate control theory is that the reticular formation of the brain can process only a certain amount of sensory imput at any one time. When the brain is exposed to excessive information, it closes the gate to small-diameter pain impulses preferentially. On the other hand, with a deficit of sensory imput, the gate for the transmission of pain is open. Interventions that use distraction in exerting their effect apply to this part of the theory.

A third conception of the theory involves the impulses of the cerebral cortex and thalamus. Emotions and memories may activate these areas, triggering pain impulses. Patient education and relaxation techniques may help inhibit this process.

ENDORPHINS

These natural opiates of the brain are currently being commercially produced for research purposes. Several of these compounds have been found and are referred to as either endorphins, dynorphins, or enkephalins, although when considered as a class they are usually all referred to as endorphins. They are incredibly potent pain killers. For example, a dynorphin is 190 times stronger than morphine. In a test of their ability to control cancer pain, fourteen men and women given only tiny amounts of an endorphin all experienced complete relief lasting from one to three days.

RELIEF MEASURES

Based on the information described above and applied to the patient through a systematic assessment, the nurse can formulate a plan for control of pain including both prescribed analgesia and noninvasive measures.

Cutaneous stimulation (utilizing gate control theory of pain)
- *Heat.* Hot packs or tub baths will apply moist heat to tense or painful areas of the body. Heat should not be used directly over tumor sites as it may encourage metastasis by increasing circulation, nor should it be used on skin treated by radiotherapy, which is more sensitive to heat damage.
- *Cold.* Cold has been demonstrated to be a more effective pain reliever than heat in many instances; however, many times patients find the emotional comfort of heat more satisfying, if somewhat less effective. It may be useful for patients to try this modality before rejecting it out of hand.
- *Massage.* Use of petrissage, stroking, and tapotement on the back will provide comfort to many patients. Severely emaciated patients, or those with metastasis to the spine, may find this type of massage irritating rather than helpful, however. Massaging hands or feet is another frequently used technique.

Be careful not to use deep massage on the lower extremities; cancer patients with decreased activity are prone to thromboses, which could be embolized through deep pressure.
• *Transcutaneous electrical nerve stimulation (TENS).* TENS works by transmitting an electrical impulse across a painful area of skin, thus blocking pain nerve impulses in favor of cutaneous ones. The small generator with cables attaching it to electrodes on the patient's skin provides a range of intensity that is controlled by the patient. Response to the TENS varies widely among patients and is most useful for mild or moderate pain relief.
• *Acupressure.* Some centers are using this modality for relief of pain, although it is more commonly seen in community holistic health centers as an alternative to medications. Its usefulness for cancer patients is probably very limited. If the nurse has been educated in the use of acupressure and the patient wants the therapy, it would be an appropriate modality to apply.

Analgesics
• *Oral.* Use of Brompton's cocktail, methadone, or morphine are the most frequently employed oral analgesics in use for mild or moderate pain relief in those able to tolerate this route.
• *Parenteral.* One of the methods experiencing the fastest growth in popularily is the patient-controlled analgesia system (PCA), which delivers morphine at a rate controlled by the patient within the limits set in the computerized, locked control pump. Twenty-four milligrams in four hours maximum, delivered at a maximum rate of one milligram per ten minutes at the patient's discretion is a typical order. This method allows constant blood levels with no oversedation. Furthermore, patients do not have to suffer while waiting for needed injections, nursing staff is freed for other activities, and patients maintain control over their relief. A disadvantage is that a patent intravenous line must be maintained with a continuous infusion for the PCA to function.

Morphine continues to be the most frequently used narcotic for the pain of cancer. It should be titrated to the minimum dose that offers good control of pain, and then increased over time as required. It should be borne in mind that sufficient intravenous doses of narcotics are usually one-half to one-third those required for intramuscular doses.

If the patient's respiratory rate falls below ten breaths per minute, the narcotic should be held and physician notified. Respiratory depression is most frequent with elderly or lung-impaired patients. Frequent stimulation of the patient, encouraging coughing and deep breathing, and moving the patient at intervals will help counteract respiratory depression.

More common than respiratory depression is constipation and nausea with morphine administration. Today, Reglan (metoclopramide hydrochloride) is frequently given with morphine to control these side effects.

Intractable Pain

When intractable pain complicates terminal cancer, various invasive methods may be employed to obtain pain relief.

NEUROSURGICAL PROCEDURES

Six common procedures are defined below:

1. *Nerve block.* A temporary regional anesthesia is effected by the injection of lidocaine or alcohol to an area. The effect lasts from a few hours to six months. Disadvantages to this method are the concomitant loss of function that may result in the body area and the occasional development of neuritis in the affected nerve once the drug effect has worn off.
2. *Cordotomy.* Destruction of the spinothalamic pain pathways is done by surgery or electric needle penetration selectively to destroy pain and temperature sensation to affected body areas. Hemiparesis and sexual, bowel and bladder dysfunction may be unwarranted side effects.
3. *Midline myelotomy.* This achieves the same effect as a cordotomy, but with less bowel and bladder dysfunction. Through more extensive surgery, the spinothalamic nerve tracts are cut at the anterior commissure of the spinal cord.
4. *Peripheral neurectomy.* Nerves to the painful area of the body are cut. Side effects include loss of all sensation, paralysis or return of pain. Small areas of pain are most easily treated by this procedure.
5. *Sensory rhizotomy.* The sensory root of a spinal or cranial nerve is cut proximal to the dorsal root ganglion. Thus, motor function is preserved while sensory function is lost. This procedure is most often used for thorax or abdominal pain.
6. *Stereotaxic thalamotomy.* The transmission of pain impulses

through the thalamus is stopped by implantation of an electrode in the thalamus. This is considered a last-ditch effort at pain control.

EPIDURAL OPIATES

Intraspinal opiate administration is done through a catheter placed for extended periods of time. Meningitis constitutes the most severe side effect. Relief is reportedly excellent in the vast majority of patients.

DEPRESSION AND ANXIETY

It remains unclear today what part depression plays in the experience of pain, and whether depression tends to produce more pain or pain more depression. In a study of 120 cancer patients, Cleeland (1984) found no difference in reported pain intensity between patients who were assessed as depressed and those who were not. Although Cleeland found no objective difference in functional status between the depressed and nondepressed groups, the depressed patients reported that their pain interfered more with activity and mood.

Nurses must be careful that depression or emotional disturbance is not confused as the source of hostile behavior that is actually pain-related. Just because analgesic measures are not successful does not mean that the problem is emotional rather than physiologic in nature. It may simply reflect the inadequacy of the modality or dose of analgesic used.

Anorexia

The patient who experiences anorexia, weight loss, weakness, anemia, increased basal metabolic rate, and taste and olfactory abnormalities is showing signs and symptoms of progressive cachexia. In the case of primary cachexia, the patient will not be able to counter the progressive effects of the syndrome by improving nutritional intake, either orally or parenterally. However, some cases of anorexia are the result of chemotherapy or radiation therapy, or result from depression, and can be relieved by improving the patient's oral intake.

Generally, these patients need all the calories and protein they can tolerate, as they may be in a negative nitrogen balance from the effects of inadequate intake and have increased body requirements related to their disease and therapies. Therefore, it is the best practice to offer "packed" food sources such as meat sandwiches, milk, nuts, and ice cream. A vitamin and mineral supplement is usually required for these patients, as they will not have sufficient appetite to get all their daily requirements through their diet alone. Raw fruits and salads are not recommended for the severely debilitated cancer patient. Their bacterial contamination is of no consequence to healthy people, but may contribute to sepsis in the cancer patient.

Grief and Loss

The grief that the cancer patient experiences has its roots in fear of loss of the future and fear of the unknown. Not knowing what the future will hold creates pessimism; cancer for many people represents a condition of suffering, pain, loneliness, and loss of love. It is useful to consider the framework described by Kubler-Ross (1959) in staging a person's response to approaching death. The diagnosis of cancer is closely associated with a premonition of death, and all cancer patients respond to the diagnosis with reactions described by Kubler-Ross to some degree. Once the patient has worked through the stages of grieving at diagnosis, adjustment may be successsful as therapy is begun and a prognosis is determined. If the cancer progresses and death approaches, the patient may experience a renewed sense of loss and again go through the stages of grieving. Kubler-Ross explains that individuals go through the stages at different rates according to their own unique personalities, and that the progression is not unidirectional, but that patients may go back and forth between stages or remain at any stage, and not progress. It should be noted that the application of these stages is not absolute nor do individuals have to experience any one in particular or in any specific order. Furthermore, nurses should be careful not to try to push a patient into a different stage; the psychological adjustments and changes are entirely self-determined. Others can support the patient and encourage the patient to deal with feelings in order to promote psychological peace associated with acceptance, but no one can will the patient into adjustment.

Since families of cancer patients may go through parallel grieving stages, their behavior in dealing with their feelings may sometimes compound coping problems for the patient. The patient and family members may be at different stages at any one time. Families who are in denial may not be able to handle the patient who is expressing anger, for example. The patient may become angry at the family for their reactions, which leads to guilt and more anger. The nurse may need to intervene between family and patient, explaining to each how the other is feeling and allowing the ventilation of feelings in a psychologically safe manner.

DENIAL

Denial should be a temporary defense, a buffer to unpleasant or unexpected news. Once the patient has a psychological coping system readied, he or she will be able to move from denial to dealing with the situation of a cancer diagnosis or death directly. The patient who feels vulnerable and without support may be reluntant to proceed psychologically with the work of other stages, so support is extremely important to patients throughout the duration of their illness, but particularly at times of diagnosis and impending death.

ANGER

Kubler-Ross found through her work with dying and grieving individuals that frequently anger is the first response after denial. The classic question asked of one's self is "Why me?" People who are young or who have who given attention through their lifetime to good health practices or cancer prevention measures may feel cheated and unfairly stricken. Others who may have practiced habits such as smoking that are linked to cancer may experience intense anger at themselves and the medical system that is unable to help them. Anger is frequently expressed toward those around the patient, so the nurse is vulnerable to direct attacks as well as indirect ones at the medical system in general. Nurses must allow patients to express anger and not avoid them because of it. Expressed empathy and continuation of caring behaviors by the nurse in the face of angry outbursts allows patients to deal with these feelings, so that they can move to other stages. The nurse's self-esteem must be sufficiently high that he or she does not become hostile and defensive toward the patient. Of course, the nurse should not ignore the feelings being expressed by the patient, but should be able to separate personal defensive feelings from therapeutic responses that are most appropriate.

BARGAINING

At this stage, patients may bargain with God or the medical staff or with themselves as a means of dealing with the realities they must face. For example, the patient may say to the nurse, "Just keep me alive through this shift," or to himself or herself, "Let me see my next birthday—that's all I want." Another means of bargaining the nurse may see is in patients who stoically insist on treatments or food intake beyond the limits of reasonable comfort, seeming to feel that in exchange for these painful experiences, they will be guaranteed cure. Masochistic behavior is sometimes seen as a means of "paying" for good results.

DEPRESSION

The fourth stage, depression, allows patients to deal with all the losses they are experiencing directly. Doubts about the meaning of their life and fears of the future for themselves and their loved ones can overwhelm patients. The nurse must take time to help patients and families deal with these very difficult subjects and to work out feelings. Because it is easy for nurses themselves to feel overwhelmed at the tragedy for the patient, care must be taken that nurses dealing with cancer patients have come to terms with their own feelings about death, so that these feelings do not interfere with their ability to provide comfort for patients.

ACCEPTANCE

The stage of acceptance is one in which psychological peace is felt, and the patient does not struggle against death. After all the emotionality of the other stages, acceptance is a quiet, passionless contrast. Patients may no longer wish to discuss their illness or review their lives, but may seem to regain strength and interest in the everyday occurences around them. Simple pleasures and comfort-giving measures can improve the quality of life for terminal patients, who focus on them more directly in the stage of acceptance.

Insomnia

Insomnia is linked to stress among the general population and particularly so among cancer patients. Recurring preoccupation with thoughts about the disease and physical discomfort can combine effectively to preclude sleep. Three measures can be employed to control insomnia. Sometimes it is most helpful for the nurse to engage in a middle-of-the-night conversation with the patient. Allowing patients to express some of the feelings that are churning inside them during a few minutes of conversation can offer enough peace to permit sleep.

Relieving pain is a necessary prerequisite to sleep. Sometimes patients need an extra amount of pain medication before they can fall asleep. A third measure that may be required is a prescribed sedative. Nurses should not wait for patients to suggest a sedative, but offer this medication if they determine that the patient is restless and is experiencing difficulty getting to sleep.

Loss of Control

Because patients generally have little knowledge of treatment alternatives, they may be dependent to a large extent on the medical system to determine their future activities in regard to their illness. With cancer patients this aspect of disease is heightened, since these individuals may be expected to undergo extended treatment regimens for months or years. If patients are not well informed about their disease, the treatment plan, and alternatives, they become particularly susceptible to cancer quakery. Initiating the process of contacting the alternative treatment centers and beginning these unproven therapies can give patients a sense of control that they may be missing in the traditional cancer care delivery systems.

Patients also may perceive a loss of control over their bodies; changes due to the disease process and therapies cannot be controlled by actions they take. The nurse caring for cancer patients must take into account these factors, which tend to alienate the patient. Allowing the patient to share in decisions about treatments, and giving the patient the knowledge required to control the equipment and understand the consequences of treatments will help reestablish the patient's control of some aspects of living with cancer. This is an important aspect of well-being that must be addressed by the nurse caring for cancer patients.

Social Disruption

The time and energy that is required of many cancer patients in the treatment of their disease can have a major impact on the social activities of the family unit. On a regular basis, the cancer patient may need to take time off from work or home responsibilities because of treatments or their side effects. During these times, other family members may be required to take a larger share of responsibilities involved in the running of the household. Physical debility may preclude the patient from participation in social activities or the work of keeping up a home. Severe debility may require that other family members curtail activities to assist the patient physically. Income that the cancer patient once contributed to the family unit may be reduced or lost completely if the disease interrupts or prevents employment. This may have the consequence of interrupting college education of children, vacations, or may even cause the family to rely on government agencies for assistance in routine expenses of living.

Emotional energy is expended by the patient and family to the point that they may be too tired for social functions they once enjoyed and may begin to focus almost entirely on the disease process. Friends of the cancer patient may feel uneasy about including the individual in social functions, both because of fear of the dampening effect this could have on the spirits of others involved, and for fear that the cancer patient would not be up to the event. Many cancer patients report that friends shy away from the individual socially, and that they themselves are often too drained to make the effort to initiate social events. A pattern of isolation may develop. This is certainly not unique to cancer patients; individuals who have suffered a stroke, for example, report similar isolation tendencies.

On the other hand, many cancer patients recover strength after cancer treatments and resume normal living patterns. These individuals tend to be those with healthy social patterns, satisfying work and homelife, and who are self-directed in their lives.

Nausea and Vomiting

Nausea and vomiting are not merely side effects of chemotherapy but are the end products of a complex, controlled, coordinated system through which the body rids itself of noxious substances. Several mechanisms appear to initiate nausea and vomiting in cancer patients. The chemoreceptor trigger zone (CTZ) of the brain can be stimulated directly by specific drugs, chemicals, and cellular by-products. The vestibules of the ears can transmit impulses through the cerebellum to the CTZ to initiate nausea and vomiting. The cerebral cortex controls the psychological stimuli of these symptoms. The hypothalamus is also involved in the initiation of nausea and vomiting through a mechanism that is unclear. The common final pathway for all these different mechanisms of stimulation is the true vomiting center (TVC) of the brain. When the TVC is stimulated, vomiting with or without nausea is produced. Nausea and vomiting are accompanied by the symptoms of weakness, pallor, decreased blood pressure, and brachycardia during vomiting.

Among cancer patients, nausea and vomiting are caused by stimulation of the CTZ by tumor by-products, tumor invasion of nerve tracts involved in the nausea and vomiting reflex, stimulation by chemotherapeutic agents, psychological conditioning, radiation of the cranium, or disruption of the integrity of the epithelial lining of the gastrointestinal tract. Other causes include pain, fatigue, gastric distention, gastrointestinal obstruction, renal dysfunction, and some electrolyte imbalances. Among cancer patients, nausea and vomiting are particularly distressful symptoms associated with the delivery of chemotherapy. These symptoms are quickly associated with chemotherapy and can become intractable problems. Anticipatory nausea and vomiting have been well documented in recent years, and are most frequently seen in middle-aged patients and those who are anxious, depressed or hostile (Ingle et al. 1984). The chemotherapeutic agents most frequently associated with nausea and vomiting are:

cisplatin	mithramycin
cyclophosphamide	mitomycin-C
dacarbazine	nitrogen mustard
dactinomycin	nitrosoureas
mechlorethamine	5-Azacytidine
methotrexate	streptozocin

The consequences of protracted emesis can be very severe. Dehydration with subsequent electrolyte imbalances and altered distribution of therapeutic agents, erosion of the distal esophagus, or esophageal tearing can occur. In addition, these patients may experience aspiration pneumonia, central nervous system bleeding (with thrombocytopenia), or malnutrition, or they may become noncompliant with therapy.

Interventions to relieve the distressful symptoms include antiemetics, manipulating the environment to exclude, when possible, those things associated with the symptoms, avoiding eating or drinking for several hours prior to and after chemotherapy, relaxation techniques, and distraction. Generally, antiemetics are necessary to control the nausea and vomiting associated with delivery of chemotherapeutic agents, and other modalities are employed to potentiate the effect of the antiemetic drug therapy.

Many different regimens are utilized to control nausea and vomiting. When antineoplastic agents that have a very high probability of causing nausea and vomiting are to be administered, frequently antiemetics and antianxiety medications are given prophylactically and continued after the drug is delivered. Metoclopramide (Reglan) is perhaps today the most frequently used antiemetic agent. With patients on cisplatin therapy, metoclopramide achieved 73 percent control of emesis with major control of nausea (Gralla 1982). It is usually administered intravenously beginning one half hour prior to the chemotherapy, and at two-hour intervals over the next four hours. Droperidel (Inapsine) or lorazepam (Ativan) with methylprednisolone (Solu-Medrol) or dexamethasone (Decadron) are combinations that have been successful at various cancer centers. With the administration of dexamethasone intravenously, there may be a sensation of generalized tingling lasting about five minutes (Powell

1985). Diazepam (Valium), thiethylperazine (Torecan), and prochlorperazine (Compazine) are other frequently administered medications to alleviate nausea and vomiting in various combinations and schedules. Benadryl is also frequently added to the regimen to control these symptoms. There has been a substantial amount of study on the effectiveness of tetrahydrocannabinol (THC) in alleviating nausea and vomiting. This substance has been shown to have an inferior effect to prochlorperazine and metoclopramide in large studies, although some nurses have reported excellent results with THC (Cronin 1982).

Cotanch (1985) found that young children who were taught to concentrate on pleasant experiences during chemotherapy and told that they would sleep well after drug therapy and awaken alert and well, experienced significantly less nausea and vomiting than children with whom no such interventions were taken. Bernstein (1985) has reported that withholding food for a few hours prior to delivering chemotherapy and afterwards may be helpful in averting the development of food aversions, which she found common in children. The nurse may be able to control the smells and sights associated with chemotherapy to some extent. To be effective, the nurse should include the patient in the care plan, asking about triggers of the response that the patient can identify and that can be eliminated, and about preferred comfort measures. In addition, maintaining good oral hygiene can be effective in reducing the sensation of nausea and should be routinely done after each episode of vomiting. As antiemetic drug therapy becomes more effective with advances in types of formulations, combinations, schedules, routes of administration, and supportive methods utilized, these most distressing side effects of chemotherapy may drop from being the most distressing symptoms experienced by patients to being an uncommon event.

Alopecia

Hair growth takes place in the hair root where amino acids from the blood first join with the dividing cells of the follicle. For reasons that are not fully understood, hair growth follows a cyclic pattern of active development and rest. At any one time, about 85 percent of the hair follicles are reproducing on the human scalp. Hair follicle cells in other areas of body skin spend much longer periods than scalp hair follicles in a resting state, so at any one time most are not actively dividing. Scalp hair follicle cells spend about 3 to 10 years in an active state, then slow growth over a three-week period before lapsing into a dormant stage for some three months. After this, the cycle is repeated. Both chemotherapy and radiation therapy can affect the hair follicle. Whether the hair loss will be permanent or temporary depends on the dose and length of exposure to either of these modalities.

CHEMOTHERAPY

Certain antineoplastic agents damage the DNA of hair follicle cells, resulting in their death. This may cause hair to become weak and brittle, easily breaking off at the scalp surface. The degree of alopecia varies from slight thinning to complete baldness. Once the course of chemotherapy is completed, regrowth usually occurs. It is not unusual for the hair that appears during regrowth to be of an altered texture and color and have a different degree of curl. The following chemotherapeutic agents are associated with alopecia:

highest probability:
cyclophosphamide
doxorubicin
vincristine

high probability:

actinomycin	methotrexate
bleomycin	mitomycin–C
cytosine	neocarzinostatin
daunorubicin	nitrogen mustard
5–fluorouracil	semustine
hexamethylmelamine	streptozocin
hydroxyurea	vinblastine
ICRF–159	VM–26
lomustine	VP–16–213

There are a few measures that may be useful in minimizing or preventing hair loss from chemotherapy. These measures may be used for all patients except for those with hematological neoplasms. In the case of leukemia and lymphoma patients, tumor cells may be present in the scalp vessels, so measures which decrease the flow of chemotherapuetic agents to the scalp during treatments may be contraindicated. Such measures include scalp hypothermia and scalp tourniquet constriction.

The use of vitamin E taken orally five to seven days prior to the administration of antineoplastic agents has recently been shown to be effective in preventing all or most hair loss in limited trials (Wood 1985). Scalp hypothermia techniques have not proven to be effective in all clinical trials, but may be helpful in minimizing hair loss when properly applied. Tourniquets applied to the scalp are sometimes successful in minimizing hair loss; generally they are used in conjunction with scalp hypothermia techniques. If the patient is experiencing thrombocytopenia, such techniques are contraindicated, as they may contribute to capillary damage in the scalp and subsequent bleeding.

RADIATION THERAPY

Radiotherapy also damages the DNA of hair follicle cells. The dose of radiation and extent of the treatment field determine the effects on hair. Hair loss may be expected to occur beginning about a week after the initiation of therapy. Only those areas of the skin surface that are included in the field are affected by radiation. Dosage effects can be considered at three levels:

1. 1,500–3,000 rad. Hair loss may be complete or partial, but is temporary in nature.
2. 3,000–4,500 rad. Variable regrowth and degree of hair loss. Some individuals will experience few effects, while others suffer complete hair loss with partial regrowth.
3. Over 4,500 rad. Permanent, complete hair loss over the treated area.

There is nothing that can be done by the nurse to prevent the effects of radiation therapy on scalp hair. Suggesting use of the general precautions described below is the best advice to offer the patient.

- Use only soft brushes when handling hair.
- Brush hair only when necessary.
- Use gentle shampoos, do not vigorously rub scalp, and shampoo only when necessary.
- Use wigs, hairpieces, and head-wear that do not cause undue scalp constriction.

Constipation

One of the most frequent side effects of morphine use is constipation. Not uncommonly, the patient who is battling cancer on physical and psychological fronts will also be dehydrated, anorexic, and anxious. These factors together tend to produce stools that are hard, dry, small, and very constipating. Although bulk laxatives such as Metamucil are frequently prescribed for these cancer patients, care must be taken with their use as they can contribute to the constipation when used incorrectly. Bulk laxatives only soften and hasten the passage of stool when used in conjunction with sufficient quantities of water. With dehydrated patients, the presence of the additional bulk supplied artificially can actually cause an intestinal obstruction. Stool softeners such as Colace, mineral oil lubricants, or laxatives may be useful for relief and should be used regularly if needed. Tap water enemas, which provide lubricating fluid and ready relief of constipation, should be used to keep constipated patients comfortable. Encouraging fluids is helpful, as is exercise as tolerated. Red wine has been found useful in relieving constipation.

Diarrhea

The presence of diarrhea in the cancer patient is usually related to the use of radiation therapy fields involving the gut or to the use of drugs, particularly antineoplastics such as the vinca alkaloids. Generally the problem is transient and self-limited once the treatments are completed. Treatment involves a bland diet, increased fluids, and the careful use of diarrhea control agents such as Lomotil. Moistened towelettes and soothing ointments may be needed to control rectal area burning and soreness. Attention to the electrolyte balance of the patient should be increased when diarrhea is present, as electrolytes may be lost in excessive amounts and require replacement.

Transfusions

To treat effects of the progression of cancer, or during chemotherapy or radiation therapy, the cancer patient may require the transfusion of a blood component. The nurse should understand the types of transfusions most frequently seen and general protocols for their administration. Because these patients are very likely to require multiple transfusions, repeated blood typing and cross-matching are extremely important. Hemolytic and nonhemolytic transfusion reactions can occur. The nurse must check for the signs and symptoms of these reactions during each transfusion: fever, chills, nausea, myalgia (muscular pain), hypotension, hematuria, and renal failure. These patients are frequently very sick prior to the transfusion, therefore early signs and symptoms of a reaction can be missed by the nurse who is not aware that subtle changes may herald a drastic event. The protocol for anaphylaxis should be available and well understood by the nurse who transfuses cancer patients.

The transfusion of packed red blood cells, granulocytes, and platelets will be covered in the following section.

Transfusion of Packed Red Blood Cells

When packed red blood cells (PC) are administered, the patient receives all the components of the blood, including platelets and granulocytes, without the normal plasma volume. When multiple transfusions are required, the patient may become sensitive to the platelets and granulocytes in the blood, and febrile reactions can occur. With many cancer patients, this presents a clinical problem. Leucocyte and platelet-poor PC, called buffy coat poor PC, minimize this risk to the patient and is often preferred for cancer patients. An additional problem that can occur with PC transfusions to cancer patients involves the frequent presence of replicating stem cells in the blood to be administered. If the cancer patient is immunosuppressed, the blood may be irradiated prior to administration to destroy these cells.

Transfusion of Granulocytes

Cancer patients may experience a deficit of one or more of the components of the granulocyte cell series. Neutrophils, eosinophils, and basophils are the types of granulocytes that are administered to patients. Granuloctye transfusions are sometimes given to patients who have a total granulocyte count of less than 500/cu mm for whom forty-eight hours of antibiotic therapy does not result in a reduction of fever, although the usefulness of such transfusions has not been irrefutably proven. In some cases, if profound granulocytopenia is anticipated as a result of therapy, prophylactic infusion of this blood component is performed. This therapy can only be done at a center where personnel experienced in the administration procedure are available to handle the complications that may develop.

Granulocyte transfusions require the presence of a donor with ABO and Rh compatibility, since some contamination of the granulocytes with red blood cells will occur. Human leucocyte antigen (HLA) compatibility increases the survival rate of granulocytes in the body, but is contraindicated in patients who will be considered for bone marrow transplantation. This precaution is taken in order to avoid the production of antibodies to HLA-compatible granulocytes prior to bone marrow transplantation, when the same cells may be given. Historically, granuloctyes were collected from individuals with chronic myelogenous leukemia (CML) as these individuals have a proliferation of granulocytic precursors. Now many of the donors are HLA-matched family members. The Food and Drug Administration requires that individuals donate no more than ten times each month. As daily administration of granulocytes for four or more days is required for completion of therapy, several donors may have to be available. As the lifespan of granulocytes in the bloodstream is about six hours, the transfusion to the patient must occur immediately after collection from the donor.

Leukapheresis of the donor's blood is done over a 2.5–3.5 hour period. During this procedure the granulocytes are separated from other blood components, which are returned to the donor. To enhance the number of granulocytes obtained through leukapheresis, the donor may receive oral Decadron eight to twelve hours prior to the procedure to increase the number of granulocytes in the blood. The donor must be in good general health with a normal hemoglobin and hematocrit. Abstinence from aspirin is required for the prior two week period. The procedure for leukapheresis involves the placement of a 16–gauge needle in a vein of each arm. Blood is drawn out of one arm into a blood separator, then returned to the donor. Donated granulocytes are rapidly replaced by the donor's own bone marrow. Following donation of granulocytes, the donor should increase fluids and eat a high protein diet for several days.

The patient receiving granulocytes must be carefully watched for signs and symptoms of a blood reaction. The risk of anaphylaxis is small, but must be considered. Transfused granulocytes have a tendency to migrate to the area of infection. If the patient has pneumonia, dyspnea may develop secondary to pulmonary consolidation with white blood cells. During and following a transfusion, patients with a compromised respiratory system should be evaluated carefully for shortness of breath, increased respiratory rate, tachycardia, or cyanosis. The use of mechanical ventilation may be required for a severely affected patient. Patients with a localized infection may complain of increased pain at the site following transfusion with granulocytes.

Transfusion of Platelets

Platelets have a very short life span (eight to nine days). Consequently there is frequent cell division in precursor cells in the blood, making them particularly vulnerable to side effects of radiation therapy and chemotherapy. A normal platelet count is between 150,000 and 300,000/cu mm. When the count drops to 10,000/cu mm or less, platelet transfusions may be administered to prevent bleeding. Any time the patient has a severely depressed platelet count, or is clinically symptomatic, platelets may be given. Once infused, platelets live for about two days, but this lifespan may be shortened by factors such as the presence of fever, hepatosplenomegaly, or sepsis.

Platelets are collected from whole blood by centrifuge or via pheresis. They are administered in individual units, as pooled concentrates, or in platelet-rich plasma. HLA typing is done, as this prolongs the life of the platelets once transfused. If the patient is a candidate for bone marrow transplantation, HLA-matched platelets are not administered. Because patients requiring platelet transfusions will be exposed to foreign cells, they are premedicated to minimize shaking chills and fever due to an incompatibility reaction. Often acetaminophen and Benadryl are used for this purpose.

Administration of platelets is done rapidly with filtered tubing. Pressure may be required on the infusion bag or milking of the tubing required to sustain the flow of platelets. Gentle agitation helps prevent clumping of platelets to the transfusion set. Throughout the transfusion, patients need to be evaluated to ensure that a blood reaction or anaphylaxis does not occur.

Patients who require frequent transfusions of platelets may develop antibodies to platelets over time. This may cause them to become refractory to platelet transfusions, minimizing their effectiveness. Histocompatible family members make the best donors, since they reduce the exposure of the patient to foreign platelets. ABO and Rh compatibility is required because some contamination of platelets with donor red blood cells will occur. Irradiation of platelets may be done to prevent graft-versus-host disease in immunosuppressed patients.

One platelet transfusion is considered equal to ten units of non-HLA matched platelets or four units of HLA matched platelets (Gannon 1983). One infusion in unsensitized patients will increase the platelet count by 70,000–90,000/cu mm.

If an allergic reaction occurs, platelet transfusions are generally continued with careful monitoring. As fever will destroy platelet cells, it is controlled with acetaminophen and premedication with Benadryl or SoluCortef.

Platelets are stored at room temperature and have a shelf life of three to five days (if refrigerated, they last only two days). Guidelines for transfusions are given in Table 4.2.

Common Oncologic Emergencies

A few situations that occur in oncology nursing constitute true emergency conditions. These are pericardial tamponade, septicemia, superior vena cava syndrome, spinal cord compression, tumor lysis syndrome, and hemorrhage. Other conditions that exist in the cancer

Table 4.2   Guidelines for Transfusions to Cancer Patients

Red Blood Cells	Granulocytes	Platelets
1. Assess transfusion history	1. Assess transfusion history	1. Assess transfusion history
2. Check ABO and Rh compatibility	2. Check ABO, Rh, and HLA compatibility	2. Check ABO, Rh, and HLA compatibility
3. Premedicate: Benadryl	3. Premedicate: Benadryl, steroids, acetaminophen, or meperidine	3. Premedicate: Benadryl, acetaminophen, steroids
4. Slow infusion, periodic observation	4. Administer immediately[b]	4. Administer immediately
5. VS monitoring[a]	5. Moderate infusion rate, close observation	5. Rapid infusion, frequent observation
	6. VS monitoring[a]	6. VS monitoring[a]
	7. Rinse transfusion bag with 30 ml of NS to remove adhering granulocytes	7. Use gentle shaking of bag and pressure to sustain flow
	8. Check for pulmonary consolidation in high-risk patients	8. Milk tubing as required to prevent clogging by platelets

[a]VS monitoring: 15 minutes prior to infusion; then Q15 min × 2; Q30 min during remainder of transfusion and Q4h × 24 hrs after transfusion completed.
[b]Administer granulocytes: 50–75 ml in first hr; then remainder (150–250 ml) over 1-2 hrs.
Source: Yasko 1983, 59.

patient in a chronic form may become acute emergencies. The latter conditions include disseminated intravascular coagulation (DIC), hypercalcemia, and syndrome of inappropriate ADH (SIADH). These paraneoplastic phenomena are discussed with other such syndromes elsewhere in this chapter. In this section, they will be approached in terms of their management in acute situations.

Pericardial Tamponade

This emergency consists of an accumulation of fluid in the pericardial sac. The pressure of the fluid inhibits the expansion of the heart during diastole, resulting in diminished atrial and ventricular filling and inadequate cardiac function. This condition is associated most often with breast and lung cancer, the leukemias, and the lymphomas.

The patient with cardiac tamponade demonstrates shortness of breath with progessively less activity until resting dyspnea results. Other signs and symptoms include tachycardia, leg edema, hypotension, paradoxical pulse, and distended neck veins. A pericardial friction rub may be heard. In the acute situation, pericardiocentesis must be done for relief. A catheter is often left in the pericardium, since cancer-related cardiac tamponade tends to be a recurring problem. A small opening, called a pleuropericardial window, may be made between the pleural space and pericardium to allow seepage of fluid out of the pericardial sac for continuing relief. Other actions that may relieve the situation include radiation of the heart or administration of chemotherapy to destroy cancer cells in the pericardium that may be directly responsible for the problem. On the other hand, radiation of the chest can cause pericarditis, which results in tamponade. This is usually seen after radiotherapy for Hodgkin's disease and lymphoma. In this case, corticosteroids may be useful in reducing the effects of the inflammatory process. A complete surgical pericardectomy is sometimes done.

This emergency situation may involve a long and difficult recovery period with symptoms that cause intense anxiety for the patient. Median survival after symptoms of tamponade develop is four months. The acute nursing care involved includes administration of oxygen, assistance with pericardiocentesis, and careful monitoring of vital signs and cardiac-filling pressures.

Septicemia

The oncology nurse must remain vigilant for the possibility of septicemia in the cancer patient. Septicemia may occur as a result of infections that would be readily controlled in other individuals but thast are can become life-threatening for cancer patients because of debility from therapies, cachexia, or the disease process. Immunity may be impaired by radiation, chemotherapy, or malignancies of the white blood cells as well as by individual factors. Advanced age, malnutrition from primary or secondary cachexia, and concurrent chronic medical problems all reduce the patient's ability to fight infection. When the skin, mucous membranes, urinary or respiratory tracts become infected, septicemia becomes a possibility for the debilitated cancer patient.

White blood counts above 11,000/cu mm indicate infection or hematologic cancer in the patient. If leukopenia is present, white blood counts may be below 1,000/cu mm in the presence of infection. Fever is usually present, but is not always seen in severe septicemia. If leukopenia exists, the patient will not respond to antibiotic therapy unless granulocytes are given (the procedure for administration of granulocytes is discussed earlier in this chapter). Other therapies for the patient with septicemia include broad-spectrum antibiotics and control of focal infection points that are present. Combinations of antibiotic drugs designed to work against staphylococci and Gram-negative bacilli are commonly used. Blood cultures are taken to monitor for the presence of microorganisms in the blood.

Nursing care for septicemia includes administration of parenteral antibiotics, wound care, supportive measures, and monitoring of vital signs. These patients require complete support in activities of daily living. The patient and family may require teaching of measures to prevent future episodes of sepsis or septicemia. Specific points of the teaching plan that should be included are the importance of handwashing, control of waste products, and attention to general health practices such as a balance of rest and activity, and adequate nutrition.

Superior Vena Cava Syndrome

Superior vena cava syndrome (SVCS) results from compression of the vein returning blood from the periphery to the right atrium or from internal obstruction of the vessel. It is rarely seen except with cancer patients. It is most commonly associated with lung cancer, where 3–8 percent of patients develop the syndrome. Other cancers frequently associated with it include undifferentiated carcinoma of the thyroid, diffuse non-Hodgkin's lymphomas, and mediastinal germinomas. With malignant tumors, obstruction or compression develops rapidly over a few weeks and flagrant signs and symptoms are present. Because the process causing the vena cava compression with benign tumors occurs over time, collateral circulation usually develops to some extent so that full-blown signs and symptoms of the condition are not seen. Sometimes displacement of right atrial catheters can also lead to SVCS. Symptoms of SVCS include edema and cyanosis of the face, neck, and upper extremities, headache, and changes in sensorium. Thorax and neck vein distention, dyspnea, epistaxis, and painless dysphagia may also be seen.

Treatment may include diuretics and high doses of corticosteroids for initial relief, although their use is controversial (Stapczynski 1984). Prompt irradiation of the superior vena cava is indicated as soon as the condition is recognized. In a majority of patients, relief from radiation therapy of 4,000–5,000 rads is seen in seventy-two hours. In some cases, chemotherapy may be used as an adjunct to radiation if the tumor involved is sensitive to drug therapy. Anticoagulants may be given to prevent clotting secondary to obstructed blood flow. As the condition is usually associated with lung cancer, for which there is little chance of cure, and debility occurs quickly, surgery is not a useful treatment. Of course, if mechanical obstruction from catheter displacement is causing symptoms, the catheter is removed.

Nursing care for SVCS includes limitation of activity, respiratory support, monitoring of vital signs, and institution of measures to control increased intracranial pressure. Fluid limits, avoidance of the Valsalva maneuver or straining, and positioning the patient in Semi-Fowler's or an orthopnic position are important nursing measures to include.

Spinal Cord Compression

Compression fractures of the spine may cause spinal cord or nerve root compression. Pressure on the spinal cord or nerve roots results in neurologic dysfunction. Although the condition is not life threatening, it can result in paraplegia, with devastating psychosocial consequences. The classic symptoms associated with this condition are pain, weakness, sensory loss, and autonomic dysfunction, including the loss of sphincter control. Early diagnosis and treatment can halt the progression of the condition, and result in fewer residual neurological deficits. The first symptom is almost always pain, which gradually increases and is felt in a specific area of the spine. It is followed by muscle weakness and/or sensory loss. Loss of anal sphincter control occurs late and indicates a poor chance of response to treatment. Examination of the patient may reveal hyperactive reflexes with a positive Babinski, bilateral sensory loss, or spastic weakness.

Most spinal cord compressions in cancer patients occur from invasion of the epidural space by metastatic cells from contiguous bone. About 70 percent of cases involve the thoracic spine, with 20 percent presenting in the lumbosacral spine and the remainder in the cervical spine. The condition is treated by surgery and radiation as palliative measures. A laminectomy and resection of tumor mass may be done, followed by radiation to irradicate any remaining tumor cells. Because normal healing rarely occurs after this procedure, a back brace may be required for the remainder of the patient's lifespan to stabilize the spine. If complete removal of the tumor is not possible, or if the spinal involvement is a result of metastasis, radiation therapy alone gives results comparable to the surgery and radiation combination therapy, and is the treatment of choice. The goal of treatment is to return the patient to the level of prior functioning, but this is not always possible.

Nursing emphasis is on detection of initial signs indicating the possibility of spinal cord compression, and support during rehabilitation of the patient who has neurological deficits after therapy. The sooner the compression is halted, the fewer the resultant deficits seen, so attention to complaints of pain in the spine are very important. Cancers of the lung, breast, prostate and kidney, and multiple myeloma are most often associated with this condition.

Tumor Lysis Syndrome

When there is rapid destruction of numerous neoplastic cells over a short period of time, a serious and sometimes fatal metabolic disturbance can result. This is most often seen in chemotherapeutic induction therapy for the leukemias and lymphomas, because these malignant cells are particularly sensitive to chemotherapeutic agents. The rapid cytoreductive therapy that characterizes the initial treatment of these cancers requires intensive nursing care. Leukemia and lymphoma patients with high white cell counts, large tumor masses, and/or renal dysfunction are at highest risk for tumor lysis syndrome.

The metabolic problems associated under the umbrella of "tumor lysis syndrome" are hyperkalemia, hyperuricemia, hyperphosphatemia, and hypocalcemia. If preventive and supportive therapy does not correct the syndrome, renal dialysis may need to be instituted for a few days to correct the serum abnormalities. The first two days of induction therapy are the time of greatest risk for developing these metabolic abnormalities.

HYPERKALEMIA

Hyperkalemia occurs when lysed cells release intracellular potassium more rapidly than renal cells can excrete the excess. If dehydration or acidosis are part of the clinical picture, the risks of excess potassium are increased, as these conditions both lead to extracellular shifts of potassium. Cardiac arrhythmias and asystole are the greatest threats in hyperkalemia. The classic signs of hyperkalemia are confusion, numbness or tingling sensations, weakness, and brachycardia. Cardiac standstill may ultimately develop. If the patient is at high risk for developing tumor lysis syndrome, cardiac monitoring should be established. Expected changes in hyperkalemia include tall T-waves, and prolonged PR, QRS, and ST segments.

The hypocalcemia often associated with the syndrome potentiates the cardiac effects of hyperkalemia. Potassium levels above 5.0 mEq/dl denote hyperkalemia; if potassium reaches levels above 6.5 mEq/dl, prompt treatment is indicated for potential cardiac standstill. The treatment includes withholding dietary sources of potassium, particularly foods high in potassium such as orange, grapefruit, or apple juice; bananas, apricots, or melons; potatoes; milk; bouillon; or fish and meat products. Kayexalate, or similar cation exchange resins, help remove potassium from the gut when adequate bowel movements are present. Administration of an infusion of 10 percent glucose with an added 50 units of insulin may be used to promote the transfer of potassium from the serum to the intracellular fluid. Strict bedrest should be maintained, and renal function should be monitored.

HYPERPHOSPHATEMIA AND HYPOCALCEMIA

When intracellular phosphorus is rapidly released during cytolysis, the kidneys may be unable to maintain normal blood levels. Hypocalcemia is thought to be a secondary effect of hyperphosphatemia, presumably due to calcium-phosphate precipitation. Since hyperphosphatemia is usually asymptomatic, signs and symptoms of hypocalcemia are the key to the presence of this metabolic abnormality. They include numbness, tingling of the extremities, irritability, tetany (painful muscular spasms), seizures, and a positive Chvostek sign (facial twitching elicited by tapping in front of the ear). Calcium values below 4.5 mEq/L constitute hypocalcemia. A critical consequence of this condition is cardiac arrhythmias. A lengthened QT interval is the EKG abnormality seen. Treatment is usually slow intravenous administration of a 10 percent calcium gluconate solution if several symptoms are present. In mild cases, oral calcium tablets may be sufficient treatment. Aluminum hydroxide gel may be administered, as it lowers serum phosphorus, consequently raising calcium levels. The parathyroid glands are responsible for maintaining phosphorous and calcium in balance, but the gland is not able to function quickly enough to maintain an appropriate balance in the rapid tumor lysis syndrome.

HYPERURICEMIA

This condition is relatively common in cancer chemotherapy. In the tumor lysis syndrome, nucleic acid purines are metabolized to form uric acid. At a normal urine pH level of 5–6, uric acid is poorly soluble and can block renal tubules, ultimately leading to renal failure. Generally, prophylactic allopurinol is begun twenty-four hours prior to beginning chemotherapy for leukemia or lymphoma patients, to block several pathways of purine metabolism. Maintenance of adequate hydration during and following the administration of chemotherapeutics helps to prevent blockage of renal tubules. Alkalinization of the urine increases the solubility of uric acid, thus improving its excretion. Oral or intravenous bicarbonate is usually given to maintain a urine pH of 7 or more if hyperuricemia is found in laboratory testing. Often patients are catheterized at the start of chemotherapy so that accurate monitoring of renal function can be accomplished. A minimum urine output of 1,500 ml over a twenty-four hour period should maintained in the presence of hyperuricemia. Agents such as probenecid (Benemid) and sulfinpyrazone (Anturane) are sometimes used to treat hyperuricemia in addition to allopurinol.

Hemorrhage

Thrombocytopenia, a frequent cause of hemorrhage in the cancer patient, is discussed earlier in the section on paraneoplastic phenomena. The most frequent bleeding sites seen are the mucous membranes, skin, gastrointestinal system, respiratory system, genitourinary system, and intracranial cavity. With the availability of platelets for transfusion, the danger of hemorrhage from thrombocytopenia has been reduced in recent years. Any patient with thrombocytopenia who exhibits frank bleeding, petechiae, ecchymosis, excessive menstrual blood flow, oozing of blood from wounds, or laboratory test values consistent with blood loss or imminent potential for spontaneous bleeding should be handled carefully, watched closely, and treated with platelet and blood transfusions as necessary.

In the face of acute hemorrhage, measures undertaken commonly include direct pressure applied to visible bleeding sites, immediate administration of platelets and blood, ice lavages for gastrointestinal bleeding, and intensive monitoring of vital signs.

Disseminated Intravascular Coagulation

Disseminated intravascular coagulation (DIC) sometimes occurs as a chronic paraneoplastic condition in cancer patients due to the release of thrombin by malignant cells. This mechanism is most often seen in cancers of the breast, lung, prostate, colon, ovary, and stomach and in leukemia. DIC may also occur as an acute event in cancer patients after multiple blood transfusions or in the presence of septicemia. The nurse should assess the patient with a potential for DIC for spontaneous bleeding, the onset of shock without other obvious causes, or for signs of renal failure. In DIC, the PT, PTT, and thrombin time are all prolonged. Fibrinogen levels, platelet levels, antithrombin III (AT-III) levels, and coagulation factors are low. The protamine sulfate test is positive. These laboratory values are important indicators of the onset of DIC. Treatment measures include heparin administration, antithrombin III, blood component replacement therapy, and antifibrinolytic therapy.

The immediate remedial measures taken in the presence of acute hemorrhage from DIC include treatment of shock, and sometimes the administration of heparin if brain, lung, or kidney damage is occurring in order to slow the abnormal clotting and give the body a chance to recover from the massive depletion of clotting factors. Usual doses of heparin are between 2,500 to 5,000 units given subcutaneously every eight to twelve hours. Results are usually apparent within four to five hours. An alternate treatment is the administration of antithrombin III concentrate, which is currently being tried at centers across the country. If the initial treatment is not effective, blood component replacement therapy may be done, usually including platelets and fresh frozen plasma, as well as the administration of antifibrinolytic therapy (episilon–aminocaproic acid—EACA). In the cancer patient, there is no evidence that regular warfarin therapy is of value in controlling the persistent DIC that may occur.

Hypercalcemia

Hypercalcemia may be present in cancer patients as a paraneoplastic syndrome, due to bony metastasis, or as a consequence of immobility and dehydration. Management of the condition is aimed at two objectives: to reduce the serum calcium level directly and to treat the underlying cause. Sometimes the underlying cause cannot be controlled, as when it is present as paraneoplasia for an unresectable tumor. The condition may be chronic or acute. Hypercalcemia will be addressed in this section with reference to its potential as a life-threatening condition requiring emergency measures.

Saline diuresis by means of saline intravenous infusions significantly increases calcium clearance. Central venous pressure measurements should ideally be taken throughout this treatment as fluid overloads and electrolyte imbalances can occur. Normal saline infusions at a rate of 250–500 ml/hr with 20–80 mg of furosemide given every two to four hours is generally effective therapy. Hydrocortisone infusions are effective in lympho-proliferative diseases and some cases of bony metastasis. The use of glucocorticoids in this manner takes several days to reduce serum calcium levels. Oral prednisone, 10–30 mg/day, is sometimes used to maintain reasonable calcium levels. The glucocorticoids are effective in treating hypercalcemia because one of their mechanisms of action is to reduce intestinal absorption of calcium, reduce renal reabsorption of calcium, and reduce the rate of bone turnover. Calcitonin (Calcimar) is a peptide hormone used to reduce serum calcium levels by infusion therapy. The effects of calcitonin end when therapy is discontinued, but moderate reductions in blood levels are seen during infusion therapy. Nausea is seen in about 10 percent of patients during the initiation of calcitonin therapy. The major nursing concern with its administration is the potential for anaphylaxis. Sometimes skin testing is done prior to calcitonin therapy to assess for allergic potential. Because calcitonin can adhere to the walls of the administration set, albumin is usually added to the infusion solution to coat it.

For patients who do not have renal dysfunction, oral phosphate supplements are useful adjuncts to the treatment of hypercalcemia. Diarrhea is often the limiting factor in the use of oral phosphate. Mithramycin (Methracin) is an antineoplastic agent that inhibits bone resorption and causes hypocalcemia. Given as an intravenous bolus, it causes significant reductions in calcium levels within about twelve hours. Doses every three to four days can maintain reasonable serum calcium levels. Generally, this therapy is used when other modalities have failed. At doses used for treatment of hypercalcemia, common gastrointestinal symptoms associated with chemotherapy in general occur with mithramycin therapy. Facial flushing and a skin rash may also occur. Nonsteroidal anti-inflammatory agents such as Indomethacin and aspirin inhibit prostaglandin activity and can reduce serum calcium levels through this mechanism. Hypercalcemia associated with cases of lung cancer and kidney cancer have responded particularly well to nonsteroidal anti-inflammatory agents.

Syndrome of Inappropriate ADH Secretion

The paraneoplastic syndrome of inappropriate ADH secretion (SIADH) may result in water intoxication with hyponatremia, which can be life threatening if not controlled. Cyclophosphamide and vincristine are antineoplastic agents that can also cause SIADH in some patients. The syndrome is seen in about 50 percent of small cell lung cancer patients as well as in a smaller percentage of cases of pancreatic cancer, Hodgkin's lymphoma, non-Hodgkin's lymphoma, and thymoma. Severe expression of this syndrome may cause somnolence, seizures and coma, and mental confusion secondary to electrolyte imbalance. Treatment of the syndrome includes fluid restrictions, administration of demeclocycline (a tetracycline derivative), or phenytoin, or infusion of hypertonic saline.

The infusion of hypertonic saline is used if the condition has developed to a severe degree. In this case, confusion, stupor, convulsions, and muscle twitching are present. Small amounts of hypertonic sodium chloride are administered slowly, with the goal of raising the serum sodium level to half the normal level within eight hours. A potential danger in this treatment is fluid and circulatory overload. Sometimes furosemide is initially given with saline infusions following. Potassium levels must also be carefully evaluated and replacements given when necessary. Hourly evaluation of serum electrolytes is undertaken to guide therapy.

Nurses must carefully monitor intake and output, observe for changes in neurological status, and for signs of fluid and electrolyte imbalance. With elderly patients, the dangers associated with this syndrome are greater, because these patients may have concurrent medical problems that compound the effects of the syndrome.

5
Clinical Management of Major Cancer Sites

The following sections provide essential information on the major cancers of the United States population. The etiology of the cancer is described, basic pathophysiology outlined, and the common clinical course of the cancer set forth. The management skills included must be incorporated by the nurse based on a complete patient assessment. The standard of practice today dictates that professional nurses are responsible for performing a complete assessment and basing their practice on that assessment.

Lung Cancer

Etiology

Lung cancer is largely a preventable disease. Data (1982) indicate that among men, 90 percent of lung cancer incidence is attributable to smoking, and that among women 75 percent of lung cancer is smoking-related. Perhaps the world's greatest cancer problem, lung cancer may now surpass stomach cancer as the most common malignancy among males worldwide. As smoking increases among women, lung cancer will become the foremost cancer problem among this group sometime during the 1980s. Although the vast majority of lung cancer cases are among the smoking population, it should be understood that most smokers will not suffer lung cancer. About 85 percent of smokers will die of other causes—often heart or lung disease also influenced by smoking.

DEMOGRAPHIC FACTORS

Geographic variation. Lung cancer is the leading form of cancer in North America and western Europe, with a significantly lower incidence rate among Indian, Chinese, and African populations. This variation may disappear in the future. The World Health Organiza-

155

tion has recently decried the large-scale export of tobacco from the United States to African nations, forseeing a lung cancer epidemic occurring in Africa in ten to twenty years related directly to increased tobacco consumption.

Within the United States, clustering of lung cancer is noted mostly among Southeastern Seaboard communities, with some clustering also seen in the urban, industrial Northeast. Other countries, notably China, have noted some excess lung cancer cases in industrialized areas. However, the number of lung cancer cases attributable to industrial pollution is probably very small. One difficulty in separating the relative risks of smoking and industrial pollution is that the rates of smoking are highest among urbanized populations. Most studies to date show no consistent gradient of lung cancer incidence with urban pollution.

Time and person variability. Lung cancer incidence is increasing in much of the world following a twenty-year parallel increase in smoking. In the United States, the fastest increasing incidence is seen among black males and white women. Smoking and lung cancer incidence are overrepresented among blacks, the poor, gays, and the mentally ill. Upper socioeconomic groups have curtailed smoking since the 1960s, and lung cancer incidence in this group is dropping correspondingly.

There is a growing body of evidence of a genetic predisposition in certain individuals to lung cancer. Smokers with a relative who contracts lung cancer are eleven times more likely to develop the disease. It has also recently been shown that a diet deficient in vitamin A may reduce the lung mucosa integrity, predisposing to lung cancer.

Evidence on the role of passive smoking inhaling "second hand" smoke is equivocal, but to date it points in the direction of increased relative risk for those exposed on a regular basis to heavily smoke-contaminated environment.

Occupational exposures. Substances with an established relationship to lung cancer are:

radioactivity (radium, uranium)	arsenic
nickel	mustard gas
chromates	chloromethyl methyl ether
asbestos	vinyl chloride
coal gas and tar	

Some of these substances potentiate the effects of tobacco in causing lung cancer as well.

Common Clinical Course

DETECTION

Presenting symptoms in lung cancer differ according to location of the primary tumor and extent of the disease. Central tumors often cause presenting symptoms of coughing, wheezing, dyspnea, or generalized chest pain. Peripheral tumors are often asymptomatic until distant metastasis or regional involvement cause symptoms to develop. Then, excruciating chest pain, superior vena cava syndrome from mediastinal node involvement, or symptoms related to increased cranial pressure from brain metastasis may develop.

PATHOPHYSIOLOGY

Bronchogenic carcinoma advances through the body by direct extension through the tissues of the chest as well as through the lymph vessels. Nerves within the thorax may become involved, causing paralysis of the larynx, which may be a key to detection.

Small-cell carcinoma has the strongest relationship to cigarette smoking. It is most common to see it among smokers with a history of ten or more "pack years," with smoking continuing within the previous ten years. Small-cell carcinoma is also associated with the poorest prognosis of all the lung cancer types. At the time of presentation, disease is limited in only 20 to 40 percent of patients. Most have metastatic spread to the lymph nodes, bone, bone marrow, brain, and/or liver. The frequency of brain involvement is approximately 10 percent at diagnosis and 30 percent at autopsy. The prognosis in various types of lung cancer is shown in Table 5.1.

Table 5.1   Prognosis in Lung Cancer

Histologic classification	Incidence (percent)	5-year survival (percent)
Central tumors:		
Squamous cell (epidermoid)	25–30	25
Small cell	20–25	1
Peripheral tumors:		
Adenocarcinoma	30–35	12
Large cell	15–20	13

Source: Modified from *Nurses Clinical Library: Neoplastic Disorders* (Springhouse, Penna.: Springhouse Corp., 1985), 143.

DIAGNOSIS AND STAGING

The following diagnostic tools are used in detecting the presence of lung cancer:

chest X-ray
sputum cytology
bronchoscopy
hematoporphyrin derivative (HpD) testing
mediastinoscopy
radioisotope scan
bone marrow biopsy
CEA levels

For lung cancer it is especially important to determine the type and extent of the disease, since 47 percent of symptomatic patients will be found to have metastasis. Chest X-rays are the usual initial diagnostic tool, but in a significant number of cases they fail to detect early disease. Unfortunately, most symptomatic individuals no longer have early disease. Thus, the usefulness of chest X-rays is mostly as a screening tool for high risk individuals.

Sputum cytology is a powerful tool for detecting lung cancer in symptomatic individuals or for detecting central tumors in asymptomatic individuals. Early peripheral tumors frequently go undetected with this test, however. The use of bronchoscopy may enable localization of a lesion in a patient with a normal roentgenogram but positive sputum test. If the bronchoscopy does not show the tumor, the use of HpD, which glows under violet light, is now used to detect occult cancers.

In past years, two techniques that are no longer routinely recommended were used in diagnosing lung cancer. The usefulness of scalene node biopsy in determining resectability of a lung cancer tumor is now in doubt. Thoracotomy has similarly been found to be a poor technique for the diagnosis and staging of lung cancer, because over 50 percent of all individuals are inoperable when they first present with symptoms and the procedure carries high mortality and morbidity rates.

Mediastinoscopy has been found to be a most valuable tool in determining the operability of lung cancer. The procedure involves general anesthesia to examine paratracheal, tracheobronchial, and subcarinal lymph nodes. Uncommon side effects of mediastinoscopy are pneumothorax, infection, and recurrent laryngeal nerve injury.

With so many symptomatic individuals initially presenting with metastatic disease, a radioisotope scan of the skeletal system, liver, and central nervous system, with bone marrow biopsy, are essential to determine accurately the prognosis and reasonable treatment alternatives. CEA levels are sometimes measured in order to monitor response to treatment.

TREATMENT

Definitive. The only treatment considered definitive for well-localized tumors is surgery. Unfortunately, of the 50 percent of patients who are resectable at diagnosis, one half will be found unresectable once operated upon, and only 7–8 percent of the total group will ultimately survive. A lobectomy, or removal of a lobe; or pneumonectomy, removal of an entire lung, are the surgical alternatives. Complications of these procedures include pulmonary embolism, empyema, cor pulmonale, respiratory failure, and cardiac dysrhythmias. In addition, incision pain may linger for months after these procedures.

Palliative. For *non-small-cell carcinomas*: Chemotherapy is a frequently used modality that promotes tumor regression. It has not been shown to affect ultimate survival, however. A three-drug combination using cisplatin, vindesine, and mitomycin has shown the best response rate to date, with some 56 percent of patients entering remission on this regimen. Other drug combinations give response rates that are nearly as good.

The use of bacillus Calmette-Guerin (BCG) with chemotherapy or postoperatively has not been shown to increase survival in recent trials. Currently, new trials are underway nationwide to determine if either chemotherapy or immunotherapy, or the combination, can increase survival in any subpopulation of lung cancer patients.

For patients with *Small-cell carcinoma*: the median survival time has increased from three months to one year since the 1960s. In virtually all cases, the disease is systemic when diagnosed, so surgery is not considered a treatment. The increased survival over the last two and a half decades comes from the use of chemotherapy and radiation therapy in combination.

The chemotherapeutic agents most active against small cell carcinoma are cyclophosphamide, doxorubicin hydrochloride, VP 16–213 (etoposide), vincristine sulfate, lomustine (CCNU), and methotrexate. Chemotherapeutic regimens normally contain three or four of these drugs, usually including cytoxan.

Several new *prospects for treatment* are being explored. Endoscopic phototherapy, the use of HpD and violet light, may eventually be used to treat superficial bronchial cancers in those who cannot tolerate surgery.

Bone marrow transplantation is currently being investigated for use as a supportive treatment of small-cell lung carcinoma. It is thought that it may facilitate more rapid hematologic recovery in patients undergoing intensive chemotherapy (Murphy 1984). The only patients who have thus far shown a benefit from bone marrow transplantation are those who were in complete remission before transplantation.

Although alpha- and beta- interferon have not proved useful in the treatment of small-cell lung cancer, recent gamma-interferon studies have shown initially positive results.

Management Skills

DETECTING METASTASIS AND PARANEOPLASTIC SYNDROMES

Metastasis either presents as a part of the clinical picture of lung cancer or is part of the clinical course for almost all patients. Lung cancer is also the malignancy most frequently associated with paraneoplastic syndromes. Because of these two facts, the nurse needs to be aware of related signs and symptoms in lung cancer patients. The following common findings are suggestive of metastatic disease:

- shoulder and arm pain; fractures of the first and second rib; sinking in of the eyeball, ptosis, myosis, decreased facial sweating, and neuritis (Horner's syndrome)–indicative progressive superior sulcus syndrome
- superior vena cava syndrome
- pleural effusion (at least 50 percent of lung cancer patients)
- epidural spinal cord compression (typical with small-cell carcinoma)
- thrombophlebitis (lung cancer is the most common cause)
- low-grade disseminated intravascular coagulation
- sterile thrombotic endocarditis

It is also necessary for the nurse to check for the following typically seen paraneoplastic syndromes:

- clubbing of the fingers
- symptoms mimicking rheumatoid arthritis (osteoarthropathy occuring in 5–12 percent of lung cancer patients)
- Cushing's syndrome
- hypercalcemia (6–16 percent of lung cancer patients-hyperparathyroidism)

EFFECTS OF TREATMENT

Because so many of these patients present with metastatic disease for which there is very little hope of survival, the effects of treatment must be weighed against the ultimate benefits derived from any therapeutic regimen.

Pulmonary insufficiency after a pneumonectomy must be carefully guarded against. Because the planning for surgery takes into consideration the amount of lung function that needs to be preserved, inadequate residual lung is rarely the cause of postoperative pulmonary insufficiency. Since risks to these patients from pneumonia are greater than for other types of surgical patients, prevention of pneumonia is an important goal of a nursing staff.

The long-term complications of radiation therapy for lung cancer include pneumonitis, fibrosis of the remaining lung, rib fractures secondary to osteoradionecrosis, esophageal stricture, pericardial and myocardial fibrosis, and radiation myelitis. Because the lung cancer patient is usually severely debilitated, these complications must be frequently considered for any post-radiation therapy patient. Physical reserves are typically small and the complications severe. Prevention of these complications through sophisticated therapy by the radiologist is more useful than subsequent treatment, which often holds little probability of success. When chemotherapy is combined with radiation therapy, the complications of esophagitis, radiation pneumonitis, and bone marrow suppression are more likely to occur.

A major drawback of chemotherapy for lung cancer is the risk of chronic toxicity, even when a favorable clinical response is achieved. Patients may be plagued by bone marrow hypoplasia, cardiomyopathy, or CNS disorders. Long-term survivors face an increased risk of acute leukemia, as well. Chemotherapy may add an extra few months to survival, at a cost of additional symptoms.

Prostate Cancer

Etiology

Adenocarcinoma of the prostate is the second most common cancer in American men and the third leading cause of male cancer deaths. It has been found that 30 percent of men have prostate cancer by the time they reach age 70, and that between ages 70 and 80, 40 percent of men will have the disease. After age 80, fully 70 percent of men harbor metastatic carcinoma of the prostate. Still, most elderly affected men will die of causes other than prostatic cancer because the disease is usually indolent in its course.

DEMOGRAPHIC FACTORS

Geographic variability. Japanese men have a particularly low incidence of prostate cancer, but when they migrate to the United States, their incidence rates rise. This cancer is rare in the Near East and less frequent in Eastern Europe than in Western Europe. The population with the highest worldwide incidence of prostate cancer is that of black males of Alameda County, near San Francisco. Whites of the San Francisco Bay area have the second highest incidence rate worldwide.

Time and person variability. In the United States, the incidence of this cancer is rising, among blacks faster than among whites. There appears to be no socioeconomic correlation, however. It has been established that there is a familial tendency towards this disease, either from shared environmental factors or through genetic inheritance. The Mormons, who abstain from tobacco, alcohol, coffee, tea, and use less animal fat in their diets than the general population, do not have prostatic cancer rates appreciably lower than those of other white males, so these factors are not considered important environmental causes of prostatic cancer.

Sexual activity and hormones. Ever-married men have been found to have a higher incidence of prostate cancer than never-married men. Furthermore, prostate cancer patients are more likely to give histories of past venereal disease than other men and are found to have had more coital activity with a greater number of partners. The relationship of androgen plasma levels and sexual activity may hold a key to understanding the etiology of prostate cancer.

It is hypothesized that low androgen levels or high estrogen levels may be protective for prostate cancer. For example, prostate cancer is not commonly found among castrated men. It has also been found that cirrhosis, which causes high levels of circulating estrogen, is associated with lower than expected rates of prostate cancer. The worldwide populations with low prostate cancer rates may reflect the higher incidence of liver damage common to those same areas. High fat diets, which influence the body's hormonal milieu, have also been implicated in prostate cancer in some trials. To date, there are no firm explanations for the variability of prostate cancer among different groups, but the hormone connection and its link to sexual activity holds great promise in preliminary studies of the relationship of prostatic cancer and environmental factors. As in the case of cervical cancer, the possibility of a sexually transmitted virus in the etiology of prostate cancer cannot be ruled out as an important etiological factor.

Common Clinical Course

DETECTION

About 85 percent of these cancers originate in the posterior lobe of the prostate, which is readily assessable by digital rectal examination. Unfortunately, however, only about 20 percent of local cancers are found by digital examination, possibly due in part to inadequate physical assessment. Most patients present with urinary symptoms of obstruction from hypertrophy of the gland and local invasion, which leads to the cancer diagnosis. About 15 percent of patients present with symptoms of general metastasis, generally bone pain or spinal cord compression, at which point cure is unlikely.

PATHOPHYSIOLOGY

Adenocarcinoma accounts for about 95 percent of prostatic cancer. Local invasion by direct extention usually involves the seminal vesicles, bladder, membranous urethra, and pelvis. The rectum is rarely involved. As the cancer progresses and the lymphatic system becomes involved, metastasis occurs to the surrounding bone of the pelvis and spine.

DIAGNOSIS AND STAGING

Diagnosis is usually based on a closed needle biopsy by either the perineal or transrectal route. Broad-spectrum antibiotic coverage is sometimes given the patient to avoid post-biopsy infection. Grading of these tumors is according to three categories—well differentiated, moderately differentiated, or poorly differentiated. Staging of the tumor usually involves blood studies of serum alkaline phosphatase and serum acid phosphatase, although even with recent improvements in performing the latter test, it is still of limited value in staging, as even early disease may yield elevated values. A bone scan is done to check for bony metastasis. Lymphangiography may be done, but often does not detect metastasis to the nodes most commonly involved in metastatic spread of the disease. The injection of technetium 99 antimony sulfide colloid to visualize lymph nodes is a new procedure that may prove more useful than lymphangiography in the future in the staging of prostate cancer.

Several systems are currently employed to define stages of prostatic cancer, but the TNM system of the American Joint Committee for Cancer Staging and End Results Reporting is the most comprehensive and is readily understood in relation to TNM stages of other cancers.

TREATMENT

Prostate cancer is relatively slow growing, and because it primarly affects elderly men, is often concomitant with other life-threatening illnesses such as heart disease, lung disease, or diabetes mellitus. When well-differentiated disease is found in the earliest stage, no treatment is generally given to patients, since the fifteen-year survival of these men is the same as for the general population of the same age. For other patients with more poorly differentiated disease or invasion of other organs, radiation therapy or radical prostatectomy are the usual treatments employed. Survival rates for patients undergoing either surgery or radiation are very similar, although with very advanced disease, surgery may be slightly more successful. The two modalities may be employed together. Frequently with advanced disease, a radical prostatectomy is followed by external beam radiation or interstitial radiation therapy.

Radical prostatectomy. This surgery involves the removal of the prostate gland, seminal vesicles, ampulla, the vas deferens, and the cuff of the bladder. When the cancer has not invaded other tissues or metastasized, this therapy alone is the treatment of choice. It does, however, result in almost 100 percent impotence. The two types of radical prostatectomy employed are retropubic and perineal. Use of the former procedure allows for pelvic lymphadenectomy and possible cystectomy if deemed necessary. The perineal route is selected for patients with compromised respiratory systems, but requires that pelvic lymphadenectomy be performed as a separate procedure.

Radiation therapy. Patients with locally invasive disease are often treated with a radical prostatectomy and external beam radiation or interstitial radiation therapy. Patients who cannot accept the possibility of impotence may be treated with external radiation, which rarely causes this complication. Interstitial implants are often used if during lymphadenectomy nodes are found to be positive. Once nodes are positive, there is no advantage to the patient in radiotherapy, as length of survival is not improved, but this therapy does give local control of disease. Radiation is also often used for palliation of painful bony metastases, pathologic fractures of bone and spinal cord compression that may result from prostatic cancer.

Hormonal therapy. Hormonal therapy has been shown to be useful in palliation for disseminated disease. Bilateral orchiectomy decreases the level of testosterone in the plasma by about 90 percent. Estrogen administration, in the form of diethylstilbesterol, accomplishes the same therapeutic goal. Symptoms of weight loss, poor appetite, and decreased energy can be reversed temporarily by these manipulations of the patient's hormonal milieu in about 80 percent of cases. Responses frequently last about one year. There is no advantage to employing both of these modalities or using one if its alternate fails to cause a symptomatic response. Two antiandrogens, cyproterone acetate and flutamide, are sometimes used in the treatment of prostate cancer to accomplish the same goal of symptomatic relief.

Chemotherapy. The use of chemotherapy is limited to very advanced disease that has failed to respond, or which has relapsed after hormonal manipulation. The use of several drugs together has not proven more useful than single drug chemotherapy, but both single drug and combination drug therapy are seen in the treatment of prostate cancer. Two agents that hold the promise of better response rates than more standard regimens are estramustine phosphate and prednimustine. Besides these two, cytoxan, bleomycin, 5–FU, cisplatin and the nitrosoureas are sometimes used. The most frequently used drug today in the treatment of prostate cancer remains doxorubicin (Adriamycin).

Management Skills

DETECTING METASTASIS

Most patients present with locally invasive disease. Therefore, changes in a prostate cancer patient's condition that may indicate metastasis usually involve the skeletal system. Watch for:

Bone pain. Fifteen percent of patients will present with this symptom and almost all who eventually die of their disease will have this symptom at some point.

Spinal cord compression. This is a devastating, yet not life-threatening complication of advancing disease. The presenting symptoms are pain, weakness, sensory loss, and loss of sphincter control of the bladder. Motor loss usually follows soon after sensory loss. Pain near the affected vertebra may be present for weeks or months prior to the establishment of the diagnosis. Sensory loss and weakness may occur early or late in the compression process. By the time autonomic symptoms are present, the possibility of response to treatment is severely decreased. Laminectomy and radiation therapy are the two modalities employed in treating this complication. Early diagnosis is the key to adequate response to treatment. Pre-treatment motor status is the best prognosticator of response; if paralysis lasts beyond one week, a very poor treatment response rate is seen.

EFFECTS OF TREATMENT

Radical surgery usually results in impotence, and about 10 percent of patients experience urinary incontinence as well. These side effects of surgery can have tremendous impact on the patient's life and self-image. Even elderly men who are not sexually active may want a penile implant. An external condom catheter or penile clamp may be used to control dribbling or incontinence after surgery. If a transurethral resection of the prostate is done for partial gland removal, retrograde ejaculation may result. This "dry climax" is not uncommon and should be described to patients as a possible consequence of surgery.

Radiation therapy preserves continence and potency. However, external beam radiation involves daily doses for as many as seven weeks, which can be a severe hardship on some commuting patients. External radiation or 125–I interstitial implantation may result in mild and temporary dysuria and diarrhea, or urethral narrowing. Radiotherapy may produce skin irritation that can cause patients to abstain from sexual activity, or neuropathy affecting sexual function. In order to avoid painful gynecomastia that may result from estrogen therapy, sometimes pretreatment radiation of the breast is given.

Estrogen therapy may result in unpleasant symptoms such as nausea and vomiting, loss of libido, and accumulation of fat in breasts and hips. Because so many prostate cancer patients are elderly, estrogen therapy with concomitant retention of sodium and water can result in congestive heart failure.

If chemotherapeutic agents are employed, the standard precautions are appropriate. The two newest drugs used in treating this disease may present complications of which the nurse needs to be aware:

Estramustine phosphate (Estracyt, Emcyt) may produce transient nausea and vomiting, congestive heart failure, gynecomastia, gastrointestinal disturbances relieved by antacids when taken with a meal.

With *Prednimustine* (a linkage of prednisone and chlorambucil) reported side effects are myelosuppression, thrush, adrenal insufficiency, congestive heart failure, peptic ulcer, and hyperglycemia.

Rehabilitation

Impotency subsequent to radical prostatectomy can be psychologically devastating to a man and is the most frequent rehabilitative need seen in this population. Semirigid penile implants or inflatable cylinders are well accepted prosthetic devices that should be described to all patients.

Incontinence after surgery can be another annoying and traumatizing development. A full explanation of leg bags, external catheters and penile clamps should be given soon after this side effect is demonstrated in the patient, so dignity and control can be maintained.

Castration of the patient to effect a prolonged comfortable life results in sterility, but not necessarily impotency. However, the psychological impact of missing testicles and the feminizing qualities that develop may cause a distinct decrease in the man's potency. The man may feel better physically, but be psychologically distraught. Teaching the patient what may be expected with antiandrogen therapy may help in adjustment as will the nurse's referral from time to time to the potential for problems, to allow ventilation of feelings by the patient.

Breast Cancer

Etiology

Breast cancer, the most frequent cancer diagnosed among women, will affect one American woman in eleven during her lifetime. It is the second greatest cancer killer of women, after lung cancer.

CHARACTERISTICS OF WOMEN AT HIGH RISK

age over 40	previous cancer of
high socioeconomic status	breast
white	endometrium
single	colon/rectum
nulliparous	salivary gland
nuns	ovary
late age at birth of first child	exposure to ionizing radiation
history of breast cancer in	early menarche
mother, daughters, sisters	late menopause
prior benign breast disease	urban
	Scandinavian, German descent

DEMOGRAPHIC FACTORS

Geographic variation. Throughout the world, the incidence of breast cancer varies considerably. Although the course of the disease is similar worldwide, the rate of disease occurrence varies from a high among Caucasian Hawaiians to a low among the Japanese and non-Jewish Israelites. In general, the most highly developed countries have the highest breast cancer incidence, with Japan as the notable exception. Recent studies suggest that young Japanese women are experiencing rates of breast cancer more in line with other international statistics, however. Dietary factors, discussed elsewhere, are being carefully studied for their role in the variability documented worldwide.

Time and person variability. Generally, breast cancer develops among women after menarche with an increasing incidence until menopause, after which the incidence rate slows. Most breast cancer occurs in women over age fifty. In the past, American black women had breast cancer rates that were lower than among whites, but their incidence rates for this disease are now beginning to approach those of whites. There is a genetic predisposition for at least one pathway of breast cancer development, as evidenced by the increased risk among women with first degree relatives with breast cancer. The overall influence of this genetic effect in breast cancer etiology among the population is probably small.

Hormones. The role of estrogen and progesterone in breast cancer etiology has been the subject of intense study for a number of years. Pregnancy and multiple births are protective against breast cancer and both increase the role of progesterone in the body. The use of exogenous estrogen in large doses or over many years tends to increase the risk of breast cancer, while oophorectomy is protective, with its greatest effect in young women. These two differing responses of the breast to hormone stimulation, less breast cancer with progesterone activity or reduced estrogen activity and more of the disease in populations with excess estrogen stimulation, have led some investigators to propose the following simplified model for the role of sex hormones in breast cancer causation.

There are both estrogen and progesterone receptors in breast tissue. Prior to a woman's first pregnancy, there is a deficiency in progesterone receptors, so the nulliparous woman lacks the protection progesterone provides. Pregnancies provide differentiation activity of breast tissue by the increased action of progesterone, which counteracts the tissue stimulation estrogen engenders. Neoplasms are more likely to develop in the milieu of ductal proliferation stimulated by estrogen than during the tissue differentiation subsequent to progesterone binding.

Additonal support for this position includes the evidence that combination estrogen–progesterone birth control pills do not increase risk of breast cancer, while estrogen alone does increase risk, although marginally. The role of progesterone as a protective factor is today generally considered of more probable significance than the disease-enhancing capabilities of estrogen.

Two areas of study that have sought to relate normal breast

functions to differing breast cancer risks in various populations involve lactation and prolactin excretion. Lactation has been studied as a possible protection against breast cancer, but results have been almost entirely negative. The role of prolactin in the etiology of breast cancer remains elusive, although its relationship to dietary fat has been a tempting target for speculation and research.

In the next few years, it is probable that the overall hormonal milieu, rather than a single hormone's influence, will be shown to be more important in breast cancer etiology.

Common Clinical Course

DETECTION

In 1982, the American Cancer Society published the results of its five-year summary of the Breast Cancer Detection Demonstration Project. Modalities utilized in the detection of breast cancer included physical examination, teaching breast self-examination (BSE), mammography, and thermography. Thermography was discontinued as a detection modality in 1977 after review disputed its usefulness. Although physical examination and mammography each identified cases not detected by the other test, the contribution of mammography was substantially greater. Mammography alone was responsible for positive findings in about 42 percent of all cancers detected in the project. Mammography was particularly impressive in its ability to detect small cancers. Recommendations of the American Cancer Society for detection of breast cancer in asymptomatic women are covered in Chapter 7.

Today, over 90 percent of breast cancer is detected by the woman herself. In 60 percent of cases, the woman feels a lump that is between 1.1 and 3 cm in diameter. Because fewer than 18 percent of women perform monthly BSE or have routine screening examinations, the length of time during which the lump is present and detectable before it is discovered probably varies considerably.

PATHOPHYSIOLOGY

Over 80 percent of breast cancers are of the ductal type; most of the remainder are classified as lobular carcinomas. Several methods of categorizing breast cancer types exist which creates confusion among clinicians. The most frequently seen breast cancer types and their incidence are listed below.

Infiltrating carcinoma—70–80%
Carcinoma of mammary lobules—10–20%
Carcinoma of mammary ducts—4–7%

Paget's disease—2–3%
Sarcomas of the breast—rare

Incidence according to location within the breast has been broken down as follows:

Upper outer quadrant—48%
Upper inner quadrant—15%
Lower inner quadrant—6%
Lower outer quadrant—11%
Multifocal—rare

DIAGNOSIS AND STAGING

Diagnostic procedures consist of the following:

chest X-ray
complete blood count
blood analysis
urinalysis
liver enzyme studies
mammography
biopsy
hormone receptor assay test

Routine procedures are undertaken to determine the extent of the primary tumor as well as to evaluate for local, regional, or distant metastasis.

Usually, a chest X-ray, complete blood count, blood analysis, urinalysis, liver enzyme studies and mammography are ordered. Common metastatic sites for breast cancer are the lungs, bone, liver and adrenals. The chest X-ray may expose abnormal lung lesions, suggesting metastasis. Blood and urine studies are indicators of the patient's general health. Liver studies generally include lactate dehydrogenase, serum glutamic-oxaloacetic transaminase, and serum glutamic-pyruvic transaminase, elevations of which may indicate liver metastasis. The mammography is ordered to clarify the lesion's form as well as to detect any other foci of cancer in the breasts.

Following these studies, a biopsy is usually indicated to establish diagnosis and determine histologic type and grading of the tumor. A needle biopsy or excisional biopsy are the usual methods of obtaining breast tissue for examination.

A hormonal receptor assay test is performed from a portion of the biopsied tissue to establish the presence or absence of estrogen and progesterone receptors. This knowledge may prove useful in determining the utility of hormonal therapy at a later time. Recently it has been found that circulating lymphocyte estradiol receptor levels may be the most accurate means available for predicting tumor response to hormones (Paietta 1985).

Following the evaluation of the above tests along with a complete patient assessment, the physician will stage the breast tumor. The usual procedure is to rate the tumor according to the TMN system between stages one and four.

Trials are underway currently in the use of monoclonal antibodies for the detection of breast cancer. This method of detection involves a blood test that would screen for certain tumor markers that are present only when breast cancer exists. (See Table 5.2).

TREATMENT

There has been no significant change in the age-adjusted death rate between 1951–1952 (26 per 100,000) and 1976–1978 (27 per 100,000) for breast cancer. Nonetheless, there are many four-year cures for breast cancer that currently exist. Fully two-thirds of the 90,000 women with newly diagnosed breast cancer each year ultimately suffer recurrence within months or years, regardless of what surgery or chemotherapy they receive. To date, four types of breast cancer therapy remain in use: surgery, radiotherapy, chemotherapy, and hormonal therapy. The sophistication in the application of these modalities has grown over the years, although the survival rate for breast cancer overall has not appreciably changed since the 1930s. Part of the reason for this poor showing may be that early detection is still not common in the general population, and therapies available today are not effective equally against all breast cancers. Treatment success to date has been limited to specific subpopulations of breast cancer patients.

Of 106,000 American women with newly diagnosed breast carcinoma each year, approximately 50,000 will have positive axillary lymph nodes at the time of initial treatment. Survival rates over ten years are appreciably higher for patients who begin treatment before lymph nodes become involved:

Table 5.2 Stages of Breast Cancer

Stage	Tumor	Nodes	Metastasis
I	local	negative	negative
II	local	positive	negative
III	extending	positive, fixed	negative
IV	extending	positive, fixed	positive

negative axillary nodes—65 percent
1 to 3 positive nodes—38 percent
4 or more positive nodes—13 percent

Surgery. The most frequently performed surgery today for breast cancer is the modified radical mastectomy (78 percent of all breast cancer surgeries). Although there remain surgeons in the United States convinced of the superiority of the classic Halsted radical mastectomy, most surgeons recommend the more limited surgery. Between 1976 and 1981 the incidence of radical mastectomies declined from 27 percent to 3.4 percent of cases. Long-term studies published around 1974 showed that the modified radical surgery resulted in survival rates comparable to the radical surgery when there was no lymph node involvement detectable. When lymph nodes were positive, the modified surgery resulted in somewhat poorer results, when used without subsequent chemotherapy. Lumpectomy, the removal of the tumor with a margin of surrounding tissue, has shown acceptable survival rates when no local extension or positive nodes are detectable. Generally, radiotherapy is employed in conjunction with this treatment. The acceptance of lumpectomy is still somewhat limited in most communities. Breast cancer surgery options include:

radical mastectomy (now rarely performed)
modifided radical mastectomy (pectoralis major spared)
quadrantectomy (quadrant removed)
segmentectomy (less than quadrant removed)
lumpectomy (tumor and tissue margin removed)

Radiotherapy. Today there are more than one thousand facilities offering megavoltage radiation treatment in the United States. The American College of Radiology, which has profiled the best cancer management now possible utilizing radiotherapy, found that small, independent institutions conformed to the standards less consistently than did large facilities. There exists today a wide variation in the quality of radiotherapy offered.

Primary treatment of breast cancer using radiation therapy is limited to Stage I or II disease. Five- and ten-year survival rates for Stage I disease with radiation have been 91 percent and 81 percent, and in Stage II disease 77 percent and 54 percent in recent trials. The two modalities employed to provide primary radiation therapy are external beam radiation and interstitial radiation after lumpectomy. External beam therapy generally is delivered in divided doses over a five- or six-week period. Hospitalization is not required unless concomitant problems complicate the situation. Interstitial irradiation involves the temporary implantation of radioactive iridium seeds in flexible nylon rods across the breast surface. Usually left in place for forty-eight hours, they necessitate radiation precautions during the therapy. In this procedure steel guide needles are first threaded through the tumor area. Nylon tubes are then threaded through the guide needles (which are removed). Finally, strands of radioactive seeds are threaded through the nylon tybes, which are secured with buttons.

Radiation therapy has played a key role in maximizing local and regional control, which is a significant problem in breast cancer. Of approximately 34,000 deaths in 1978 from breast cancer, about 4,800 were estimated by some investigators to be the result of local and regional failure. Other researchers dispute the role of local failure in ultimate death from breast cancer. Today, the routine use of postoperative chest wall radiotherapy has been challenged. Radiotherapy is now utilized for this purpose when local recurrence occurs rather than prophylactically.

There is widespread research today aimed at modifying radiosensitivity. Efforts have largely been directed at improving radiation's effect on hypoxic tumor cells.

Radiation has a longer history in breast cancer as a palliative modality than as a primary therapy. It is often used in this manner for symptomatic control of obstructing tumors or of debilitating bone pain, which may occur with breast cancer.

Chemotherapy. Systemic chemotherapy generally follows surgery when lymph nodes are positive. If lymph nodes are negative, the use of chemotherapy is generally not advised since resistance may develop and chemotherapy prove impotent if needed for later disease recurrence. There is evidence that adjuvant chemotherapy is of only marginal benefit to the vast majority of postmenopousal women who develop breast cancer. When Bonadonna and Vilagusie (1976) reported their success in Milan with Stage II patients given adjuvant chemotherapy, the subsequent embrace of the regimen in this country was overwhelming. Cyclophosphamide, methotrexate, and 5–fluorouracil (CMF) became the cornerstone of chemotherapy. CMF plus vincristine and prednisone, as advocated by Dr. Richard G. Cooper of Buffalo (1979), is today the gold standard of chemotherapy. The best success of this regimen is among Stage II premenopausal women. Adjuvant chemotherapy is most effective when the patients receive at least 85 percent of their targeted dose. If less than 65 percent of the dose is received, no appreciable benefit is noted.

Today, research findings are that nodal status is the overwhelming prognostic factor in breast cancer. If a patient has many positive nodes, none of the currently available chemotherapeutic treatments will have much effect. In patients with relatively small numbers of positive nodes, all of the available regimens are probably equally effective.

When chemotherapy is used to treat metastasis, the average response rate is 50 percent, with a median duration of response of six to twelve months. Ultimate survival is not enhanced with chemotherapy, however: the average life span with breast cancer metastasis is eighteen to thirty-six months.

Hormonal therapy. Endocrine regulation in breast cancer treatment is today a rapidly expanding field. The cellular effects of hormone receptors are being clarified and manipulation of their effects in treating cancer is becoming a reality. Today, hormonal therapy is clinically used in estrogen-receptor positive (ER+) patients and is usually useful in the postmenopausal populations. Among ER+ patients, about 65 percent will respond to tamoxifen citrate, the mostly widely used antiestrogen, with a two-year remission. In the premenopausal population, oophorectomy results in a disease remission of about one year in 50–60 percent of ER+ patients. However, among these premenopausal women, there has been no difference in recurrence rate or mortality between castrated women and uncastrated women after radical surgery. Evidence is accumulating that progesterone receptor (PR) status is a better predictor of how patients will respond to tamoxifen than ER status. The use of androgens, progestins, or aminoglutethimide are second-line therapies that are less effective than either tamoxifen citrate or oophorectomy in treating metastatic breast cancer.

Management Skills

DETECTING METASTASIS

All breast cancer patients should be routinely assessed for metastatic involvement of the lungs, bone, liver, and adrenals. Remember to watch for the following:

* pleural effusions—seen in 50 percent of breast cancer patients; survival time from diagnosis of the malignant effusion is 7–13 months.
* pathologic bone fractures; hypercalcemia; skeletal pain
* liver failure; hepatic encephalopathy
* adrenal insufficiency

EFFECTS OF TREATMENT

The surgical patient particularly needs to be assessed for infection at the incision site and lymphedema in the arm on the affected side. In light of current early discharges from the hospital, many patients will go home with dressings that may need changing. Be prepared to give the patient or family members opportunities to practice any skills they may need. Patient teaching is a critical need.

Radiotherapy's most debilitating effects are on rapidly dividing cells. Adenocarcinoma of breast epithelia has a fairly low relative radiosensitivity. A total dose of 5,000 rads is common post-mastectomy, while 6,500 rads is common when radiation is used in conjunction with lumpectomy. In advanced disease, 8,000 or more rads may be used for local control or control of symptoms. Fibrosis or necrosis of breast tissue is possible at these doses, as is pneumonitis related to lung damage.

Hormonal therapy may result in specific problems for which the nurse must be alert. Tamoxifen citrate therapy may cause hypercalcemia within a week of therapy if there is bony metastasis. In addition, hot flashes, nausea, and blurred vision as well as transient increased pain may be observed. All these symptoms usually subside within a week. The transient pain is sometimes called "tamoxifen flare" and is associated with high response rates.

The CMF plus vincristine and prednisone regimen most frequently seen in breast cancer treatment may cause the following common toxic problems (reference to a drug manual for comprehensive information is necessary during administration of chemotherapy):

- cyclophosphamide (Cytoxan, Endoxan): leukopenia, nausea, and vomiting, alopecia in 50 percent of patients within three weeks, hemorrhagic cystitis (extravasation does not cause local irritation and thrombophlebitis has not complicated intravenous administration)
- methotrexate: leukopenia, thrombocytopenia, mouth ulcers, severe diarrhea, liver dysfunctions after one year, pneumonitis
- fluorouracil (5–FU, 5–fluorouracil): granulocytopenia, stomatitis, dermatitis in 10–20 percent of cases
- vincristine (VCR, Oncovin-R): constipation, peripheral neuropathy, alopecia (extravasation results in cellulitis and phlebitis)
- prednisone: euphoria, congestive heart failure, peptic ulcer, hyperglycemia, acute adrenal insufficiency with sudden withdrawal or severe stress

Rehabilitation

Current modalities in the rehabilitation of the breast cancer patient include the following:

exercise for function
follow-up medical examinations
"Reach for Recovery"
external prosthesis
breast reconstruction
infection precaution
lymphedema control

Shoulder dysfunction is a frequent complication following treatment for breast cancer. About 30 percent of patients will complain of some degree of this complication. Most textbooks covering breast cancer rehabilitation describe the common exercises to promote full extension of the affected arm, including "climbing the wall," "arm swinging," and "rope pull." As many of us know who try to maintain an exercise program, exercise for its own sake is often difficult to sustain. Better success may be obtained with many women by explaining the need for full arm extension to prevent muscle shortening, promote lymph and blood circulation and maintain muscle tone, and then encouraging the woman to use extension in usual activities. Hair combing, dressing, household activities, and leisure pursuits can become useful exercises if the woman consciously includes arm extension when doing them.

Reach for Recovery was started in 1952 and in 1969 became an American Cancer Society rehabilitation program. The program is carried out by volunteers who have had a mastectomy. Recent research has shown that about 58 percent of patients found a Reach for Recovery visit to be very helpful, 31 percent found it somewhat helpful, 7 percent thought it of no consequence and 4 percent rated it as not at all helpful (Rogers et al. 1985). The data also found that the volunteer's visit had no effect—either favorable or unfavorable—on emotional state or return to former activities, yet one year later patients for the most part perceived the visit positively.

For most women today who undergo modified radical mastectomy for breast cancer treatment, the option is available for breast reconstruction. Research in 1980 found that whether or not a woman opted for reconstruction, she wanted the option for surgery available for some time in the future (Kirkpatrick 1980). Thus, the availability of reconstruction is comforting to women whether or not they ever commit themselves to the procedure. Across the nation, more and more insurance companies are paying for the procedure, which in most cases is a relatively simple one.

Because most women today will have heard of reconstruction through general public media, a woman may be interested in discussing the surgery with her nurse. General descriptions of the surgery are appropriate and the nurse should encourage the woman to ask about her specific case with her surgeon.

Many women decide that a prosthesis is the best option for them. A prosthesis is not utilized until the chest incision is well healed and the woman ready to proceed with rehabilitation. It should never be considered a second-best alternative, but is the method of choice for most women to regain a natural sillouette.

Infection control is important in the ipsilateral arm because of the impaired lymph and blood circulation usual after a mastectomy. The patient must be assertive in assuring that for the remainder of her life she protects her arm. During visits to laboratories or during future hospitalizations, employees may attempt to use the affected arm for blood-drawing or venipuncture. Only the patient will be able to consistently halt the inadvertent use of her affected arm. The patient must also be conscientious about using gloves during gardening, a thimble for sewing, and other protective measures against cuts or other injuries.

To control lymphedema, the best measures to date include regular range of motion exercises, an elastic sleeve, control of obesity, and pneumomassage by a physical therapist. Lymphedema occurs in about 40 percent of women following mastectomy and is often considered a normal sequela of the surgery. Early and consistent use of the modalities mentioned above is necessary to help control this debilitating effect.

Uterine Cancer

Etiology

The uterus is composed of two parts, the cervix and the endometrium (uterine corpus). Cancers of the two parts are distinct entities with different etiologies and prognoses. Epidemiologic study of the two cancers has been complicated by the fact that until recently countries reported them together as uterine cancer. Only relatively recently have their different etiologies begun to be unraveled. Together, these cancers account for about 11 percent of female cancer incidence and about 5 percent of cancer deaths among women.

CHARACTERISTICS OF WOMEN AT HIGH RISK

Cervical cancer:
    early age at first coitus
    multiple consorts
    use of oral contraceptives
    history of venereal infections
Endometrial cancer
    nulliparity
    late menopause
    early menarche
    high socioeconomic status
    obesity
    history of breast cancer
    estrogen use

DEMOGRAPHIC FACTORS

Geographic variability. For *cervical cancer* there is great geographic variability. Jewish women of America have a much lower lifetime risk for cervical cancer than do women of Colombia or Brazil, where the highest rates prevail. Most American women have intermediate rates.

Rates for *endometrial cancer* are higher in prosperous countries than in poorer countries. Incidence rates in Israel are much higher than in China, for example, and Switzerland, a very prosperous country, has very high rates.

Time and person variability. Worldwide, the incidence of invasive *cervical cancer* has been declining. In this country, much of the decrease in the morbidity and mortality since 1950 is probably due to the use of cervical cytology (Pap smear). In countries where good records are kept it has been shown that cervical cancer deaths can be dramatically decreased by the institution of cervical cytology in public screening programs. However, some of the worldwide decrease in the incidence of this disease cannot be attributed to screening cytology. Other factors that help to account for this decline have not yet been identified.

Women between the ages of thirty and fifty are at greatest risk for preinvasive cervical cancer. Invasive cervical cancer tends to occur among women in the perimenopausal or postmenopausal years, and is more common among married than among single women. It is exceedingly rare among virgins. There is also an increasing risk of the cancer with lowering of social class. In the United States, blacks have a twofold greater risk compared to whites, which is most likely due to historic social class differences rather than racial differences in susceptibility. Promiscuity and increased venereal infections are other factors linked to increased risk for cervical cancer. After World War II, the transient increase in cervical cancer deaths noted in England has been linked to the greater promiscuity prevalent during wartime. It is interesting to note that recent evidence links smoking with an increased risk of cervical cancer.

The highest incidence of this *endometrial cancer* in North America is among San Francisco whites. Populations with a tendency toward obesity, such as the Maoris and Hawaiians, also show high incidence rates for the disease. Urbanization has been shown to have no consistent effect, seeming to follow prosperity gradients rather than urban-rural gradients. Affluence generally shows a close parallel to endometrial cancer incidence.

Throughout the world, the incidence of endometrial cancer appears to be increasing. Two factors suggested for this increase are the observed increasing wealth and subsequent obesity among many populations, such as the African Bantu of Johannesburg, heretofore nearly unaffected by endometrial cancer; and the more frequent use of exogenous estrogen for treatment of menopausal symptoms. Because endometrial cancer has a 75 percent survival rate at five years, the increased incidence has increased cancer deaths only by a relatively small amount. When uterine cancer death rates are reported, the decrease noted in cervical cancer deaths tends to outweigh the increase in endometrial cancer deaths, with an overall decline noted for the organ as a whole.

There appear to be two peaks in the incidence of endometrial cancer over time; one peak among high risk individuals at ages fifty-five to fifty-nine and a second peak at sixty-five to sixty-nine years for lower risk women (deWaard 1982). The menopausal peak for high risk individuals has moved the American Cancer Society to recommend endometrial tissue biopsy for these women at menopause, regardless of lack of specific symptoms suggesting the presence of the cancer.

Venereal disease and cervical cancer. Herpes genitalis (HSV–2), trichomonas vaginalis, chlamydia, cytomegalic virus, and papilloma virus have all been associated with increased risk for cervical cancer. Women who have been infected with multiple agents have a greater risk for cervical cancer than those with a history of infection from only one agent.

Hormones and endometrial cancer. The evidence implicating the use of sequential oral contraceptives in endometrial cancer supported the notion that excess stimulation by estrogen, without the protective effect of progesterone, promoted endometrial cancer. Other evidence supporting this contention included (1) animal studies in which estrogen alone induced endometrial tumors, while the concomitant use of progesterone was protective; (2) rising cancer incidence following prescribed estrogen at menopause; (3) increased serum estrogen levels with increasing obesity; and (4) the occurrence of endometrial cancer in some transsexuals who were on estrogen therapy after sex change surgery. Early onset of menses with late menopause causes prolonged estrogen stimulation of body tissues and is also a risk factor for endometrial cancer. This is one cancer type in which a single hormone's role is quite clear. The biological evidence that estrogen stimulates tissue proliferation while progesterone causes tissue differentiation coincides with the epidemiologic evidence.

Common Clinical Course

DETECTION

Cervical cancer. There is longstanding evidence that dysplasia and carcinoma in situ (CIS) exist prior to the development of invasive cervical cancer. Women with evidence of CIS were followed after biopsy in the 1950s without any treatment because the progression of CIS to invasive cancer was not appreciated (Petersen 1956). Researchers found that 40–75 percent of these CIS cases progressed to invasive disease. Richart and Barron (1969) found that about half of women with dysplasia progressed to CIS by four years. Thus there is research to support the notion that a preclinical condition exists that can be treated to prevent the development of cervical cancer. Studies of the use of the Papanicolaou smear show that its use correlates with a decrease in cervical cancer mortality because early disease can be detected and successfully treated.

Women with early stage cervical cancer are usually asymptomatic or may experience some abnormal bleeding. Often this bleeding is associated with minor trauma from a douche or coitus and is characterized as watery, blood-tinged discharge. As the stage of cancer progresses, the symptom of bleeding often increases. In addition, a purulent and foul-smelling discharge may be noted. By the time pain becomes a symptom, the disease is usually metastatic. If the disease spreads to local organs, symptoms of bladder or bowel obstruction may also occur. If pelvic lymphatic vessels become involved, generalized lower truck edema may develop.

Endometrial cancer. The peak occurrence of endometrial cancer is in the sixth and seventh decades of life for most women. If the uterus is not enlarged by tumor growth, it is often difficult to detect early cancers except if abnormal bleeding occurs. Cervical cytology can detect some cases of endometrial cancer, however 60 percent will be missed by this technique alone. Sampling the vaginal secretions may increase the detection of this cancer in high risk individuals. Biopsing the endometrium at menopause is the recommended procedure for high risk individuals in order to find early stage cancer, which is readily treatable.

PATHOPHYSIOLOGY

Cervical cancer. Cancer of the cervix is the most common malignancy of the female reproductive system. Lesions from the epithelium on the external surface of the cervix that are of the squamous variety comprise about 95 percent of cervical cancer cases. These preinvasive lesions are referred to as cervical intraepithelial neoplasia (CIN). Adenocarcinomas comprise about 5 percent of all cervical cancer. These are associated with diethylstilbesterol (DES) exposure in utero.

CIN is characterized as mild, moderate, or severe dysplasia, corresponding to grades 1, 2, or 3. The difference between CIN grade 3 and CIS is not distinct. Some CIN or CIS lesions will not progress to invasive disease, but the majority will eventually do so. The rate at which CIN progresses through CIS to invasive cancer probably varies widely, from a few months to several decades.

Endometrial cancer. Ninety percent of all endometrial neoplasms are adenocarcinomas. The degree of histologic differentiation of the tumors is closely related to the extent and prognosis of the disease. Well-differentiated tumors have a better prognosis than poorly differentiated ones. Adenocarcinomas of the endometrium tend to be relatively slow-growing tumors that remain localized for long periods of time.

DIAGNOSIS AND STAGING

Cervical cancer. If a cytologic smear test (Pap smear) is abnormal for a woman but no lesion can be seen, diagnosis of cervical cancer is done by endocervical smears and curettage of the endocervix. Colposcopy and biopsy of any abnormal regions is advocated subsequent to any abnormal Pap results. The colposcope provides a lighted, magnified stereoscopic view of the cervix. This relatively expensive equipment, which requires specific training for its use, is becoming more common in the practice of general clinicians rather than being used only by specialists. If colposcopy does not visualize the entire lesion, or it is thought that microinvasion may have occurred, then a cone biopsy is usually done. Staging of cervical cancer extends from Stage 0, or carcinoma in situ, to Stage IV, with distant organs involved.

Endometrial cancer. Curettage under anesthesia with sampling of the endometrial tissue should be done if symptoms of this cancer are present or if the woman is at especially high risk around the time of the menopause. Staging of endometrial cancer is from Stage 0 (CIS), to Stage IV with cancer extension into the pelvis or involvement of the bladder or rectum. In about 80 percent of women presenting with endometrial cancer, their disease is confined to the uterine cavity without cervical involvement (Stage 1). Caucasians tend to present with early disease more frequently than black women, who may delay seeking medical advice in the presence of symptoms.

TREATMENT

Cervical cancer. Only a few women are treated for cervical cancer with drugs, because this type of cancer is resistant to presently known chemotherapeutic agents. CIS is often treated by conization, particularly if future pregnancies are desired by the woman affected. Otherwise, a hysterectomy, sometimes with removal of the upper portion of the vagina, is the treatment of choice. If the lesion is well contained and has not become invasive, sometimes simply cryosurgery, electrocautery, or laser surgery is all that is necessary to remove the cancerous cells. If these latter techniques are used, the patient must be carefully followed for years subsequent to treatment. Once cervical cancer has become invasive, even if only at a micro level (Stage 1A), then a radical hysterectomy and pelvic lymphadenectomy are usually recommended. Pelvix exenteration usually is reserved for recurrent disease for the small proportion of patients with a resectable lesion. Most clinicians recommend treatment by radiation therapy alone.

If radiation treatment is elected, the patient usually requires a course of external irradiation as well as intracavitary radium therapy. These may be done separately or concurrently. If the lesion is found early, then sometimes intracavitary radium placement utilizing colpostats and tandems is sufficient. With large, invasive cancers wholepelvis irradiation is essential. Sometimes, radiation therapy is used prior to surgery to help debulk large tumors.

Endometrial cancer. Hysterectomy with removal of the fallopian tubes and ovaries, as well as part of the vagina, is the principal treatment for this cancer. Preoperative or postoperative radiation therapy may be included in the treatment plan. The cure rate for Stage 1 disease, which is the stage at which most women present, is over 75 percent. Chemotherapy is not used, as the endometrium, like the cervix, is resistant to the drugs presently available. Sometimes doxorubicin (Adriamycin) is used in metastatic disease, but little increase in survival has been noted with this treatment.

Some clinicians prefer to use radiation therapy alone for endometrial cancer, although early studies have shown that surgery alone is generally superior (Bichenbach et al. 1967). Once endometrial cancer is advanced, radiation is the usual method of treatment, including both external irradiation and internal pelvic radiation. Exenterative surgery is useful for a few patients with resectable lesions; however, five-year survival rates are not good following this modality.

Progestational agents, such as megestrol acetate (Megace), may be prescribed for metastatic endometrial cancer. The response rate averages about 30 percent, and is poorer when used to treat pelvic recurrence. Pulmonary metastases are most likely to respond to this hormone treatment. Remissions last about one and one half years overall after progesterone therapy.

Management Skills

DETECTING METASTASIS

Uterine cancer usually spreads by direct extention, with metastasis occurring only in late state disease. The organ most at risk for cancerous involvement is the vagina. Lymphatic spread also occurs involving the whole pelvic lymph node system. With late disease, the bladder or rectum is commonly involved. Distant organs at greatest risk for metastasis are the lung, liver and bone. Watch for:

- change in character of vaginal discharge, especially foul, odorous fluids
- abdominal pain, which may indicate pelvic involvement
- change in bowel or bladder habits, a sign of advanced disease.

EFFECTS OF TREATMENT

Cervical cancer treated by local surgical modalities rarely results in complications. Hysterectomy for uterine cancer infrequently results in fistulas, infection, and hemorrhage. Radiation therapy can result in uretal strictures, cystitis, fistulas, bowel perforation, dermatitis, and diarrhea.

REHABILITATION

Perhaps the biggest rehabilitation problem of uterine cancer is that occuring in young women who still desire children. These women may elect to avoid hysterectomy and utilize local modalities of treatment. This requires that they undergo periodic examinations, usually every six months, for many years following treatment in order to assure that there is no recurrence of cancer. The knowledge of the possibility of a cancer recurrence, which could be largely eliminated with a hysterectomy, can be very wearing psychologically. It can also be a deciding factor in choosing to have children. Even if other social and psychological factors weigh against becoming pregnant at a particular time, a woman may decide to go ahead with a pregnancy because of the past uterine cancer. This can create particularly difficult situations for the mother and new infant.

In the past, there was great emphasis put on the psychological ramifications of a hysterectomy on a woman's self-image. Today, affected women less frequently feel that they have lost their most important attribute following the surgery. Many women still fear, however, that the surgery will age or change them detrimentally. Health providers should routinely question women about their fears following a hysterectomy in order to help them rehabilitate to their pre-surgical activities.

Epithelial Ovarian Cancer

Etiology

Ovarian cancer is the fourth most frequent cause of cancer deaths among women. Although the ovarian cancer incidence rate is lower than for other gynecologic cancers, the mortality rate is the highest. Significant progress has been made in the last decade in the diagnosis and treatment of women with epithelial ovarian carcinoma. However, only in the last several years have these improvements begun to be reflected in the survival rates for the disease.

The large majority of ovarian tumors are epithelial in origin. Although germ cell tumors and sex cord-stromal tumors of the ovary are etiologically different from epithelial tumors, much data reported on this disease relate to the ovary as a whole, thus complicating epidemiological study. Further, when ovarian cancer has metastasized, it may be very difficult to diagnose as the primary site. In spite of these difficulties, there exist some important clues to the etiology of epithelial ovarian cancer.

CHARACTERISTICS OF WOMEN AT HIGH RISK

fewer than three full-term pregnancies
history of breast or endometrial cancer

family history of cancer, especially breast, ovary, colon
nulliparity
talc use on sanitary napkins
herbicide exposure

DEMOGRAPHIC FACTORS

Geographic variability. The highest rates of ovarian cancer are found among white women of Europe and North America. Generally, Asian, black, and hispanic women have a relatively low incidence of these tumors. San Francisco Bay area whites, Jewish women, and Hawaiians have particularly high incidence rates.

Time and person variability. Black women tend to have incidence rates for epithelial ovarian cancer that are lower than whites after age forty, whether they reside in Africa or the United States. Chinese and Japanese women who migrate to the United States show incidence rates that are intermediate between those of Asia and those of white American women. Over the last two decades, the incidence of ovarian cancer has not changed appreciably among North American white women.

Hormonal factors. Multiple sources of information suggest that pituitary gonadotropin (FSH, LH) stimulation increases the occurrence of ovarian cancer (Weiss 1982). The ovaries produce both estrogen and progesterone; if the production of these hormones falls, there is a concomitant rise in the body levels of FSH and LH, which in turn predisposes the woman to ovarian cancer. Multiple pregnancies reduce the relative risk of ovarian cancer, each pregnancy incurring more protection. Pregnancy and the use of combination oral contraceptives both protect against ovarian cancer. Some clinicians suggest that oral contraceptives containing both estrogen and progesterone may someday be used in high risk individuals to decrease epithelial ovarian cancer incidence.

Miscellaneous factors. The evidence implicating the use of talc on sanitary napkins needs verification before public health measures to stop the practice are undertaken. However, several studies have now demonstrated that the practice is associated with an increased relative risk of ovarian cancer (Cramer 1982). Nurses should consider suggesting a halt to this habit as it serves no health purpose and eventually may be substantiated as a cancer risk factor by multiple supporting studies.

Preliminary evidence exists implicating herbicide exposure and ovarian cancer (Donna 1984). Because herbicides are implicated in the etiology of several cancers, caution with their use would be prudent.

Common Clinical Course

DETECTION

Most ovarian cancer occurs in women between the ages of forty and sixty. Unfortunately, there are no symptoms indicative of an early stage of ovarian cancer. One woman in every twenty will develop a benign or a malignant ovarian neoplasm during her life (Horton and Hill 1977). Most will be benign, but a lack of symptoms will be common to both types of tumors. Therefore, regular physical assessment, including bimanual abdominal examination, is particularly important. The most common symptom associated with ovarian cancer is enlargement of the abdomen, whether due to tumor growth or the formation of ascites. Some women experience vague abdominal discomfort or changes in bowel and bladder function as the first symptoms of this insidious disease, which is very difficult to diagnose. Approximately 60–70 percent of women will have advanced disease by the time it is diagnosed. This fact, more than any other, accounts for the poor prognosis for epithelial ovarian cancer. With advanced disease there is little hope of long-term survival. Pap smears are not a good method for early detection of ovarian cancer, as they are positive in only about 40 percent of cases.

PATHOPHYSIOLOGY

Over 85 percent of ovarian tumors are epithelial in origin. The most common routes of metastasis associated with this cancer are direct extension and lymphatic spread. Sites of metastasis commonly include the peritoneum, omentum, and bowel surfaces. Spread to the pelvic organs, liver, lung, kidney, spleen, and bone is also frequently seen.

DIAGNOSIS AND STAGING

Diagnosis is usually based on a positive pelvic evaluation, followed by ultrasound, fractional dilation and curettage, and laparotomy. The initial workup usually includes chest X-ray, barium enema, GI series, intravenous pyloregram, and proctosigmoidoscopy.

Four stages of ovarian cancer are commonly described, from local disease in Stage I to widely disseminated disease in Stage IV. The median survival time after diagnosis of ovarian cancer is 1.4 years, with women under forty-five surviving about 5 years, and women over seventy-five surviving about nine months.

TREATMENT

Surgery. This is the usual management technique employed for ovarian cancer, except in Stage IV disease, when it serves little purpose. A total hysterectomy is done as well as bilateral salpingo-oophorectomy, appendectomy, and omentectomy. When tumor is visualized anywhere in the surgical field, it is removed to the greatest extent possible. Recent evidence shows that if residual tumor masses are no more than 3 cm at their greatest diameter, response to chemotherapy is greatly enhanced. Debulking surgery has been confirmed as a major determinant of overall response to therapy.

Chemotherapy. Both combination chemotherapy and single agent drug therapy are used in treating ovarian cancer. Single drug regimens are generally reserved for palliative care of unresectable patients. In the last ten years, the usual agents used for this purpose are Cytoxan, melphalan, doxorubicin, and cisplatin. Used singly, they produce a response in about 40 percent of patients that lasts about a year. Although melphalan was once considered the most active drug in ovarian cancer treatment, cisplatin is now considered to be most efficacious, either on its own or particularly when combined with other drugs.

Combination chemotherapy has been purported to be potentially curative for some Grade I ovarian cancers when used as an adjunct to surgery. Several regimens are currently being used with excellent response rates and a good percentage of complete remissions. Generally, response is greatest if the patient has not been treated previously by chemotherapeutic agents.

Hexa-CAF consists of hexamethylmelamine, cyclophosphamine, methotrexate and 5–fluorouracil. Response rates as high as 75 percent have been reported and complete remissions noted in 30 percent of patients on this regimen. CHAD, a combination of cyclophosphamide, doxorubicin, cis-platinum and hexamethylmelamine, has shown very similar results in recent trials. PAC, which consists of cisplatin and doxorubicin, has good efficacy with advanced ovarian cancer for a period of time.

Sometimes a second laparotomy is done when a chemotherapy course of treatment is completed, usually six to twelve months after the initial drug dose. This allows the physician to determine if all tumor has indeed been irradicated or if chemotherapy should be continued in the case of potentially curable disease. The usefulness of second-look surgery in terms of prolonging ultimate survival has not yet been established.

Radiation. Total abdominal radiation, as opposed to pelvic radiation, has been shown to be effective in prolonging survival in late stage disease when used after surgery removing most of the tumor present. Total abdominal radiation has been shown to be similar in effectiveness to chemotherapy. However, recent success in inducing response with chemotherapy has caused many clinicians to reduce the role of radiation therapy in the treatment of ovarian cancer (Piver 1984). A process for delivering radiation used in ovarian cancer is the moving strip technique, which has lately been shown to be no more effective against metastatic pockets than whole abdomen irradiation, but to produce significantly more bowel complications following surgery. This technique is now being abandoned at many institutions.

Miscellaneous therapeutic techniques. Hormonal therapy has been found to be of little value in ovarian cancer. Advanced, low-grade tumors sometimes show a response to tamoxifen, but hormonal manipulation is not used in other situations. Intraperitoneal infusion of Corynebacterium parvum, a nonspecific immune system enhancer, after surgical and drug therapy, has been effective in prolonging life in some cases. Monoclonal antibodies have been developed to ovarian carcinoma tumor cells and may show promise in future years as they become more commonly used.

Management Skills

DETECTING METASTASIS

Because more than 70 percent of women have disseminated disease at the time of diagnosis, detecting metastasis is not generally a foremost consideration. Even if an ovarian cancer is detected early, there are no signs that indicate early metastasis once treatment is completed. A common problem related to metastasis in patients with advanced ovarian cancer is intestinal obstruction. Unfortunately, by the time this problem is seen, general peritoneal metastasis has occurred, and obstructions in multiple sites are present or imminent. Therefore, surgery is frequently unsuccessful in effecting relief. Ascites is another common late metastatic problem in ovarian cancer. Check for symptoms of

- intestinal obstruction: persistent nausea and vomiting, abdominal distress, constipation
- ascites: gradual increase in abdominal girth; taut, tympanic abdomen

EFFECTS OF TREATMENT

The common effects from surgery and chemotherapy are described in the following paragraphs.

After surgery to remove the ovaries, related organs, and any peritoneal tumor masses, bowel function may not return to normal for quite some time, or the patient may require techniques of dietary management to maintain bowel function. Including high fiber foods and prune juice in the diet may be helpful. Stool softeners or mild laxatives may also be useful to maintain bowel function.

Side effects associated with chemotherapy include the following:

1. *Hexa-CAF therapy*
   - hexamethylmelamine (HXM): continuous nausea throughout therapy, CNS effects of agitation, depression, and Parkinsonian symptoms—particularly with long-term treatment
   - cyclophosphamide (Cytoxan, Endoxan): leukopenia, nausea, and vomiting, alopecia in 50 percent of patients within three weeks, and hemorrhagic cystitis.
   - Methotrexate: leukopenia, thrombocytopenia, mouth ulcers, severe diarrhea, liver dysfunctions after one year, pneumonitis
   - 5–Fluorouracil (5–FU, 5–fluorouracil): granulocytopenia, stomatitis, dermatitis in 10–20 percent of cases
2. *CHAD therapy*
   - cyclophosphamide (Cytoxan, Endoxan): see above
   - doxorubicin (Adriamycin): ulceration with extravasation, liver damage, myelosuppression peaking in fourteen days, nausea and vomiting in about 50 percent of patients, alopecia beginning two to five weeks after beginning of therapy, recall of radiation skin reactions, cardiomyopathy and congestive heart failure, phlebitis of injection vein
   - cisplatin (Platinol, cis-platinum): kidney damage (forced hydration is required after drug administration), vomiting beginning one hour after the start of treatment, ototoxicity, and anaphylaxis after several doses
   - hexamethylmelamine (HXM): see above

Colorectal Cancer

Etiology

Cancer of the colon and rectum are the commonest visceral neoplasms in the United States. Although it is not yet entirely understood what causes this cancer in the population, changes over time and among different populations have given clues to possible environmental factors in the etiology.

CHARACTERISTICS OF INDIVIDUALS AT HIGH RISK

prior colon cancer
colon adenomas
age over 50
familial polyposis syndromes
chronic ulcerative colitis
Crohn's disease
familial colon cancer
prior cancer of the endometrium, breast or bladder
low fiber, high fat diet

DEMOGRAPHIC FACTORS

Geographic variability. Uncommon in undeveloped countries of Africa, Asia, and Central and South America, this disease shows significantly greater incidence in North America and Europe. Interestingly, those countries with a high incidence of stomach cancer tend to have low rates of colorectal cancer, and vice versa. Countries with high colorectal rates are positively correlated with pancreatic, breast, kidney, and prostate carcinomas.

Populations with low colorectal rates tend to subsist on diets low in animal and vegetable fat and protein, and high in fiber. The typical North American or European diet tends to be very high in fat and protein with low concentrations of fiber, with constipation a frequent problem.

Time and person variability. Since 1930 in the U.S., the incidence of colorectal cancer among men has been gradually increasing, while rates of stomach cancer have dramatically dropped. Among women, over the same time period both colorectal and stomach cancer rates have declined, although much more signficantly in in the case of stomach cancer. Today, men show a slight excess of both colorectal cancer incidence and mortality (American Cancer Society data, 1980).

Blacks and hispanics in the United States have shown a steady and sharp increase in colorectal mortality over the last thirty years. Today their rates are very similar to those of whites.

Within the United States, the greatest colorectal mortality is in the Northeast. High-death-rate areas include New Jersey, Massachusetts, southern New York State, and areas around the Great Lakes (Schottenfeld and Fraumeni 1982). Countries with high rates tend to have larger populations, higher education and income, and more are of Irish, German, or Czech descent (Blot et al. 1976). In Hawaii, rates of colon cancer are low among Hawaiians and Filipinos compared to the rate among whites, but Chinese males have the highest rate of this cancer in Hawaii.

The risk of colorectal cancer generally increases steadily with age. Migrant studies have shown that either males are more susceptible or have greater exposure to factors causing colorectal cancer, raising the possibility of occupational risk factors. Studies also suggest that the environmental factors at work in the etiology of colorectal cancer invoke a short latency period.

Associated bowel diseases and syndromes. Ulcerative colitis of over twenty years duration incurs a twenty-fold increase in the risk of colon cancer. There is an increased risk of colon cancer in patients who have Crohn's disease, but not as high as for ulcerative colitis.

Syndromes of familial polyposis include inherited adenomatosis of the colon and rectum, Gardner syndrome, and Turcot syndrome. With these syndromes, the risk of developing colorectal cancer is extremely high, approaching 80 percent by age forty for untreated individuals with inherited adenomatosis syndrome. There exist "cancer families" for whom the chance of colorectal cancer is very high and tends to occur in the right side of the colon. Within these families, rates for breast, endometrium, and stomach cancer are also greatly increased. In other families, colorectal cancer cases tend to accumulate, whether because of environmental or genetic factors remains to be determined.

Common Clinical Course

DETECTION

Change in bowel habits can signal colorectal cancer. Many patients complain of alternating diarrhea and constipation, which is also a symptom of common irritable bowel syndrome and may frequently be seen in patients with other bowel diseases associated with colorectal cancer. Pain is a presenting complaint in 50–75 percent of cases (Marino 1981). Often related to right-sided colon cancer, it signals partial obstruction. Iron deficiency anemia from occult blood loss secondary to a growing colon cancer may be detected and is especially indicative of right-sided cancer. Left-sided cancer may present with gross rectal bleeding and obstruction. Rectal cancers may cause gross bleeding, obstruction, or diarrhea, and tenesmus.

The value of fecal occult blood testing (FOBT) is only as good as the patient's preparation prior to testing. Vitamin C, iron tablets, aspirin, and nonsteroidal anti-inflammatory drugs should be avoided for four days prior to testing. Rare red meat, Golden Delicious and

Gravenstein apples, bananas, pears, peppers, celery, lettuce, grape-fruit, cauliflower, broccoli, and cantaloupe are examples of foods that should be avoided for three days prior to testing. The patient will need to understand the importance of following the directions accompanying the test packet explicitly. Even under the best of circumstances, FOBT may not detect bleeding from colorectal cancers. It is well recognized that bleeding from adenomas and cancers is sporadic; several days can go by without the occurrence of bleeding. Periodic use of the test is therefore necessary to catch these slow-growing cancers early.

Flexible sigmoidoscopy and colonoscopy. Flexible sigmoidoscopy (35 cm range) and colonoscopy (60 cm range) are beginning to replace rigid sigmoidoscopy because these techniques allow examination of more of the colon and better visualization. The 35 cm instrument can be used by primary care physicians for a relatively comfortable examination. This detection modality is the best available means of finding early cancers and premalignant polyps within the limits of the instrument.

Sigmoidoscopy is derived from a technique that is at least as old as America. In the 1700s, patients were asked to bend over a simple table, whereupon a cigar-sized tube was inserted rectally and a candle used to illuminate the rectal area for the practitioner (Shealey 1985). Today, patients generally lie prone on a movable examination table positioned to an appropriate angle, or they may simply assume a lateral knee-chest position for the examination. The flexible sigmoidoscope has a four-directional tip, with fiber optic components and source of illumination, which transmits magnified images to the lens viewed by the practitioner. Attachments are available to take tissue samples or photographs, inject air to aid in visualization, or perform other procedures. Since about 1982, medical schools have been teaching students to use the flexible instrument, and many established physicians are retraining in sigmoidoscopy to replace the rigid instrument in their practice. In many areas, however, only specialists are proficient in flexible sigmoidoscopy or colonoscopy. Colonoscopy involves the visualization of the entire colon, rather than just the sigmoid portion.

PATHOPHYSIOLOGY

Over 98 percent of colorectal cancers are histologically categorized as adenocarcinomas. Recognition of the neoplastic adenomatous polyp as a premalignant precursor of colorectal carcinoma has been controversial but is now generally accepted. With the use of endoscopic polypectomy utilizing the flexible colonoscope, such patients can be treated at a premalignant stage. For reasons that are unclear, over the past twenty years the distribution of colorectal cancer has moved from being predominantly in the rectosigmoid colon and rectum to more proximal areas, beyond the reach of the sigmoidoscope. Today it is found that over half of large bowel cancers are above the rectosigmoid colon and another third are found in the right colon. With this very different picture, clinicians may find that palpation and colonoscopy will not offer the same detection capabilities they have in past years.

Many authorities adhere to an adenoma-to-carcinoma sequential progression in colorectal cancer. Adenomas less than one cm in diameter are rarely invasive; those between one and two cm are invasive in about 10 percent of cases, and when they are greater than two cm, 50 percent of cases are invasive. Size has been found to be the most important factor associated with carcinoma, although the more villous a polyp, the more likely the development of cancer. Fortunately, only about 10 percent of adenomas are villous in nature. The number of polyps present is also a factor in cancer risk. If three or more are present, the greater the risk of colon cancer.

DIAGNOSIS AND STAGING

The fifty-year-old Dukes system of staging colorectal cancer is no longer the only method used. More recent classification systems frequently utilized today are Astler-Coller and the TNM system, which offer more prognostic information and correspond in terminology to similar systems for other cancers. These two systems recognize five different stages. The earliest is associated with an 80 percent five-year survival rate, dropping steadily to 25 percent survival at five years for the last stage.

Diagnostic studies commonly undertaken by the clinician include a barium enema, sigmoidoscopy, carcinoembryonic antigen testing to determine the extent of disease, and tests for metastasis. These latter tests include computed tomographic scans (CT scans) of the pelvis and liver function blood tests. Sometimes an air contrast enema is substituted for a regular barium enema as it detects polyps particularly well. This is particularly useful because of the reduced effectiveness of barium enemas if the bowel is inadequately cleansed, as is frequently the case.

TREATMENT

Surgery. Standard surgical treatment of colorectal cancer involves removal of the tumor mass as well as a generous margin of normal bowel on either side of the tumor. Radical procedures involving the removal of extensive bowel have not proved effective in prolonging survival from this type of cancer, so are not generally warranted as they increase morbidity and mortality from the surgery itself. If the tumor mass has extended to adjacent tissues in the pelvis or abdomen, metallic clips are attached to the involved organs so that radiotherapy can be used as an adjuvant therapy and accurately directed.

If the tumor presents as an obstructing left colon mass, a three-stage procedure is often necessary for adequate surgical treatment. First a diverting transverse colostomy is formed, followed by resection and a colostomy closure. If the rectum is involved, all efforts are made to preserve the sphincter. If the tumor is in the distal portion of the rectum, a permanent sigmoid colostomy must be established. Depending on how much bowel must be removed, the patient who requires a colostomy will have one from the ascending, transverse, descending, or sigmoid colon, or require an ileostomy from the small intestines. In all cases, an anastomosis is performed instead of a colostomy whenever it can safely control the cancer.

Radiation therapy. Endocavitary irradiation for adenocarcinoma of the rectum may be used for patients with early stage disease without lymph node involvement. The tumors should be well differentiated and no larger than 5 cm in diameter. Due to the limitations of the equipment used in radiation therapy, the lesion can be no farther than 12 cm from the anal verge. About 20 percent of patients with cancer of the rectum will fit these criteria (Sischy et al. 1984).

The treatment requires a Fleets enema about two hours prior to therapy and is done on an out-patient basis. Endocavitary irradiation is tolerated very well by patients. The main side effect noted is transient diarrhea.

Radiation therapy may also play a role as an adjuvant to surgery. In about 10 percent of cases, post-surgical radiation will reduce the incidence of local recurrence. Preoperative radiation is usually reserved for inoperable rectal tumors and precedes surgery by about a month to six weeks. Radiation is used for palliation of obstructing tumors in any part of the colon or rectum. It is also used to reduce the size of tumors when massive metastasis is already present.

Chemotherapy. After twenty-five years of testing, it has been found that fluorouracil (5–FU) remains the most effective agent against colorectal cancer. Combination therapy as well as other single agents have been used, but none surpasses fluorouracil used alone for effectiveness. Unfortunately, the response rate is only about 25 percent, and complete remissions are rare when fluorouracil is used. Survival is prolonged by about six months with chemotherapy. A typical schedule is a loading intravenous dose over five days followed by monthly therapy over five days, or weekly therapy.

If liver metastasis has occurred, intermittent hepatic artery infusion may be used, or continuous infusion with a permanent catheter and portable pump, to deliver chemotherapy. These routes are commonly used if patients fail on systemic chemotherapy. They do not produce sufficient improvement in survival to warrant their use on a routine basis.

Because response is so poor with any chemotherapeutic regimen, patients may be advised that there is no proven effective adjuvant chemotherapy and none recommended for colorectal cancer. Various centers across the country are involved in trials of different agents in the hope of discovering a useful drug or regimen for future use.

Recent advances. The Eastern Cooperative Oncology Group has recently begun a trial on individually tailored vaccines for colon cancer. In initial studies, the vaccine has proven effective in reducing the recurrence of colon cancer after resection for the disease. Not a preventive against the development of cancer initially, it is derived from the patient's own tumor cells as a means of combating recurrence.

Management Skills

DETECTING METASTASIS

Pain in the pelvic, perineal, or buttock area is a common complaint that signals metastasis in the associated area after surgery. A colonoscopy every two or three years after surgery is recommended to detect new polyps, which develop in about 5 percent of patients. Carcinoembryonic antigen studies twice yearly may be recommended to detect metastasis, if such detection would lead to therapeutic intervention for the particular patient. Chest X-rays are often recommended to detect metastatic lung lesions. If such lesions are small and solitary, resection may be undertaken to control the spread of disease. The most frequent point of metastasis for colorectal cancer is the liver. Blood test for LDH, SGOT, bilirubin, and alkaline phosphate are useful for determining if hepatic metastasis has occurred. Once it has, the patient generally has about six months to live.

To assess the presence of metastasis in the colorectal cancer patient, the nurse should watch for the following:

- pain, particularly of the pelvis, peritoneum or buttocks.
- liver enlargement or signs of hepatic failure (indicative of extensive liver metastasis and very poor prognosis)

EFFECTS OF TREATMENT

The most distinctive effect of surgical treatment is the potential for the creation of a colostomy. This subject will be covered from the rehabilitative standpoint in the following section. Immediate postoperative care of the fresh colostomy involves assuring that circulation to the colostomy bud remains good and that it is not traumatized by ill-fitting appliances.

Transient diarrhea is common after radiation therapy. Ensure that patients are well hydrated and that electrolyte imbalances, particularly excess potassium loss, do not occur.

Fluorouracil treatment should be delivered with an understanding of the potential for the following conditions: leukopenia (the presence of this toxic reaction is associated with increased response), and stomatitis. Between 10 and 20 percent of patients develop dermatitis while on 5–FU.

Rehabilitation

THE COLOSTOMY PATIENT

Around 60,000 people will require a colostomy in the United States each year. Although some will be temporary, all the placements have a life-long impact on these cancer patients, adding enormously to the burden of rehabilitation in colorectal cancer.

The most important principle to consider when initiating rehabilitation of the new ostomy patient is to increase gradually the patient's involvement in self-care. The shock of a diagnosed cancer, routine postoperative debilitation, and distaste for dealing in this manner with body waste products is overwhelming for many patients. Patients also fear that they will be left to tend to their own needs once they leave the hospital without understanding the procedures involved. The nurse who competently and calmly cares for the ostomy and appliance on new patients without making it seem complicated or distasteful does much, without directly saying a word, toward patient acceptance. Assuring the patient that there is community help and support available through ostomy clubs and practicing enterostomal therapists as well as thorough in-hospital teaching prior to discharge will help the patient relax about learning new techniques, and subsequently allow him or her to learn better.

The most important facets of rehabilitation of the ostomy patient are: diet and fluid considerations; appliance handling and irrigations; esthetics; and effects of the ostomy on interpersonal relations. Each will be considered in the following paragraphs.

Diet and fluid considerations. In the past, rather exact recommendations were given to colostomy patients in order to improve control of the colostomy or reduce odor and flatus. In recent years, however, rigidity has been abandoned. Having a colostomy is not the same as having a chronic disease such as diabetes or heart decompensation, which require dietary modifications in order to put the patient in the best health possible. A colostomy is simply an alternate means by which feces and flatus are eliminated. Ostomy associations have studied diets and their effects for many years and have found that patients who adjusted best to their colostomy ate a diet of their own choosing (Rowbotham 1981).

Recommending the avoidance of certain foods that may cause increased odor or flatus in some individuals does not contribute to enjoyment of a regular diet or a sense of normalcy. In addition, foods do not cause the same effects in all individuals. It is best to let patients discover what foods tend to cause disagreeable effects in their own systems. Colostomy patients should be able to enjoy tasty and nourishing meals, while eliminating foods that, through experimentation, they have found cause unacceptable gas, odor, or bulk. Foods that patients enjoy but cause odor or gas can be avoided on social occasions.

The deliberate manipulation of a diet to aid in achieving control of a colostomy has been found through the years to be unsatisfactory for many individuals. Inherent capabilities among individuals to achieve good control vary widely. Although a low roughage, low residue diet may decrease the number of times a sigmoid colostomy empties, with no sphincter to stop expulsion, the goal of complete control is too difficult for most people to achieve. A few individuals with a natural tendency toward constipation may be able to avoid wearing an appliance, but this is an unrealistic goal for many colostomy patients. In essence, there is no "colostomy diet" to which these patients should adhere. Encourage experimentation and a healthy, varied diet of their own choosing.

Colostomy patients should be reminded to avoid dehydration. With an ascending or transverse colostomy placed, more fluid is lost from the body than before the surgery and patients may need to increase their daily fluid intake on a regular basis. With a sigmoid colostomy, severe constipation may result from inadequate hydration, although no extra loss of water occurs from this low colostomy.

Appliance handling and irrigations. If a patient with a sigmoid colostomy chooses to attempt colostomy control with manipulation of the diet and periodic irrigations, he or she should be encouraged and taught proper procedures. Control usually means that only small amounts of fluid or feces are expelled between scheduled irrigations.

Although a gauze pad may be all that is required over the stoma between irrigations for some individuals, most people will require a small appliance under the best of circumstances.

An irrigation is simply an enema, usually 1,000 cc of warm water, given every other day to sigmoid colostomates. It is not a required procedure, as normal peristalsis causes expulsion of feces automatically. Irrigations are not a sure means of controlling the timing of such expulsions, but for some individuals they do work quite well. If the patient desires to do irrigations, he or she should be cautioned to use a short conical tubing tip to avoid the possibility of colon puncture, which is possible with a regular enema tip. The entire procedure requires about one hour.

The choice of an appliance should be made with the help of a trained enterostomal therapist. The placement of the stoma, the type of colostomy, and the patient's anatomy, dexterity, and individual preferences should all be considerations. Individuals often find that they wish to use different appliances on different occasions. Many products in various price ranges are now available through pharmacies and ostomy organizations.

Esthetics. As stool moves through the colon it tends to increase in its characteristic odor. Ileostomies expel very irritating substances, but less offensive odors than the less irritating, but malodorous feces produced after sigmoid colostomies. Four means are commonly used to control sigmoid colostomy waste odors. First, oral bismuth subcarbonate QID reduces fecal odor considerably. It is an inert substance that is not absorbed and may act only to slow down bowel action.

Secondly, manufacturers have created odor-proof disposable pouches and permanent appliances. When these are handled hygienically, they are very effective. A third measure that may be taken to eliminate odors is the use of topical deodorants for use in pouches. Banish is the most widely recommended brand of topical deodorant. Finally, the colostomate can avoid foods that result in increased fecal odors when going out in public.

Since colostomates do not have sphincters, control of flatus is not possible. Therefore, although odors can be controlled, noise cannot. Most flatus is actually from swallowed air, not from gas-forming foods. It should be impressed upon patients that the less attention they pay to their own gas passing, the less others will be embarrassed for them. Anxiety can cause the increased swallowing of air, so many ostomates notice that noise becomes less of a problem with the passing of time and increased adjustment.

Effects of the ostomy on interpersonal relations. A small percentage of men may become impotent following resections of rectal cancers. However, impotence is a problem with some men although no nerve damage is evident. The changes in self-image and debilitation from the disease and surgery both may serve to increase the chances of such difficulties. The incidence and nature of sexual difficulties among women ostomates is not well documented. Women can conceive and deliver babies normally following such surgery, however. Among both men and women the psychological effects of an ostomy are much more significant than physical limitations in influencing sexual functioning.

A natural inclination among new ostomates is to withdraw from social contacts following their surgery in order to spare others from the perceived offensive effects of their ostomy. With time, a majority of patients find that this is unnecessary and re-engage in normal activities. Initially, however, most patients will need to be assured that their surgery is not obvious to others and that they are in no way offensive. The United Ostomy Association and American Cancer Society are both extremely useful organizations for the rehabilitation of the person who has had a colostomy or ileostomy.

Leukemia

Leukemia is not a single disease, but a heterogeneous group of neoplastic disorders involving the cells of the blood-forming organs. A characteristic that the leukemias share is that they all arise from cell systems that circulate in peripheral blood and originate in large part in the bone marrow. The leukemias are usually broadly categorized as either of lymphocytic or myelogenous form. Some authorities characterize the leukemias as lymphocytic or nonlymphocytic for the acute forms because of the tremendous heterogeneity seen in the latter type. Leukemias are further categorized as either acute or chronic; but today, treatment regimens are blurring the difference between the clinical courses historically seen in the two classifications. Acute leukemia patients can survive for prolonged periods of time. The "acute" designation indicates that the disease involves immature (blast) forms of myeloid or lymphoid precursors. Chronic myelogenous leukemia (CML), also referred to as chronic granulocytic leukemia (CGL), is characterized by a tremendous proliferation of granulocytes at all stages of development. Chronic lymphocytic leukemia (CLL) involves increased numbers of adult lymphocytes in the peripheral blood and bone marrow.

The leukemias only account for about 5 percent of all annual cancer incidence. They are one of the rare cancers that show a peak in childhood; childhood leukemia is overwhelmingly of the acute type. Overall, the leukemias are about evenly divided between the acute and chronic forms. In the acute form, most adults evidence the myelogenous subtype, while 80 percent of children present with the lymphocytic subtype. CML rarely occurs in childhood and has a peak incidence in the middle forties. CLL, which is almost unknown in childhood, shows an increasing incidence with each decade of life with an average age at presentation of about sixty-five years.

Etiology

The mechanism by which radiation and certain mutagens cause leukemia is uncertain. It is known that retroviruses are capable of cauing leukemia in cats, mice, and gibbon apes, and evidence has been found that the HTLV-I virus is capable of causing leukemia in man. Very few cases of leukemia can be linked to radiation exposure or specific mutagens, so prevention has been handicapped by lack of knowledge of environmental determinants of the diseases that may exist. The role of retroviruses in leukemia needs to be further elucidated.

DEMOGRAPHIC FACTORS

Geographic variation. Unlike most other forms of cancer, the leukemias show very little geographic variability around the world. Differences are usually no more than twofold between different populations and may be partly attributable to variations in reporting accuracy. One striking exception to this is the exceedingly rare occurence of CLL among Oriental people compared to other populations.

Time and person variability. From 1900 to 1940, a dramatic increase in the incidence of leukemia was noted among industrialized societies. Since the 1940s, no further increase has been noted, and in fact, a decline in rates, particularly among whites, has been documented. The increase noted in the early part of the century may be partly due to improved reporting of mortality data as well as improved diagnosis. Some of the increase, however, is perhaps the result of increased exposure to radiation and chemicals (particularly benzene) in industrial countries, at levels that have not changed to any great extent since.

Males generally are affected more often by leukemia than females. The sex difference is most pronounced in CLL, where there is a two-to-one ratio. Some data suggest that this difference is due to the varying exposure rates of males and females to radiation and chemicals, and is thus a factor of occupational exposure and not a true sex-linked difference. Whites show a consistent excess of disease over blacks and Jewish populations, for unknown reasons. Because Orientals who move to new geographic locations retain the same low incidence of CLL as in their country of origin, it is hypothesized that true genetic differences in susceptibility may exist in this case.

Chromosomal aberrations. Leukemia has been linked to conditions characterized by chromosomal aberrations, known chromosomal disorders, and certain immunologic diseases. The aberrations noted in the leukemic cell chromosomes vary widely from case to case. One chromosomal abnormality specifically linked to CML is the Philadelphia chromosome seen in marrow cells of these patients. It has been known for a long time that leukemia incidence is greatly increased in Down's syndrome patients and those with Klinefelter's syndrome. Leukemia is also linked to genetic disorders such as Bloom syndrome and Fanconi anemia. Some immunologic disorders predispose to leukemias. These include ataxia telangiectasis and Bruton-type X-linked agammaglobulinemia.

The Hiroshima and Nagasaki experience. Follow-up studies have been done on the Japanese population surviving the 1945 atomic bomb explosions on Hiroshima and Nagasaki. The ionizing radiation to which the populations were exposed caused an increase in all forms of leukemia except CLL. The incidence of leukemia began to increase over normal levels about two years after the bombing. Peak excess was noted at five to ten years after the blast, and incidence at forty years post-explosion continues to be slightly elevated. The excess leukemia noted appears to be dose-related, particularly at higher dose levels.

Common Clinical Course

DETECTION

Acute leukemias are usually detected by the signs and symptoms of fatigue, malaise, and anorexia or after they progress to anemia, pallor, and signs of hemorrhage associated with thrombocytopenia. Oozing gums, epistaxis, ecchymoses, and excess bleeding with injury are common initially recognized manifestations. At the time of diagnosis the organs most commonly involved are the liver, spleen, and superficial lymph nodes. On physical examination, about 50 percent of patients are initially found to have diffuse adenopathy and hepatosplenomegaly. Sometimes bone pain is a symptom, caused by the migration of cancer cells to the joints or by direct infiltration.

Funduscopic examination may demonstrate hemorrhages or lesions representing retinal infiltration.

In the chronic forms of leukemia, symptoms of weight loss in spite of an excellent appetite, low-grade fever, night sweats, and fatigue may be initially reported. Splenomegaly is characteristic of CML and may cause a sensation of fullness in the left side of the abdomen. Often in CLL there are no early symptoms and the disease is discovered by routine blood work. The most common initial complaints of those who have CLL are fatigue and glandular neck masses.

PATHOPHYSIOLOGY

The molecular basis of the leukemic transformation of cells is unknown. The fundamental defect in the acute leukemias is an unregulated proliferation of cells that cannot differentiate in response to normal hormonal signals and cellular interactions. Normal and abnormal cells coexist, competing for space within the bone marrow. Acute leukemias are extraordinarily heterogeneous, with many types existing in both the myelogenous and lymphocytic forms. AML is increasingly referred to as acute nonlymphocytic leukemia (ANLL), in acknowledgment of the heterogeneity.

CML is characterized by many abnormal granulocytes and few normal cells. The Philadelphia chromosome is associated with the common forms of this condition and is found in immature granulocytes, and in megakaryocyte and erythroid precursors. CLL is usually a monoclonal proliferation of immunoglobulin-producing B lymphocytes with a block in cellular maturation. In 5–10 percent of cases, CLL is of T-cell origin.

DIAGNOSIS AND STAGING

Laboratory analysis of blood is necessary to establish a diagnosis of leukemia. In all the leukemias, diagnosis and staging are done by peripheral blood smear evaluation and bone marrow aspiration. In acute lymphocytic leukemia (ALL), white blood cell counts of 5,000 to 30,000/cu mm are most common. Decreased adult neutrophils and platelets are seen in peripheral blood smears, with many blast cells evident. The diagnosis is confirmed by bone marrow aspiration. CML often presents with a white blood cell count of 50,000 to 500,000/cu mm. More than 90 percent of white blood cells are noted to be in the granulocytic series. The diagnosis of CML is confirmed by a low leucocyte alkaline phosphatase score and the presence of the Philadelphia chromosome. CLL is also diagnosed by peripheral blood smear and bone marrow aspiration. It is staged according to the presenting of abnormalities beyond lymphocytosis alone, which is

Stage 0. Stage IV is characterized by lymphocytosis with thrombocytopenia, with or without anemia and organomegaly.

TREATMENT

Approximately 50 percent of patients less than fifteen years old with ALL are now experiencing long-term leukemia-free survival. This is largely due to improved induction to complete remission, administering chemotherapy during remission, and prophylactic treatment of the central nervous system (CNS). Vincristine (Oncovin) and prednisone produce complete remission in 90 percent of pediatric patients with ALL. Other drugs, usually L-asparaginase, daunomycin, or adriamycin, are also used to effect complete remission. Since the 1960s, CNS irradiation and/or intrathecal methotrexate administration have been used as prophylaxis for central nervous system involvement. Radiation doses of 1,800 to 2,400 rads over two and one half weeks are commonly used in CNS radiotherapy. A poor prognosis is associated with a high WBC, extramedullary infiltration, age of less than two years or greater than nine, a mediastinal mass, and T-cell markers on the leukemia cells.

Methotrexate and 6–MP are most often used in maintenance therapy for ALL. The induction and maintenance regimens are producing apparent cures in about 50 percent of children. The best time to stop maintenance therapy is not yet known; generally clinicians continue treatment for two and one half to five years. Most relapses are in the bone marrow, although increasingly the testes are involved as the initial point of relapse in males. Relapse during therapy heralds an ominous prognosis; relapse after therapy can be controlled for considerable periods.

Successful remission induction is possible in 60–80 percent of pediatric patients with AML (ANLL) and about 40 percent of adults. Individuals who develop AML subsequent to drug treatment for other neoplastic disorders, radiation treatment, or immunosuppressive drug therapy have remission rates of only 20–30 percent. Doses of drugs required to effect remission are very close to those needed to kill all marrow cells, so prolonged bone marrow aplasia is often seen after therapy. Significant morbidity and mortality are seen in treating AML. Ara-C, and adriamycin or daunomycin are the usual drugs employed to establish remission. The use of maintenance chemotherapy does not result in any improvement in survival length in AML. The only factor that affects survival is age: patients forty years or older at diagnosis tend to live a few years longer than younger patients. A median duration of remission is one to one and one half years. Only 10–20 percent of patients survive for five years or more.

These patients may particularly benefit from bone marrow transplantation, which significantly prolongs life if done during the first year of AML.

Treatment does not alter the natural course of the chronic phase of CML. Myeleran or hydroxyurea, or splenic irradiation are sometimes employed to reduce the spleen size. Median survival in patients with chronic myelogenous leukemia is from three to four years. Patients usually die from a blast crisis that typically develops at some time in the disease's course and can be only infrequently controlled.

CLL demonstrates a wide variety of clinical courses. The median survival is about five years, although a third live for ten years. Because CLL is so frequently seen in older individuals, many deaths are not directly attributable to it. Therapy is usually aimed at controlling anemia or thrombocytopenia or is begun if adenopathy develops. Chlorambucil or cytoxan along with steroids are often used for this purpose.

Management Skills

EFFECTS OF TREATMENT

Acute tumor lysis syndrome is often associated with induction therapy for ALL (see page 149). To avert the hyperuricemia related to tumor lysis syndrome in ALL, patients are started on allopurinol before induction is started. Sometimes antibiotics such as trimethoprim 160 mg or sulfamethoxazole 800 mg (adult doses) are used to prevent severe infections. Bleeding or infection may arise during the induction or maintenance phase due to the disease process itself or from drug-induced cytopenia or immunosuppression. Mucositis, anaphylaxis, neurotoxicity, cardiotoxicity, hepatic or pulmonary fibrosis, and secondary neoplasms are complications that may result during treatment.

Facilities to support the patient through three to five weeks of profound leukopenia and thrombocytopenia must be available before therapy for AML (ANLL) is started. Nursing support is critical during this period. Death from infection and bleeding is still common. Besides these life-threatening problems, cardiotoxicity, mucositis, alopecia, and nausea and vomiting are significant complications that can occur.

It is doubtful that treatment results in prolonged survival in CLL, except in cases where the disease has entered a blastic phase. Therapy is aimed at symptom relief but may prolong life in some individuals by a few months or years once the blastic phase occurs. Anemia, granulocytopenia, and thrombocytopenia may result from the disease process or therapy.

CML, sometimes referred to as chronic granulocytic leukemia (CGL), occurs primarily in patients between the ages of thrity and sixty. Treatment is aimed at symptom relief or, during the blastic phase, complete remission. Therapy is chosen on the basis of morphology and biochemical markers, but is effective in only about 25 percent of cases. Common chemotherapeutic regimens result in side effects such as bone marrow depression, wasting, amenorrhea, and pulmonary fibrosis. Dermatologic reactions and gastrointestinal distress are also often seen.

Rehabilitation

Rehabilitation of the family with a leukemic child is often difficult. Parents must cope with the psychosocial and economic aspects of a chronic illness as it affects the family, relatives, and the community. Parents often experience depression, frustration, emotional exhaustion, and anger. Their ability to deal with crises, disease-related or otherwise, is often marginal. Parents are expected to deal with feelings of guilt and anguish, while treating other siblings and the leukemic child sympathetically and honestly.

The child who comes home from the hospital in remission is one who has the potential to become sick, requires frequent medical check-ups, and has to take medications that are constant reminders that all is not as it once was. Although the normal flow of daily living may return, each time there is a break in the leukemic child's equilibrium, there is an immediate resurgency of the familiar fears and anxieties, which remain just under the surface of consciousness at other times. How much the child should be told about his or her condition depends on the particular family, the age of the child, and the physical and psychological state of the child. Children generally pick up a great deal of knowledge about their illness in hospitals, although they may not be able to express it.

The leukemic child at home often expresses anger—anger at feeling ill, at not being able to keep up, at being treated differently, and at having to return again and again for medical check-ups and treatment. Other siblings may evidence attention-getting behaviors, not always socially acceptable ones, if they feel relegated to the background of the family. Managing the family unit to provide for happy times and normal experiences sometimes is difficult for the struggling parents.

Community supports include local branches of the American Cancer Society and the Leukemia Society of America. These groups can provide transportation to the hospital, financial aid for the purchase of drugs, and literature about the cancer. The National Cancer Institute also can provide literature about the cancer process and means to cope with it. The Candlelighters, an organization of parents of young cancer patients formed in 1970, can offer emotional support. Make Today Count is another nonprofit organization dedicated to helping cancer patients and their families.

A child's concept of death changes with advancing age. It is felt by experts that young children take comfort when approaching death by conceptualizing it as a peaceful or happy alternative to the life they lead. Anticipatory grieving may be a process that parents go through when a child is terminal. Sometimes parents and others may be inclined to withdraw from the child once they are reconciled to the impending death. Others may withdraw from the child because the pain is too great when they are in the child's presence.

The impact of a sibling's death has enormous impact on remaining children in the family. They may feel grief, guilt that they are in some way responsible for the death, and that their own lives are threatened. Their sense of invulnerability is forever gone. Many families, both adults and children, become much more concerned about health after the death of a leukemic child. In some ways, there is a sense of relief that life can return to some normalcy that is not threatened.

Those caring for the child and family through the process of remission, maintenance, and sometimes death need to understand the reactions they can expect to see from all those involved, as well as understand the usual clinical course so they can effectively intervene as needed.

Bone Marrow Transplantation

Bone marrow transplantation (BMT) can be accomplished by using an HLA matched donor (allogeneic), an identical twin (syngeneic), or the patient's own marrow (autologous). Allogeneic BMT is the most common method used, syngeneic BMT has been found to result in more relapses clinically than the other types of BMT, and autologous BMT is the newest approach. Autologous BMT for treatment of leukemia is now possible because methods have been developed to purge the harvested bone marrow of residual tumor cells (clonogenic cells), prior to reinfusion into the patient.

Allogeneic bone marrow transplantation may be a treatment modality chosen for the acute forms of leukemia. The procedure is offered at large cancer centers for patients in their first or second remission of AML (ANLL) or ALL. The procedure has been responsible for a 60 percent disease-free survival for more than one year in selected patients under thirty years of age with AML. In patients with ALL, survival rates above 90 percent are achieved using BMT during a first remission. One current opinion holds that individuals with acute leukemia should be considered for transplantation while in their first remission rather than subsequent remissions, because inferior responses are observed with the later use of BMT (Huang 1984). However, many clinicians hold that use of BMT should be reserved for second remissions, except in high risk patients (T- or B-cell leukemia, for example).

BMT has also been shown to be useful in the chronic phase of CML; reports of around 60 percent survival following the procedure have been accumulating. Whether to jeopardize a three-year controllable survival period prior to the anticipated accelerated phase in order to undergo BMT, with its associated risks, is currently a dilemma. Results of BMT during the accelerated phase are poor.

When autologous BMT is undertaken, the patient's marrow is first harvested from the anterior or posterior iliac crest under general or spinal anesthesia. A 150-lb patient will have about 700 cc of marrow removed (some 10 percent of the total), after which it is frozen. The harvesting procedure is the same for allogeneic and syngeneic BMT, and involves only minor risk to the donor (Applebaum 1984).

The BMT patient receives large doses of cyclophosphamide, BCNU, or other drugs singly or in combinations, and usually total body irradiation prior to undergoing the reinfusion of marrrow cells in order to eradicate leukemic cells and to impair the ability of the patient to reject donor marrow cells. Total body irradiation is performed several days after chemotherapy is given to the patient undergoing BMT. The radiation procedure takes about an hour, and is done twice daily for three days. During therapy the patient is monitored by closed circuit television. Immediate side effects possible include nausea and vomiting, diarrhea, and headache. Later, fever, skin reactions, hair loss, sterility, stomatitis, and further bone marrow suppression may occur. At this point, the patient is very susceptible to infection, and nursing measures and teaching are of vital importance to prevent complications. Reverse isolation protocols are utilized, and plants, flowers, and visitors with upper respiratory infections are not permitted in the room.

Between twenty-four and seventy-two hours after this preparation, an HLA-identical relative or twin's marrow cells, or the patient's own treated cells, are administered intravenously. Dimethylsulfoxide (DMSO) is used as a protectant during the freezing storage of marrow cells, and the patient will experience a characteristic garlic taste in the mouth and obvious breath odor for several days after marrow cell infusion. Complete recovery with normal blood counts is usually apparent within four to six weeks. Graft versus host disease and interstitial pneumonitis have accounted for the major morbidity and mortality in these patients.

The month after reinfusion of marrow cells is one requiring intensive nursing support. There is severe immune deficiency, with resultant susceptibility to a variety of life-threatening infections. Infections of fungus, protozoa, and viruses (particularly herpes simplex, cytomegalovirus, and varicella zoster) all occur. *Pneumocystis carinii* infection has been largely controlled with the use of trimethaprim-sulfamethoxazole, and amphotericin B helps control fungal infections. Acyclovir is currently being tested as an agent to control herpes simplex and varicella zoster infections. Cytomegaloviral (CMV) infections remain problematic at most cancer centers, however. Prophylactic treatment of patients with CMV hyperimmune globulin has been promising in recent studies. Graft versus host disease is currently being treated with cyclosporine, an immunosuppressant agent, with promising initial results.

Lymphomas

Lymphomas are clinically related diseases caused by neoplastic proliferation of lymphoreticular portions of the reticuloendothelial system involving lymph nodes, bone marrow, spleen, or liver. The vast majority of these patients present with disease of the lymph nodes or spleen, but disease may be present in extranodal sites. The most common types are Hodgkin's disease and non-Hodgkin's lymphomas (NHL), which will be discussed here.

Etiology

Hodgkin's disease is responsible for about 5,000 to 6,000 cancer cases each year in the United States. The dramatic improvements in the survival of patients with Hodgkin's disease have been a signal in the accomplishments of cancer research. Non-Hodgkin's lymphoma accounts for 7,000 to 8,000 cancers diagnosed annually.

DEMOGRAPHIC FACTORS

Geographic variation. Generally, childhood Hodgkin's disease occurs most frequently in undeveloped countries, while Hodgkin's disease associated with young adulthood occurs most often in Western industrialized countries. One exception to this pattern is the extreme rarity of young adult disease in Japan. There is also a north-south gradient in Hodgkin's disease in the United States. In young adults, more mortality is seen in the northern states. In Japan there is also a north-south gradient, but in the reverse direction to that of the United States. When Japanese migrate to the United States, their incidence of Hodgkin's disease begins to approach the rates prevailing in America, suggesting an environmental influence in the disease.

Non-Hodgkin's lymphoma has been increasing in prevalence in Western countries since 1960, particularly affecting older individuals. Singapore Chinese have experienced a very large increase in incidence, while the Japanese record a decrease in the same time period.

Time and person variability. It has been suggested that conditions affecting children, young adults, and older adults are made up of three different diseases with different etiologies. It is suggested that the disease of youth is in reality infectious in nature, although of very low infectivity, while that of old age is a true malignant neoplasm. Although the research is compelling, this needs to be studied further. Males tend to experience a greater incidence of the disease than females, particularly in youth. Some research has suggested that pregnancies are protective against middle-aged Hodgkin's disease, but the research is only preliminary. Hodgkin's disease is much less common among blacks than among whites in the United States, and the Jewish population tends to be at higher risk than other populations. Hodgkin's patients tend to be better educated and of higher socioeconomic status than the general population, although this pattern may be changing. There is a definite relationship between Hodgkin's disease and being an only child. The more siblings in a family the less likely is the risk of Hodgkin's disease. There has also been a noted relationship between infectious mononucleosis and HD, which has been confirmed by several studies.

NHL is relatively uncommon in the United States, with about 15,000 cases reported annually. There is a slight excess of disease among males, and among whites over blacks. There is a positive association between socioeconomic status and NHL. Recently, the incidence of NHL has been increasing in Connecticut, and also among native Hawaiians. The incidence of NHL among adult women is increasing at a rate second only to lung cancer in the United States. Individuals who are immunodeficient are much more likely than the general population to develop NHL. Transplant recipients have an increased risk of NHL, as do patients with rheumatoid arthritis and systemic lupus erythematosus. There is much preliminary evidence of an association between occupational exposure to a variety of chemicals and an increased risk of NHL.

Familial aggregation. There have been numerous studies of multiple occurrences of Hodgkin's disease (HD) within families. Siblings of the same sex as cases have a risk of HD almost twice that of siblings of the opposite sex. As same sex siblings are more likely to share rooms, an environmental exposure is hypothesized. There is also evidence from some research of person-to-person transmission of HD among school-aged children, although other studies have not shown any aggregation of cases.

There is an increased incidence of NHL among siblings of cases. Two types of high risk families have been identified to characterize the familial aggregation. One group consists of preadolescent male siblings with extra-nodal NHL, primarily of the gastrointestinal tract (Greene 1982). The other involves adult siblings, mainly females, with nodal NHL.

Common Clinical Course

DETECTION

Most patients with HD present with lymphadenopathy, usually of the supraclavicular or cervical area. In about half of cases, the disease appears confined to lymph nodes above the diaphragm, but lymphangiography or laparotomy detects occult nodal sites below the diaphragm. Computerized tomography and lymphography are complementary modalities employed to detect sites of nodal involvement initially, with laparotomy often used to detect extranodal involvement. HD rarely presents in extranodal sites. Epitrochlear nodes are very rarely involved with HD compared to NHL. Approximately one third of patients will complain of fever, night sweats, or weight loss, which usually herald a more aggressive form of the disease. NHL in localized form is present in about one third of patients presenting with symptoms of fever, sweats, or weight loss.

PATHOPHYSIOLOGY

In HD, contiguous spread of tumor from node to node is the rule, and most patients present with disease limited to the lymph nodes and are therefore candidates for curative radiation therapy. In contrast, most NHL patients present with advanced disease. HD is curable at any stage, but in NHL only certain histologic types are curable when disseminated. Lymph nodes may obstruct or compress adjacent structures, resulting in conditions such as the superior vena cava syndrome.

HD tissue is heterogeneous and pleomorphic; composed of lymphocytes, eosinophils, plasma cells, fibroblasts, mononuclear cells, and occasional reticulum cells known as Reed-Sternberg cells. The disease is classified by four histologic patterns: lymphocyte predominance, nodular sclerosis, mixed cellularity, and lymphocyte depletion. Alcohol ingestion in HD makes swollen nodes painful for unknown reasons. Asymptomatic mediastinal masses occur commonly in HD and may reflect abdominal infiltration.

NHL was referred to as lymphosarcoma and reticulum cell sarcoma in earlier literature. About 75 percent of NHLs are of B-cell origin, 15 percent are from T-cells, and the remainder are of monocyte origin or are unclassifiable. NHL is classified by nodal form: nodular or diffuse, and cell type: lymphocytic, histiocytic, small, or large cell. The nodular form of the disease carries a better prognosis than the diffuse form.

DIAGNOSIS AND STAGING

The sine qua non for diagnosis of HD is the presence in tissue samples of Reed-Sternberg cells, which are considered to be the end stage cells in this disease. Lymph node biopsy is used to diagnose HD and NHL as well. The extent of both the lymphoma types is established through laboratory tests, X-rays, computerized tomography (CT), and bone scans. If necessary, futher techniques such as laparotomy and lymphangiography are used to stage the disease more accurately.

Staging for HD and NHL is necessary for effective treatment. Four stages are currently recognized, progressing from Stage I, where disease is limited to a single lymph node chain or single, confined extralymphatic organ, to Stage IV, where one or more extralymphatic organs or tissues show diffuse involvement, with or without lymph node involvement. Each stage is subcategorized into A and B forms; A denoting an asymptomatic condition, and B indicating the presence of fever, sweats, and weight loss.

TREATMENT

Overall ten-year survival rates for patients with Stage I to III HD vary from 65 to 95 percent, with a disease-free survival of 85 to 90 percent for Stage I, 70–85 percent for Stage II, and 40–60 percent for those with Stage III disease. Stage IIIB and IV HD patients treated with chemotherapy have a ten-year survival rate of 43 percent. Rates are somewhat higher if the patient is asymptomatic on presentation.

The prognosis for NHL patients is related to histology and stage. Median survival after radiotherapy for Stage I or II disease is 7.5 years (3.5 years disease free) with nodular lymphomas compared to 2.6 years (0.9 years disease free) with diffuse lymphomas. Prognosis is considerably worse for Stage III and IV disease.

The lymphomas frequently cause oncologic emergencies. Superior vena cava syndrome; spinal cord compression; obstruction of the urinary, biliary, or gastrointestinal tract; hypercalcemia, and leukemic transition all occur.

Radiation therapy. In HD, radiation is potentially curative for Stages I, II, and selected cases staged at IIIA. Megavoltage radiation is delivered by cobalt 60, teletherapy, or a linear accelerator. To determine treatment fields, the lymphatic system is divided into the mantle, which represents the lymph node areas above the diaphragm; the para-aortic region, which includes the lymph node areas to the level of L4; and the pelvic region, which includes all the lymph node regions below L4. Using a one-field, two-field, or three-field technique to irradiate the lymph node regions described above, the radiologist delivers 4,000–4,400 rads in four to four and one half weeks to the involved areas as well as 3,600 rads to adjacent regions. Lead blocks are used to shield the lungs, a portion of the heart, and the ovaries. Careful field shaping is done to protect other organs, particularly the spinal cord, from excess radiation. Pelvic irradiation is avoided if laparotomy is negative. Patients with Stages IIB disease are often treated with both radiation and chemotherapy, although the most effective form of therapy for this presentation continues to be debated.

The approach to NHL remains considerably more varied than that for HD. For the small group of patients for whom disease is confined to one or two lymph node areas, radiotherapy may be employed for cure. Radiation therapy may also be employed in NHL to palliate; whole body irradiation has proved to be an effective form of palliation in patients with Stage III nodular lymphocytic lymphoma and well-differentiated lymphocytic lymphoma. Radiotherapy may also be employed to debulk patients with late-staged disease, although this has not proved consistently effective.

Chemotherapy. Chemotherapy is the primary form of treatment for Stage IIIB and IV HD patients. Complete remission and cure is possible with combination chemotherapy as devised in the last ten years. Although there are eight or more chemotherapy combinations in general use today to treat HD, the MOPP program is the most widely selected. MOPP consists of nitrogen mustard, Oncovin, procarbazine, and prednisone. Chemotherapy for HD usually consists of a six-month program, although prednisone is only given during the first and fourth monthly cycle. Complete remission occurs in 75–80 percent of patients with advanced disease, of whom about 50 percent are cured. Patients whose disease relapses more than a year after therapy with MOPP may be treated with additional cycles of the same drugs. If patients have received radiation, it is often difficult to deliver therapeutic doses of chemotherapy because of the compromised bone marrow reserve. After chemotherapy, radiation therapy is problematic because of resultant leukopenia and thrombocytopenia.

Chemotherapy is the main treatment for NHL. If radiation is employed in early stages of the disease, care must be taken to preserve adequate bone marrow function. Because relapse with diffuse extranodal spread is common, marrow function must be maintained at a level competent to handle chemotherapy. A common regimen employed is the use of a single alkylating agent with or without vincristine and prednisone for Stage II to IV disease. Although excellent control can be achieved for months or years, cure is rare. Occult residual foci of slowly proliferating small lymphocytes eventually cause relapse. Several other combination chemotherapy programs are also available for treating advanced NHL.

The incidence of central nervous system involvement in NHL has been increasing in recent years, particularly with late stage disease. Malignant cells may be identified in spinal fluid, or focal brain masses may occur. Therapy for this complication includes the use of corticosteroids, cranial irradiation, and intrathecal methotrexate or Ara-C. High dose methotrexate with leucovorin rescue is an effective treatment strategy. In refractory cases, the use of an Omaya reservoir with daily injections of methotrexate may be employed.

Surgery. Occasionally, surgery is employed in NHL to treat localized disease in an isolated lymph node, skin lesion, the spleen, gastrointestinal tract, or other area of the body. Prolonged remission and even cures have resulted from this modality in selected patients. In general, however, surgery plays a minimal role in the management of HD and NHL.

Management Skills

EFFECTS OF TREATMENT

Chemotherapy for HD frequently results in depressed blood counts. Alopecia also occurs regularly, but is reversible. Because so many HD patients are surviving for many years, long term effects of chemotherapy are now becoming apparent with this population of patients. Late effects of chemotherapy are infertility, premature menopausal symptoms, and occasionally prolonged bone marrow depression. If radiation is also used in treatment programs, the risk of a future leukemia or other malignancy is slightly increased.

The drugs commonly used in treating NHL may result in reversible myelosuppression, leukopenia, and thrombocytopenia. Granulocyte and platelet transfusions are frequently necessary. Other common toxicities seen with these patients are hemorrhagic cystitis from Cytoxan use, cardiac arrhythmias and congestive heart failure from high doses of Adriamycin, and hyperpigmentation related to use of Adriamycin and bleomycin. Bleomycin should not be given to patients with preexisting lung disease, as lung infiltration can occur with doses above 200 to 300 mg. Amenorrhea usually occurs and reserves itself in a few months after completion of chemotherapy.

Supportive measures are increasing the numbers of patients with HD or NHL who achieve remission or cure. Broad-spectrum antibiotics and amphotericin-B for fungal infections have minimized mortality associated with sepsis from therapy-induced debility. Amphotericin-B is a highly toxic drug that is given intravenously for potentially fatal fungal infections. It frequently produces fever and chills, irregular heartbeat, hypokalemia, and phlebitis in the infusion vein. Signs to watch for that could indicate hypokalemia include muscle cramps or pain, unusual tiredness, or weakness. Sometimes small doses of adrenocorticoids are given just prior to or during intravenous administration of this drug to reduce febrile reactions. With intrathecal use, headache, nausea and vomiting, and unusual weight loss occur fairly frequently. Bactrim (trimethoprim-sulfamethoxazole) is sometimes given prophylactically during withdrawal from steroids to reduce the incidence of *Pneumocystis carinii* pneumonia, a severe protozoan infection.

Rehabilitation

A long-term difficulty facing individuals cured of Hodgkin's disease is the disinclination of employers to hire them. HD is one of the few cancers that can now result in a high ratio of cured cases, but many lay people still view a past diagnosis of any cancer as a prognosis of disability or early death. An additional problem these individuals may face is an inability to get life insurance. Many of the individuals cured of HD are in young or middle adulthood and need to be self-sufficient and gainfully employed for a satisfactory life. Nurses can do little to intervene directly, but may take action by informing the public they serve about the curability of HD and the potential for a long, productive life. Furthermore, nurses can influence the legislators of their states to pass laws making discrimination on the basis of a cancer for which a cure has been effected illegal. In many cases, physicians have to support an individual cured of HD with letters of explanation or personal contacts with potential employers for years after the patient's disease has been eradicated. This is a most frustrating potential consequence for the cured cancer patient.

Pancreatic Cancer

Pancreatic cancer is responsible for 5 percent of cancer deaths among both men and women. It accounts for a smaller percentage of new cancer cases in each sex, but has a very low survival rate and so accounts for proportionally more deaths. The incidence of pancreatic cancer has been slowly rising over the last several decades in the United States and worldwide, but recently seems to have leveled off. In the United States, the increase in incidence over the last forty years has been almost 100 percent. In Japan the increase has been even steeper.

Etiology

DEMOGRAPHIC FACTORS

Geographic variability. The highest rates of pancreatic cancer occur in northern Europe and in countries populated by migration from those areas. The incidence in southern Europe is relatively low. In the United States, incidence seems to be higher in the South and is especially common around the Mississippi Delta (Blot et al. 1978).

Time and person variability. In the United States, blacks have about two times the chance of developing pancreatic cancer as whites. In Africa, the reported incidence is low; however, questions about the reporting and diagnosis of cases have been raised. Hawaiians and Maoris have especially high rates of this cancer. The Polynesians show an excess of cases among young adults and males, whose rates are almost double those for whites in the same populations.

The most reliable and important known predictor of pancreatic cancer incidence is age. After age forty, incidence increases steadily, being approximately forty times more likely at age eighty than age forty. Pancreatic cancer is about 50 percent more common among men than among women worldwide, the division lessening as age advances. There appears to be an excess of cases among Jewish men, verified by several studies (Wynder 1973). Seventh Day Adventists have shown lower rates. Pancreatic cancer appears to occur more frequently among single men and women, although the effect is not strong. An urban–rural gradient has been seen in several, but not all, studies (Mack 1982). Occupational risk factors have been too confusing to ascertain relevant elements of concern to date. A familial tendency toward pancreatic cancer has been noted, although the overall importance of this factor is slight in the general population. Chronic pancreatitis with calcification is a probable risk factor for this cancer, but the relationship has not been thoroughly established. Surprisingly, perhaps, diabetes mellitus does not seem to be a risk factor for pancreatic cancer. It is associated with the cancer, but diagnosis of diabetes usually occurs within one year of diagnosis of pancreatitis, so a causal relationship is not inferred although they are associated. An excess of cirrhosis has been noted in pancreatic cancer cases in the United States. Smoking is another factor associated with a 2 to 4–fold increase in pancreatic cancer risk, although it accounts for only a small proportion of the cancer cases. In general, current knowledge of the etiological risk factors for pancreatic cancer is weak. Current studies are underway to determine the role of alcohol and diet, particularly fat and coffee, in the etiology of pancreatic cancer, as these seem to be the most likely factors based on preliminary studies.

Common Clinical Course

DETECTION

The pancreas is inaccessible to palpation or easy radiologic examination. Therefore, detection is usually through recognition of symptoms associated with advanced disease. The classic symptoms for carcinoma of the head of the pancreas are pain, weight loss and progressive jaundice. In its early stages, symptoms tend to be vague. Compression of adjacent organs such as the common bile duct and duodenum may lead to anorexia and increasingly severe pain. Pain associated with cancer of the head of the pancreas tends to be epigastric in origin and is relieved when the patient bends forward or assumes a sitting position. Over time, it may radiate to the right upper quadrant and change from an episodic nature to a continuous one. Weight loss is often severe due to anorexia, malabsorption related to the absence of exocrine enzymes, and pain experienced when eating. Diabetes mellitus is seen in about 30 percent of patients within one year of the cancer diagnosis, and jaundice is almost always present with cancer of the head of the pancreas. If complete biliary tract obstruction has occurred, bulky, clay-colored stools may occur.

PATHOPHYSIOLOGY

About 75 percent of pancreatic tumors originate in the head of the gland, but by the time of death, most of the gland is usually involved. Tumors of the body and tail of the pancreas usually remain asymptomatic for long periods until the time of presentation, when distant metastasis has occurred and the patient complains of symptoms of severe epigastric pain with weight loss. The vast majority of all types of pancreatic tumors are duct cell adenocarcinomas.

The most frequent sites of metastases are the regional and paraduodenal lymph nodes, peripancreatic lymph nodes and the nodes in the hilum of the liver. The liver is almost invariably involved in end-stage disease. Direct seeding of the abdominal cavity is also common.

DIAGNOSIS AND STAGING

Nine out of ten patients with pancreatic carcinoma are beyond prospect of cure by the time of diagnosis, and the five-year survival rates are 1–2 percent for this deadly disease. The TNM categorization of pancreatic cancer established by the American Joint Committee for Cancer Staging and End Result Reporting gives four stages, from locally confined disease through advanced disease with distant metastasis. In many instances, the disease is not staged as it is not helpful in assigning treatment or determining prognosis.

A glucose tolerance test is abnormal in about one-third of pancreatic cancer patients. If biliary obstruction has occurred, serum bilirubin and alkaline phosphatase levels tend to be high, and transaminase determination may reveal moderate elevation. Retrograde pancreatography helps in the diagnosis of pancreatic cancer, but is usually not considered except in the presence of symptoms, at which time the disease is commonly advanced. Ultrasound, computerized tomography, arteriography, lymphangiography, and barium studies are sometimes used to aid in diagnosis. A biopsy may be taken by needle biopsy, laparoscopy, or laparotomy for conclusive evidence of pancreatic cancer.

TREATMENT

Surgery. A radical pancreatoduodenectomy (Whipple procedure) is a potentially curative modality that can be employed in the treatment of this cancer. Unfortunately, operative mortality is high, the proportion of explored patients with resectable disease is low, and the five-year survival in resected patients is only about 5 percent.

Recently, it has been shown that the use of postoperative radiation therapy may increase the length of survival by several months.

Chemotherapy. Chemotherapy is compromised by the debilitated condition of most of these patients at the time treatment is begun. Fluorouracil, streptozocin, mitomycin, and doxorubicin all show a response rate in the neighborhood of thirty percent and are the most active singly used agents found to date. Combination chemotherapy has been tried recently. The combination streptozocin, mitomycin, and fluorouracil (SMF) has recently been shown in trials to yield response rates of 30–45 percent, resulting in a ten-month survival period. Fluorouracil, doxorubicin, and mitocycin (FAM) together have resulted in response rates of about 40 percent, with survival extending for one year.

Radiation therapy. Radiation with concomitant administration of fluorouracil is the most useful treatment found to date for patients who are inoperable. The best group in recent trials of this program survived for 39 weeks, a result similar to that of patients having radical surgery. Many patients undergo surgery first to determine resectability prior to the initiation of external radiation treatment.

In recent years, radiotherapists have worked with surgeons to develop techniques for delivering a larger dose of radiation to the pancreas than that which can safely be delivered by external beam irradiation. Permanent radioactive seed implantation of iodine–125, or intraoperative electron beam radiation supplementation are two such techniques.

Management Skills

DETECTING METASTASIS

Usually the pancreatic cancer patient dies before physical findings of metastasis are found. Frequently the diagnosis of metastasis is made at autopsy. Check for:

- enlarged liver—the most frequent organ of failure responsible for death from this cancer
- palpable gallbladder—seen in about 30 percent of patients with tumors of the head of the pancreas (Courvoisier's sign).
- abdominal mass—most frequently related to tumors of the tail of the pancreas
- splenomegaly—caused by compression of the splenic vein.
- arterial bruit over the left epigastrium—caused by compression of the splenic artery (Bauerlein's sign)

EFFECTS OF TREATMENT

Pancreatoduodenectomy is frequently followed by obstruction of the pancreatic duct and pancreatic enzyme deficiency. Under these conditions, steatorrhea often develops and patients will require supplemental pancreatic enzymes before each meal. If the entire pancreas is removed, enzyme supplementation is mandatory and diabetes with insulin dependency will invariably result. The amount of insulin required to maintain these patients is not excessive. Sometimes dietary fat is controlled in these patients so that steatorrhea does not develop; however, because these individuals often are losing weight rapidly, fat should not be unduly curtailed. Chemotherapy with SMF and FAM regimens may result in myelosuppression with both leukopenia and thrombocytopenia. Therefore, sepsis or bleeding may become management problems.

Perhaps the greatest problems for these patients, however, are those of coming to grips with the fatal prognosis for this form of cancer and coping with the tremendous physical debility that is part of the final clinical picture. Nurses should be knowledgeable about the grieving process, and able to relate comfortably with patients and families dealing with one of the most painful and rapidly fatal forms of cancer known. Satisfaction in providing nursing care for the patient with pancreatic cancer lies in being able to relieve physical pain and discomfort, along with the psychological support provided to the patient and surviving loved ones.

Care of the Patient with AIDS

When the virus associated with Acquired Immune Deficiency Syndrome (AIDS), designated HTLV-III, infects the human host, it invades helper T-cells, blocking their ability to recognize foreign substances and modulating the cell's functions from immunological surveillance to viral replication (Lane 1985). Research indicates that the HTLV-III virus can replicate itself approximately 1,000 times faster than other kinds of viruses, hence consumption of the body's helper T-cells can be rapid. Once helper T-cells are consumed, the virus can no longer replicate in the host and it may disappear from peripheral blood. The immunological damage to the host is severe and recovery does not appear to occur. It is not certain that everyone who becomes infected with the AIDS virus will develop the disease, however. Scientists are aware that presently most HTLV-III-infected individuals show no symptoms or a mild form of the disease referred to as AIDS-related complex (ARC). Based on blood transfusion recipient studies, it is estimated by some researchers that about 10 percent of those infected through blood transfusion will eventually contract the disease (Bennett 1985).

The confirmed routes of transmission of the HTLV-III virus are sexual, intravenous, blood and blood product transfusions, and mother to fetus or newborn. Although the HTLV-III virus has been found in all body fluids including urine, tears, and saliva, the only routes documented as capable of transmission of the virus are those mentioned above. High risk groups include homosexual males, intravenous drug abusers, and persons with hemophilia A. It is estimated that the present population of homosexual males is from 30–68 percent seropositive for HTLV-III (Bennet 1985). Based on studies of existing AIDS patients who contracted their disease through blood transfusions, it is suggested that the incubation period for the disease ranges from several months to more than four years.

Because nurses and other direct care professionals are at risk for diseases such as hepatitis B that are thought to be spread through blood products, there is understandable concern among these individuals about their own risk of contracting this disease for which there is no known cure. Precautions to be used when giving direct care to patients are only now being developed, but generally include wearing gloves when in direct contact with body secretions, when delivering oral care, or when performing dressing changes or venipuncture. Needles should not be recapped after use, but immediately placed in a plastic contaminated needle holder. If a nurse has broken skin, the area should be covered with an occlusive dressing, and gloves should be worn if the injury is on a nurse's hand. Linen should be routinely double-bagged, and specimens should be clearly labeled with the patient's diagnosis. While a single room is not necessarily required, it is suggested if the patient is coughing or has questionable personal hygiene. If there is a possibility of a nurse being splattered with blood, protective covering, such as goggles, gowns, shoe covers, and caps, should be worn. Hand washing before and after patient care, of course, is mandatory. Because AIDS patients are frequently carriers of other opportunistic infections, such as cytomegalovirus (CMV), pregnant women are advised not to work with them.

Risk-reducing behaviors regarding AIDS that should be considered for all individuals, both men and women, homosexuals and heterosexuals, include knowing one's partner's potential for infection, and eliminating the exchange of body fluids or contact of body fluids with mucous membranes (Bennett 1985). All body fluids should be considered in the above guidelines: semen, urine, saliva, feces, tears, or blood. Risk-reducing behavior is probably important even among those who are already infected; foreign body fluids contain foreign antigens that tend to stimulate the immune system, enhancing HTLV-III replication.

The cost of treating AIDS patients will become a social issue for most communities as the disease inevitably spreads. Current costs range from $50,000 to $150,000 per patient. Local resources will probably be unable to meet these costs and the federal government will have to assume a larger role. The social problems associated with this disease are heightened as the prospect of a cure or prevention of AIDS remains elusive. Prevention of AIDS by development of a vaccine is stymied by the mutagenicity of these cells, similar to the mutagenicity seen in most cancer cells. The problem of heterogeneity of the AIDS-infected cells is compounded by the rapid replication rate they demonstrate; vaccines that can currently be developed are only effective against a proportion of cells that can quickly recover in numbers. A number of antiviral medications, such as HPA–23, are currently under study; many have severe side effects that limit their long-term use, however. Alpha interferon, which in vitro is seen to support T-cell proliferation, is being used clinically with AIDS patients; results of this therapy are not yet available.

Nurses working with AIDS patients must be prepared to handle the emotional lability experienced by those on experimental therapy and the fear of death and grieving these patients will experience. Nurses should feel confident about the containment of disease, which is made possible by following isolation procedures that are currently suggested, and be willing to help these patients through an emotionally wrenching experience.

Communicable Agents in Cancer Care

Although it is Acquired Immune Deficiency Syndrome (AIDS) which has been attracting recent attention concerning the connection between viruses and cancer, other malignancies, such as leukemia and cervical cancer, are known to be linked to viral infections. There are reports in professional journals and in the general media of nurses contracting hepatitis, cytomegalovirus (CMV), Epstein-Barr virus, HTLV-III virus, and herpes viruses from patients. Documentation is sparse, but this problem will probably loom larger for nurses in the future than seems apparent today. Cancer patients may not only have malignancies that are linked to viral infection, but may be suspectible to newly acquired viral infections by virtue of debility, therapies, or depressed immune status. Although viral infections associated with malignancies are not highly contagious, care should be taken by nursing personnel when handling body secretions.

Gloves should be worn by those providing oral care for all cancer patients. Likewise, perineal care should be done while wearing examination gloves. The care provider may have small breaks in the skin of which he or she is unaware that could be potential entry sites for viruses. Communicable viruses are most likely to be found in body fluids, including urine, saliva, mucus, tears, semen, vaginal secretions, feces, and blood. Of course, viruses may not be preent in these fluids at all times, but it is presently unknown when viruses are likely to be present. Whenever handling linens and objects contaminated with body secretions, good aseptic technique should be maintained and open areas of the skin protected. Viruses generally die rapidly in a dry environment; therefore, spills and droplets from body fluids should be promptly cleaned up with solutions effective against viruses.

In the past, it has been suggested that delivering nursing care with gloves on was somehow a psychologically distancing practice. However, warm, personal care can most assuredly be delivered while wearing gloves if the nurse cares to project a warm, personal attitude. More emphasis should perhaps be given to personal qualities and less to practice techniques as the crux of interpersonal harmony between patient and nurse, and the means of establishment of therapeutic relationships.

6

Overview of Less Common Cancers in the United States

Bladder Cancer

Etiology

About 4 percent of all cancer deaths are due to bladder cancer. Certain industrial chemicals, tobacco use, and chronic inflammation are thought to be the most important causes of bladder cancer. About three times as many men are diagnosed with baldder cancer as are women. About one-third of those who have bladder cancer will die of their disease within five years.

Common Clinical Course and Treatment

Surgical resection, instillations of thiotepa and epodyl, and hyperthermia are usual treatment modalities for bladder tumors. Cystectomy may be used if metastasis has not occurred, but is not helpful in prolonging life if the tumor is deeply invasive. Most patients make a satisfactory adjustment to the urinary conduit stoma and collection bag required after cystectomy. Male impotence after this surgery is a significant problem, however. Systemic chemotherapy and radiotherapy, although used in some cases, in general are not very effective against bladder cancer.

Brain Cancer

Etiology

The peak incidence for intracranial tumors occurs in adults between ages 40 and 60. The cause of primary brain and central nervous system tumors is completely unknown at this time. More than 10,000 deaths from brain and central nervous system tumors were expected to occur in the United States in 1985.

Common Clinical Course and Treatment

The clinical course for malignant brain tumors varies widely depending on the histological type. Some are very slow-growing, while others spread quickly through brain tissue. Primary intracranial tumors rarely metastasize outside the central nervous system. Headache, especially upon awakening, vomiting, visual difficulties, personality changes, or seizures are often the first symptoms noted and are usually related to increasing intracranial pressure due to brain tissue displacement by a growing tumor mass.

Surgery and radiotherapy or radiation alone are the best available treatments. Benign tumors may be excised completely if they are surgically accessible. The role of chemotherapy in the treatment of brain tumors is not at the level of success that exists for other cancer types. Survival rates for primary brain cancers vary from 35 percent at twelve months for high-grade gliomas, to 50 percent at five years for the radiosensitive medulloblastomas. Survival rates for metastatic brain tumors are generally lower, ranging from 20 percent at one year to 10 percent at two years.

Esophageal Cancer

Etiology

A distinctive characteristic of esophageal cancer is its high incidence in only a few geographic areas. In the United States, it has been increasing over the last twenty years, especially in the Southeast. The incidence in black males in this country is much higher than among other groups, averaging some 13.3 cases per 100,000 men. The relationship of tobacco and alcohol to the disease has been well documented.

Common Clinical Course and Treatment

Because more than half of patients present with esophageal cancer which has already metastasized, current treatment of this tumor is primarily surgical palliation. A frequent goal of treatment is to restore or maintain the swallowing mechanism so the patient can live a relatively normal life. The skill of the surgeon has a great effect on the outcome of the technically intricate surgical methods required. Radiation alone is also sometimes used, although the esophagus is quite susceptible to perforation at relatively low radiation doses.

Unfortunately, in the course of the disease many patients develop severe swallowing problems, sometimes being unable to swallow even saliva. Blenderized food and liquid supplements are often used to increase caloric intake so that oral feedings can be maintained as long as possible. Severe weight loss, aspiration pneumonia, and tracheoesophageal fistulas occur frequently. The psychological and physical demands of esophageal cancer are great, both for the patient and for those who care for him.

Kidney Cancer

Etiology

About 83 percent of kidney cancers are renal cell carcinomas that peak in the sixth decade of life. These cancers represent about 2 percent of all malignancies in the United States. Men have an incidence rate twice that of women, and white men have slightly higher rates than black men. The causative factors for this cancer type remain obscure.

Common Clinical Course and Treatment

The survival rate for renal cell carcinoma has been improving steadily since the 1940s. Today, the five-year survival rate is about 67 percent. The most common presenting symptom is painless hematuria, which is not necessarily associated with early disease. Once pain, hematuria and a palpable mass are present, metastasis has usually occurred. Sometimes unexplained weight loss or fever are the initial signs of kidney cancer.

The only curative treatment for renal cell carcinoma is surgical excision. Some patients may require temporary or permanent dialysis subsequent to treatment for kidney cancer. Hypercalcemia is found in 10 to 20 percent of patients as a complication of progressing disease and may be rapidly fatal. Prognosis is directly related to the histological type, site within the kidney, and extent of the disease at diagnosis. Contralateral tumors are not uncommon; follow-up plans include intravenous pyelography on a regular basis. This is one cancer type where the aftermath of treatment may be a chronic, medically dependent state.

Liver Cancer

Etiology

In the United States primary liver cancers are most uncommon, accounting for only 1 to 2 percent of all malignancies. Hepatic angiosarcomas are particularly rare but are closely associated with polyvinylchloride exposure, so are potentially avoidable. Hepatic metastases, on the other hand, are quite common, especially as a result of gastrointestinal cancers, cancers of the lung, and cancer of the breast.

The most common form of liver cancer, hepatocellular carcinoma, has been linked to a number of compounds, including aflatoxins, carcinogens in herbal medications, nitrosamines, and azo compounds, including butter yellow, cycasin, and methylcholanthrene. Both androgens and oral estrogenic compounds have also been implicated in the development of hepatomas, both benign and malignant. Patients with cirrhosis are a recognized high-risk population.

Common Clinical Course and Treatment

Liver cancer seldom produces observable symptoms in its early stage. Alpha-fetoprotein serum testing was considered as a possible screening tool but proved disappointing, since many false negatives result with its use. No one symptom predominates in patients presenting with liver cancer, but weight loss, severe abdominal pain, anorexia, and fever of unknown origin are regularly seen. About 10 percent of patients are diagnosed only at autopsy. Five-year survivals among patients with hepatomas are few; the usual duration of life after diagnosis of liver cancer is nine months.

Treatment of liver cancer is generally palliative chemotherapy. Surgery and radiotherapy play minor roles except in the case of early, solitary lesions. Regional infusion chemotherapy after placement of an arterial catheter is gaining in popularity because it results in fewer systemic side effects than other chemotherapy delivery systems. Unfortunately, no method of treatment is particularly successful in prolonging life.

Malignant Melanoma

Etiology

The malignant melanomas may be grouped into four histological types. Most common of the four is the superficial spreading melanoma, accounting for some 70 percent of cases. This form is characterized by a long growth phase in the epidermis before spread to the dermis and general metastasis. The relative rarity of the malignant melanomas has made their study difficult. Some 7,000 deaths were predicted to occur in the United States from melanoma in 1985. Among blacks, the rates of melanoma are extremely low. Those at greatest risk are fair complexioned, light or red haired, and tend to react to sun exposure with sunburn. The role of sun exposure in the development of melanoma is not clear-cut, as melanomas occur in both sun-exposed and unexposed areas of the body. Sun exposure probably has an important place in the overall causal pathway, however. Over the last twenty years, the incidence of melanoma among U. S. whites has increased steadily, for unknown reasons.

It is now clear that melanomas do not necessarily arise from preexisting nevi, but can originate anywhere on the skin surface. Because melanocytes are concentrated in nevi, about 40 percent of melanomas originate at these sites, but the majority of cases arise de novo from melanocytes elsewhere on the skin.

Common Clinical Course and Treatment

Wide surgical excision is the treatment of choice for malignant melanoma. Patients with thick primary lesions or palpable regional lymph nodes have five-year survival rates of 30 to 40 percent, while patients who present with less extensive disease have comparable survival rates of 60 to 80 percent. Prophylaxtic excision of suspicious lesions is the best way to date to deal with the problem of malignant melanoma.

Multiple Myeloma

Etiology

Multiple myeloma is a proliferative disease of plasma cells, usually involving the bone and bone marrow. Less than 1 percent of all malignancies are due to multiple myeloma. The cause of this malignancy is unknown.

Common Clinical Course and Treatment

Normocytic normochromic anemia is a common presenting sign of multiple myeloma. Multiple myeloma is usually diagnosed by bone marrow aspiration of the elderly patient with suspicious clinical findings such as anemia, back pain, or a high erythrocyte sedimentation rate. The treatment employed is usually administration of intermittent doses of melphalan and prednisone. Response is generally slow, and complicated by toxic effects of the drugs. If bone invasion has occurred, intense pain results that can continue for many months, which requires regular narcotic administration. Methadone or a narcotic cocktail on a regular basis is generally required for pain control. Pathologic bone fractures and hypercalcemia can occur as the disease progresses and bone mass is depleted.

Oral Cancers

Etiology

It has been clearly established that alcohol and tobacco use are causative factors in the development of oral cancers. Although tobacco use results in more oral cancer than alcohol, the two factors have a combined effect that is greater than their summation. Other causes of oral cancer remain obscure. Oral cancers comprise about 2 percent of all malignancies in the United States.

Common Clinical Course and Treatment

Careful examination of the oral cavity, hypopharynx, larynx, nose, and neck can result in detection of oral cancers at a stage when they are highly curable. Up to 90 percent of these cancers result in five-year cures if detected early. Surgery and radiotherapy are most commonly employed for primary treatment. Recurrent cancers of the oral cavity are usually treated with chemotherapy, but have a poor prognosis. Second primary oral cancers are quite common, since the same etiological factors that caused the first oral cancer affect the rest of the oral mucosa.

Sarcomas of the Bone

Etiology

These rare cancers account for less than 1 percent of all malignancies in the United States. High-dose radiation of the bone can result in bone sarcoma, but other causes of the sarcomas are generally unknown. The role of genetic heritage may be important in a minority of cases. These tumors often occur in teeanagers and have a peak incidence around the age of 20.

Common Clinical Course and Treatment

The presence of a mass, chronic pain, functional deficit or pathologic fracture of a bone are the usual complaints that bring the patient to a physician for diagnosis. Radical surgery is the general approach to a diagnosed bone sarcoma, which frequently means amputation of a limb. Radiation therapy is a frequent primary treatment modality used for Ewing's sarcoma. Chemotherpy is often used after primary treatment for Ewing's sarcoma or osteosarcoma and has improved five-year survival rates to about 50 percent. Functional deficits after treatment remain a major rehabilitative problem with the sarcomas.

Nonmelanoma Skin Cancer

Etiology

Skin cancers most frequently occur among individuals with lightly pigmented skin who live at latitudes near the equator, on areas of the body chronically exposed to ultraviolet light. The common basal cell or squamous cell cancers are highly curable and are readily detected. Over 400,000 cases of nonmelanoma skin cancer occur yearly in the United States.

Common Clinical Course and Treatment

Treatment consists of surgery, radiation therapy, electrodesiccation (heat destruction), or cryosurgery. Successful treatment is virtually certain with early detection and treatment. Any unusual skin growths or changes in the appearance of the skin should be promptly assessed for malignancy. The best treatment is prevention, which consists of avoiding the sun during peak intensity and protecting exposed skin with sunscreen preparations.

Stomach Cancer

Etiology

Over the last fifty years, the incidence of adenocarcinomas of the stomach have decreased dramatically in the United States and worldwide, for wholly unknown reasons. The role of diet is being carefully studied by epidemiologists. Diets high in lettuce, celery, citrus fruits, and milk are characteristic of low-risk populations, while the use of pickled, salted, and nitrate-rich foods is seen in high-risk groups. Persons with group A blood type have a greater incidence than those with group O. In the United States, stomach cancer still accounts for about 14,000 deaths annually, making it a continuing significant health problem.

Common Clinical Course and Treatment

After pancreatic and lung cancer, stomach cancer has the poorest five-year survival rate among cancers. Because almost half the patients are diagnosed with metastatic disease, the overall survival rate is only about 12 percent. Unfortunately, early signs of the disease do not exist, and complaints of indigestion and epigastric distress usually portend metastasis if gastric cancer is diagnosed. The treatment of choice remains surgical excision. Adjuvant chemotherapy may prolong survival, but does not usually promote cure.

Cancer of the Testis

Etiology

Less than 1 percent of all malignancies in the United States are the result of testicular tumors. These highly malignant and rapidly progressive tumors are quite readily detectable as scrotal masses. They occur most commonly among men aged 20 to 34, with the vast majority occurring between ages 15 and 44. Men with undescended testes are at higher risk than other men.

Common Clinical Course and Treatment

Radiation therapy following radical orchiectomy is highly effective when local disease is diagnosed. Even when metastasis is present, with adjuvant chemotherapy, cure rates at five years approaching 80 percent are now seen. Retrograde ejaculation and infertility remain rehabilitative problems associated with testicular cancer.

Thyroid Cancer

Etiology

Fewer than 1,200 deaths are expected from thyroid cancer on an annual basis today in the United States. The malignancy is associated with radiation to the neck during childhood, but is not associated with benign thyroid conditions such as goiter.

Common Clinical Course and Treatment

The disease usually presents as a solitary nodule on the thyroid gland. Treatment plans and prognosis vary considerably, depending on the histology of the thyroid cancer. Surgical excision of the lobe with the malignant nodule is often sufficient to achieve cure with differentiated thyroid cancers. Undifferentiated thyroid cancers, such as the giant cell form, generally cannot be cured regardless of stage at diagnosis or treatment. Some experts do not advocate routine total thyroidectomys as this course of treatment does not increase patient survival rates and does result in a high incidence of hypoparathyroidism with attendant metabolic problems. Some patients require a permanent tracheostomy after extensive surgery or complications. In tracheostomy, use of a Tucker valve, which enables the patient to inhale via the tracheostomy but exhale through the mouth and thus phonate adequately, is an immeasurable aid to the rehabilitation of these patients.

7

General Cancer Screening Assessment

The general cancer screening assessment encompasses the basic elements of data collection and physical examination, but analysis is aimed at eliciting and recognizing various facets of information that may indicate increased cancer risk or suggest the presence of an undetected cancer. When a general assessment is done for an individual previously diagnosed with cancer, the purpose is to determine if metastasis is detectable or a second primary cancer is present. On a cancer unit within an acute care facility, nurses also perform general cancer assessments in order to plan patient management competently. Together with information derived from results of diagnostic testing, the assessment will enable the nurse to feel confident that critical findings have not been missed and that the patient will be managed on the basis of complete information. After completing a general assessment, the nurse will be able to perform patient teaching that is appropriate, individualized and pertinent.

Generally in nursing, a cancer screening assessment is done by an oncology clinical nurse specialist in private practice or working in a primary care clinic. A general assessment is part of a cancer unit's staff nursing protocol; these professional nurses are looking for clues that will enable them to manage nursing care competently as well as proficiently address prescribed treatments or medical measures. Opportunities abound for nurses skilled in cancer screening and assessment.

In order to accomplish a cancer assessment effectively, the nurse needs to be aware of the usual clinical findings associated with major cancers as well as important risk factors for the major cancers. Unusual findings that do not fit general patterns are evaluated on an individual basis. Elsewhere in this book information is provided that is important for the nurse to know before proceeding with the assessment process. Armed with knowledge, the correct equipment, and motivation to assess detailed as well as general aspects of the patient's condition, the nurse can lay the foundation for top quality care. This is what any patient is entitled to from a professional nursing staff.

Nurses practice at different levels of specialization as well as in different settings. The procedure for the general cancer screening assessment that follows is applicable for the clinical nurse specialist and may have to be modified for nurses practicing in other roles. (The overall process and basic format for cancer screening assessment are shown in Figs. 7.1 and 7.2.) Ordinarily, the generalist in cancer nursing will be familiar with equipment and procedures excluding internal examination portions of the complete assessment. Nurses performing a complete cancer examination do so within the confines of their health facility's policies.

Preparation

It is always preferable to complete an assessment in a treatment room with a proper examination table. If the individual must be assessed in a patient bed with another patient in the room, assure that visitors are asked to leave for about forty-five minutes and take all measures possible to provide for confidentiality and privacy. In this situation vaginal examination will have to be postponed until an examination table is available. Be sure that interruptions will not occur and that meals or tests are not scheduled during the examination period.

It is impractical for the nurse to schedule more than forty-five minutes to complete the screening assessment. In the real world, nurses must use their time efficiently for their services to be viable within the time and economic constraints of today's health services organizations. Focusing the patient interview and diplomatically putting limits on patients whose anxiety may cause them to seek extended attention are issues the nurse must be prepared to handle. All health providers are faced with the situation of having to restrict interviews that both the provider and patient would like to extend if other responsibilities and commitments did not stand in the way. It must be recognized, however, that quality need not be sacrificed to efficiency and, in fact, is frequently enhanced.

By initially describing the process of the assessment and the time allotted, with the assurance that an opportunity will be provided to answer questions and provide information within the assessment period, the nurse can establish control and a friendly atmosphere. Sometimes, beginning the assessment by listening to those things that the patient seems eager to explain helps establish that the nurse is interested in the patient as an individual. This helps instill a sense of trust in the nurse. The nurse must be able to cap or divert this discourse if necessary in a tactful manner without rushing the pa-

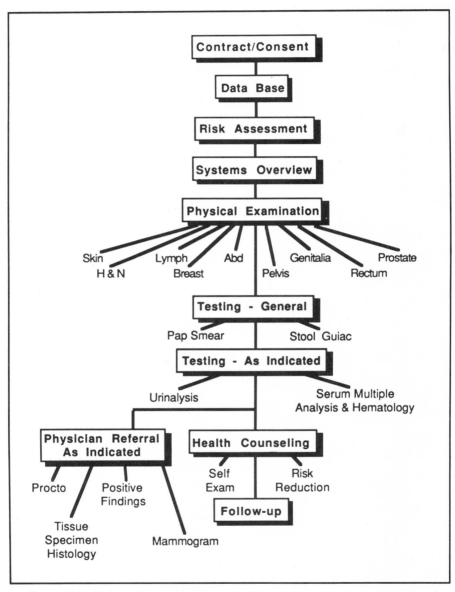

Figure 7.1   Cancer Screening Assessment

DATA BASE

- biographical information
- symptom analysis
- personal health history
- family health history
- lifestyle

RISK ASSESSMENT

SYSTEMS OVERVIEW

- general survey
- skin survey
- head & central nervous system survey
- neck survey
- breast survey
- hematologic survey
- respiratory survey
- gastrointestinal survey
- urinary survey
- genital survey
- musculoskeletal survey

PHYSICAL EXAMINATION

ANALYSIS AND EVALUATION

HEALTH COUNSELING

- patient's cancer risk from data
- seven warning signs of cancer
- self-examination
- risk reduction

REFERRALS AND FOLLOWUP

Figure 7.2   Format for Cancer Screening Assessment

tient's speech. If this patient-generated area of attention seems to lead into part of the assessment, proceeding immediately in more depth with the subject makes good logistical sense and can allow the assessment to shift to a nurse-directed format in a smooth manner.

Although it is best to proceed in assessments in a routinized fashion so that sections of the assesssment are not inadvertently omitted, and so that back-tracking and the appearance of inefficiency are avoided, flexibility must be maintained. If the patient can't stop talking about pain in the left knee, he or she will generally prefer that the examiner check that first before proceeding onward. This is more responsive to the patient than assurances that the examiner will eventually check the bothersome symptom.

During the assessment process, avoid redundantly using phrases such as "You seem good so far," or "That's just fine." Phrases such as these will stand in stark contrast to the nurse's sudden silence if a significant finding is observed. It may also lead to unwarranted anxiety unless endlessly perpetuated once started. Anxious patients may unconsciously consider the nurse's positive assurances during an examination to be a promise of good results. Switching from "You're doing fine" to sudden silence, or to observations like "We will need to examine this mole more closely," is a more painful mental shift than proceeding from no expectations to a specific concern. In any event, the nurse will not want to make premature evaluations and should base any appraisals on the complete assessment.

Instead of offering evaluations during the assessment, the nurse can inquire as to the patient's tolerance of procedures and general comfort, and give assurances when appropriate in response to patient inquiries. These, coupled with assessment questions, should allow for a comfortable atmosphere. Studies have shown that patients, although preferring a friendly nurse, value competency above friendliness. Creating too casual an atmosphere in hopes of easing tensions will probably not be effective and may result in the patient's feeling that he or she is not being taken seriously. No one can make a cancer screening assessment a completely tension-free event, and a serious, calm attitude on the part of the nurse is an appropriate one that will be appreciated by the patient.

Throughout the assessment, finding must of course be carefully documented. Relying on memory is a poor substitute for the assured accuracy possible through the immediate recording of data.

Data Base

The basis format for this aspect of examination is shown in Figure 7.3.

BIOGRAPHICAL OVERVIEW

- name
- age
- sex
- race
- marital status over lifetime
- occupations
- domiciles

PERSONAL HEALTH HISTORY

- childhood illnesses
- chronic illnesses
- hospitalizations/operations
- injuries/illnesses
- past health check-ups
- radiation exposure
- obstetrical history

SYMPTOMS ANALYSIS

- location
- description
- intensity
- when occurs
- precipitating events
- chronic/acute
- duration

FAMILY HEALTH HISTORY

- cancers
- diabetes mellitus
- other chronic diseases
- obesity
- genetic disorders

LIFESTYLE

- alcohol
- tobacco
- diet
- sexual history
- long-term habits

Figure 7.3   Format for Cancer Screening Data Base

Biographical Information

Begin the interview with a general biographical sketch. Information on age, race, sex, marital status, parity, and work history will provide clues to some cancer risks.

Symptom Analysis

Have the patient describe any symptoms or problems of which he or she is aware. Inquiry again before you complete the physical examination as an individual may recall some symptom as attention is focused on the particular body part. There are two frequent responses to assessment questions that may be encountered among patients during a cancer screening assessment. Many patients resist bringing up issues that they feel will be regarded as trivial. Therefore, it is crucial that all information given be considered seriously so that the patient does not omit information that would have proven valuable. The nurse can sort through information after the completed assessment to screen out irrelevant material. A second common reaction to screening questions is for the patient to place great importance on all symptoms, both trifling and major. This is a normal reaction and requires the same general approach by the nurse as described above. Allow the patient to vent all complaints without judging their importance during the assessment.

Help the patient describe symptoms by offering severity scales and questioning as to onset, duration, location, radiation, or cyclic nature of the particular symptom. Ask what measures bring relief and what factors initiate the symptom. Offer the patient various descriptors to help clarify meaning. For example, pain may be described as throbbing, sharp, dull, burning, aching, deep, stabbing, or vague.

Personal Health History

It is important to ask about any past health problems and treatments received. Radiation prescribed, dental work requiring multiple X-rays, or the extensive use of medications of any sort should be noted. It may be experiences many years prior to development of symptoms that are of interest in determining cancer risks. For example, drugs implicated in cancer causation may have been extensively used in years prior to the interview. Over time, the nurse may become aware of a pattern of drug use in the development of a specific cancer that needs to be researched by an epidemiologist.

Family Health History

Familial aggregation of certain cancers has been well documented over a long period of time. Whether the clustering represents genetic predispositon or common familial exposure is still being debated for some cancers. Breast cancer, stomach cancer, nonpolyposis dependent colon cancer and cancer of the uterine corpus are cancers demonstrating a familial pattern of occurrence.

A few relatively rare conditions are accepted examples of inherited cancer: retinoblastoma, xeroderma pigmentosum and polyposis-dependent colon cancer are the three that are best established. Retinoblastoma is a highly curable childhood cancer affecting the retina of the eye. Xeroderma pigmentosum is characterized by multiple carcinomas affecting the patient's skin, particularly in response to sunlight. Polyposis-dependent colon cancer develops from multiple polyps lining the individual's large intestine. The first two types of cancer are usually recognized early in life. Because the polyposis condition also is readily detected in high risk individuals, members of the family with a history of this type of cancer are followed closely for medical interventions as necessary.

Investigations are underway to determine if cancers of the breast, stomach, colon, and uterine corpus are in fact not single diseases, but that each represents at least two distinct cancer types. One type may develop in response to genetic mechanisms and another in response to environmental factors. Detecting a positive family history for any of these cancers may be suggestive of genetic predisposition.

Lifestyle

It is important to document diet practices of the individual, both recent and throughout life. Since some researchers suggest that dietary factors probably act as promotors, consumption patterns over time are important to note.

Dietary history may be useful in suggesting increased risk for several cancers. Directing the interview to specific areas such as vitamin use and consumption of meats, fish, cereals, fruits and vegetables, and fat (butter, margarine, oil) will probably give the most useful information in a limited interview.

Sexual practices, both past and present, are important to note. They suggest the possibility of exposure to sexually transmitted viruses, several of which are considered risk factors for cancer. It may be helpful to ask about multiple partners, or early coital history, anal intercourse, and homosexual acts in a matter-of-fact manner to help patients acknowledge these behaviors. Letting patients know that sexual practices play a role in helping determine overall risk of certain cancers may help them feel more inclined to express themselves on the subject. Menarche, menstrual history, and menopause should be noted for women. Males with a history of undescended testicles have an increased risk for testicular cancer; this can be picked up during the physical examination.

Habits such as alcohol intake and smoking or chewing tobacco are important to note to determine cancer risks. Any such behaviors occurring frequently over long periods of time should be noted. The use of recreational drugs may be important, especially as it may indicate a hepatitis or HTLV-III viral exposure if intravenous routes are used.

Geography plays a role in cancer risk. Ask the patient where he or she has lived and about travel, particularly overseas. Find out whether the patient has been primarily an urban or rural resident, lived near significant industry or in malaria-infested areas, or been exposed to blood or liver flukes. These latter three are related to the incidence of Burkett's lymphoma, bladder cancer, and liver cancer, respectively.

Risk Assessment

Practitioners need to perform a systematic risk assessment based on current epidemiologic data. By completing this portion of the cancer screening assessment prior to the systems overview and actual physical examination, the examiner is able to elicit information that may guide the emphasis placed on various details of the later examination. The risk assessment will also help patients perceive their risk profile in a clear manner, as the practitioner will have the organized data on which to base counseling at the conclusion of the general assessment.

In the hospital cancer unit, nurses may not find this portion of the overall procedure applicable. However, it is a useful reference for patient teaching on a more limited scale.

The risk assessment guide given in Table 7.1 is organized according to the steps of the data base of the cancer screening assessment: biographical data, personal health history, family health history, and lifestyle. The nurse's record of this assessment should note each factor that contributes to the patient's risk of developing specific kinds of cancer. Once the risk assessment guide has been completed, the practitioner may move on to the systems overview.

Systems Overview

As shown in Figure 7.4, the general appraisal of an individual should proceed in a logical manner which can be systematically duplicated with many patients and over time. This type of approach helps eliminate inadvertent omissions and facilitates efficient use of time.

Table 7.1   Risk Assessment Guide

BIOGRAPHICAL DATA

Factor	Cancer risk
Race	
White	Skin (nonmelanoma and melanoma), thyroid, breast, endometrium, testes, leukemia, bladder, ovary
Black	Lung, colorectal, cervix, prostate, stomach
Oriental	Stomach, thyroid
Socioeconomic level	
High	Melanoma, breast, colorectal, endometrium, testes, leukemia
Middle	Bladder
Low	Lung, cervix, stomach
Nationality	
Australian; N. European	Skin
N. America; N. European	Lung, breast, colorectal, endometrium, prostate, testes, bladder
Chinese	Oral, thyroid
Columbian	Breast
Eastern Europe	Stomach
Eskimo	Salivary gland
Indian	Oral
South America	Cervix
Age[a]	
Over 50	Endometrium, leukemia, thyroid, skin, (nonmelanoma)
Over 45	Lung, colorectal, bladder
Over 40	Oral, prostate
Over 35	Breast
15–40	Thyroid, testes
30–50	Cervix

Table 7.1   Continued

BIOGRAPHICAL DATA

Factor	Cancer risk
Occupational & Environmental Exposures	
Substances:	
Aniline dyes	Bladder
Aromatic amines	Bladder
Arsenicals	Skin (nonmelanoma), liver, lung
Asbestos	Mesothelioma, lung, colorectal, larynx
Benzene	Leukemia
Chromium	Lung
Coal tar & pitch	Lung
Heavy metals	Lung
Paint	Bladder
Petroleum	Lung, oral
Rubber	Leukemia, bladder, brain, lung, prostate, stomach
Soot	Skin, lung, multiple other sites
Textiles	Colorectal, oral
Vinyl chloride	Liver, brain, lung, blood system
Wood dust	Oral, Hodgkin's disease
Occupations with particular cancer risk:	
Dairy farmers	Bladder (?)
Foundry workers	Lung
Hair dressers	Ovary, endometrium, lymphoma (?)
Miners	Lung, oral, stomach
Outdoor workers	Skin (non-melanoma)
Professional artists	Colorectal
Radiologists	Leukemia, skin (non-melanoma), lymphoma, thyroid
Shipyard workers	Lung
Tanners	Leukemia

Table 7.1   Continued

PERSONAL HEALTH HISTORY

Factor	Cancer Risk
Associated conditions	
Cancer of lung	Lung, larynx, oral, bladder
Cancer of colon	Breast, another colon cancer, ovary, prostate
Cancer of breast	Colon, another breast cancer, uterus, ovary
Cancer of oral cavity	Lung, larynx, bladder
Cancer of uterus	Rectum
Cirrhosis of the liver	Liver
Colonic, polyps	Colon
Dermatomyositis	Viscera
Epstein-Barr virus infection (mono-nucleosis)	African Burkitt's lymphoma, Hodgkin's disease, nasopharyngeal cancer
Fibrocystic disease	Breast
Hepatitis-B virus carrier state	Liver
Herpes simplex-2 virus infections	Cervix (?)
Iodine deficiency	Thyroid
Lichen planus	Oral
Liver flukes (Asia)	Cholangiocarcinoma
Malaria	Burkitt's lymphoma
Molar pregnancy	Choriocarcinoma
Nevi (multiple, especially on arms)	Melanoma
Paget's disease of the breast	Breast
Paget's disease	Osteogenic sarcoma
Pernicious anemia achlorhydria	Stomach

Table 7.1   Continued

PERSONAL HEALTH HISTORY

Factor	Cancer risk
Schistosomiasis (Africa, Asia)	Bladder, colorectal
Scleroderma	Bronchiolar carcinoma
Sipple's syndrome	Thyroid
Sjorgren's syndrome	Lymphoma
Undescended testes	Testes

Drugs and other therapies

Amphetamines	Hodgkin's disease (?)
Androgens (therapy)	Liver
Anti neoplastics	Leukemia, bladder
Chemotherapy	Leukemia, lymphoma
Chloramphenicol	Leukemia; aplastic anemia
Diethylstilbesterol	Testes; vaginal, cervical cancer risk in offspring
Estrogens (therapy)	Endometrium
Immunosuppressives	Reticulum cell sarcoma
Iron dextran injections	Local sarcomas
Metronidazole (Flagyl)	Lymphoma, lung (?)
Phenacetin	Kidney, bladder
Phenylbutazone	Leukemia
PUVA	Skin
Radiation therapy	Leukemia, lymphoma, thyroid
Radio pharmaceuticals	Leukemia, bone sarcoma
Reserpine	Breast
Hydantoin	Lymphoma
Tar products	Skin
Phenobarbitone	Liver (?)

Table 7.1 Continued

PERSONAL HEALTH HISTORY

Factor	Cancer risk
GYN history	
Few pregnancies (full term)	Endometrium, breast, ovary
Late first pregnancy (after age 30)	Breast
Early menarche	Endometrium, breast
Late menarche	Ovary
Early menopause	Ovary
Late menopause	Endometrium, breast

FAMILY HEALTH HISTORY

Factor	Cancer Risk
Cancer of breast (in mother or sister)	Breast
Cancer of colon (right)	Colon
Cancer of lung	Lung
Melanoma	Melanoma
Cancer of ovaries	Ovary
Cancer of prostate	Prostate
Cancer of stomach	Stomach
Cancer of uterus	Uterus
Diabetes	Pancreas
Genetic syndromes	
Albinism	Skin (nonmelanoma)
Bloom's syndrome	Leukemia
Cryptochidism	Testes

Table 7.1   Continued

FAMILY HEALTH HISTORY

Factor	Cancer risk
Dysplastic nevus syndrome	Melanoma
Fanconi's anemia	Leukemia
Gardner's syndrome	Colorectal
Klinefelter's disease	Breast
Multiple endocrine neoplastic syndrome	Thyroid, neuroendocrine
Peutz-Jegher's syndrome	Colorectal
Polycythemia vera	Leukemia
Polyposis coli	Colon
Xeroderma pigmentosum	Skin (nonmelanoma and melanoma)
Von Recklinghausen's neurofibromatosis	Central nervous systems, skin (nonmelanoma)

LIFESTYLE

Factor	Cancer Risk
Alcohol	Stomach (?)
Alcohol and tobacco	Oral, larynx, esophagus
Chronic irritation to skin	Skin (nonmelanoma)
Beer	Rectum
Burn injuries	Skin (nonmelanoma)
Early and/or multiple partner-coitus	Cervix
High fat, low fiber diet	Breast, colon, ovary
Nulliparity, late parity	Endometrium, breast
Obesity	Endometrium, breast
Poor nutrition	Stomach, lung
Poor hygiene	Oral, cervix, penis

Table 7.1 Continued

LIFESTYLE

Factor	Cancer risk
Smoked foods/salted foods	Stomach
Solar radiation	Skin and melanoma
Tobacco use	Lung, larynx, oral, esophagus, pancreas, kidney, bladder, stomach
Urban living	Lung

[a]The risk of acquiring most cancers increases progressively with age.

General Survey

Unexplained weight loss of ten pounds or more in an otherwise healthy adult is often the first sign of malignancy, particularly for cancer of the pancreas, esophagus, stomach, and lung. Unfortunately, all of these conditions carry a low possibility of cure, particularly by the time the weight loss has occurred. However, weight loss may signal Hodgkin's disease or renal cell carcinoma, both highly curable diseases. Obesity signals an increased risk for cancers of the ovary, uterus, breast, and colon.

Poor hygiene is a risk factor in cancer of the penis or cervix and in oral cancer. Fetid or foul odors may signal necrotic malignancies. Foul odors may be generalized, seeming to emanate from the body overall, or may be noticed on the breath or urine. A change in urine odor may be an early sign of bladder cancer, occurring before hematuria. Most foul odors occur with advanced cancers, however.

Fatigue usually signals advanced cancer. Two exceptions are right-sided colon cancer, which may cause fatigue associated with chronic blood loss at an early stage, and Hodgkin's disease and other lymphomas, which may result in anemia at a curable stage. Malaise and anorexia often occur in leukemia months or weeks before any other clinical signs of this disease develop.

Pain is most frequently associated with advanced disease. Sometimes in sarcomas, dull pain precedes a mass by a short period of time. The pain of a sarcoma is usually first described as mild and is often associated with a specific injury. Patients may state that it increases at night and does not decrease with rest.

1. **GENERAL SURVEY**
   apparent health
   weight changes
   hygiene/odors
   malaise/fatigue
   pain
   sweats/fever

2. **SKIN**
   changes in moles
   edema
   lesions
   masses
   pruritus
   texture changes

3. **HEAD AND CENTRAL NERVOUS SYSTEM**
   arm or leg ataxia
   headaches
   unilateral facial weakness/numbness
   eyes: diplopia, paralysis of convergence, visual deficits
   ears: unilateral hearing loss
   nose, nasopharynx: bleeding, lesions, pain
   mouth, throat: altered taste, difficulty chewing or swallowing,
                 bleeding, hoarseness, lesions, voice changes

4. **NECK**
   lymph node enlargement
   masses

5. **BREAST**
   masses
   nipple discharge
   nipple retraction

6. **HEMATOLOGIC OVERVIEW**
   anemia
   unexplained thrombophlebitis

7. **RESPIRATORY**
   chest pain
   cough
   hemoptysis
   shortness of breath
   wheezing

8. **GASTROINTESTINAL**
   anorexia
   ascites
   changes in bowel habits
   changes in taste
   dysphagia
   food idiosyncrasies
   hematemesis
   indigestion
   nausea/vomiting
   rectal bleeding

9. **URINARY**
   bleeding
   hesitancy/frequency/dribbling
   odor

10. **GENITAL**
    females: lesions, masses, menstrual changes, pain, post-coital
             bleeding, pruritis
    males: penis lesions, testicular masses

11. **MUSCULOSKELETAL**
    pain
    weakness

Figure 7.4 Format for Systems Overview

Virtually all patients with a malignancy will experience fever at some time during the course of their illness. Fever usually occurs when cancer is widespread or involves the liver. However, it may be an early symptom of Hodgkin's disease, non-Hodgkin's lymphoma, atrial myxoma, or renal cell carcinoma. Approximately one-third of lymphoma patients experience early fever, night sweats, or weight loss, which usually indicates an aggressive form of the disease.

Skin Survey

Malignant melanoma is the leading cause of death among diseases of the skin. The mortality rate from melanoma is increasing faster than any other cancer today except lung cancer. In addition, by the year 2000, the incidence rate for melanoma is expected to increase to one person in every hundred in the United States, and melanoma deaths will rise accordingly. While asking about any recent changes in moles or the development of new moles is important in the detection of melanoma, many patients will not be aware of these deviations from normal because they do not routinely assess their skin. This important activity is discussed under health counseling.

The most frequently found skin cancers are basal cell carcinomas and squamous cell carcinomas, both of which are highly curable and usually occur on sun-exposed areas of the body. Although the physical examination includes a complete skin assessment, patients should be quizzed about lesions they have observed. Any lesion that shows biological activity as evidenced by changes in size, shape, or color should be considered suspicious. Patients should be quizzed about pruritis associated with any mole or lesion. A lesion that forms a scab and fails to heal within two weeks represents the most frequent presentation of skin cancer.

Head and Central Nervous System Survey

Complaints of headache (particularly in the morning), arm or leg weakness, vomiting, personality changes, convulsions, or unilateral facial weakness or numbness may signal brain cancers or brain metastasis. A headache is the most common initial symptom seen in brain cancer patients. Vision complaints suggestive of brain cancers include diplopia and impaired extraocular muscle movement. Unilateral hearing loss may be an auditory symptom of brain cancer. If the pituitary gland is involved in a malignancy, hormonal changes resulting in signs such as Cushing's syndrome or amenorrhea-galactorrhea may occur.

Over 90 percent of malignant oral tumors arise from the lining membrane, often from leukoplakia. Oral cancers usually present as solitary patches of uncharacteristic skin and are frequently painless. Ear pain without obvious cause may be referred pain from an oral cancer. Oropharyngeal cancers are usually asymptomatic in their early stages, but a persistent unilateral sore throat may be an indication of this cancer. Nasopharyngeal cancers, which are extremely rare in North America, are usually asymptomatic until they obstruct the airway, bleed, or compress cranial nerves.

Cancer of the larynx may present with the initial sign of hoarseness. Later on dysphagia, stridor, hemoptysis, and pain with a palpable lesion may occur.

Nasal bleeding may be a sign of paranasal sinus carcinoma. Swelling of a cheek, unilateral sinusitis, toothache, or eye pain may be manifestations of sinus cancer. These cancers, which are very uncommon, are most often seen in woodworkers and nickel workers.

Altered taste sensation is common in many malignancies, although its etiology is unknown. It is thought to stem from biochemical changes involving progressive symptoms of cachexia.

Neck Survey

The presence of masses, sensations of fullness, or lymph node enlargement may indicate various head and neck cancers or lymphomas.

Breast Survey

Patients should be questioned about any changes of the breasts they have noted, particularly the presence of masses, nipple discharge, or nipple retraction.

Hematologic Survey

Mild or moderate anemia is a common finding in cancer patients. A marked increase in the total white cell count, usually neutrophils, is also common in patients with a malignancy. Lung cancer, Hodgkin's disease, and myeloproliferative disorders are commonly associated with thrombocytosis, or platelet counts greater than 400,000/cu mm. Chronic disseminated intravascular coagulation may predominate in the clinical picture of cancer progression. None of these hematologic surveys would be a routine part of a cancer screening assessment, but a patient who reports previous blood testing with any of these results should be carefully assessed for underlying cancer. An understanding of the potential for these hematologic changes when malignancies are present can lead the screener to appropriate referral of patients who show signs of a hematological problem. Unexplained thrombophlebitis is sometimes an indication of an undiagnosed cancer and should be considered in the systems survey.

Respiratory Survey

By the time the common signs and symptoms of lung cancer and mesothelioma are seen, the diseases are usually well advanced. Because the vast majority of lung cancer patients are smokers, indicators of bronchogenic cancer are easily confused with chronic smoking signs such as cough, shortness of breath and wheezing. Chest pain, fever, and hemoptysis may also be presenting indications of lung cancer.

Gastrointestinal Survey

There are no early symptoms of esophageal cancer, but painless dysphagia is usually the first symptom reported by patients. Stomach cancer is a "silent" cancer, usually not detected until it has metastasized. Vague complaints of indigestion may be the only indication of the presence of this cancer, which is most common among Japanese men. Stomach cancer incidence in America has dropped more than fourfold since the 1930s, for unexplained reasons. Unfortunately, its five-year survival rate is only 10 percent. The first symptoms reported are often upper abdominal pain, weight loss, and jaundice. Likewise, there are no early signs of pancreatic cancer to assess. Signs of liver deterioration characterize liver cancer. If cirrhosis is present, it is very difficult to diagnose a hepatoma, since early manifestations are masked. A dull, aching right upper quadrant or epigastric pain is often the earliest symptom of this disease and is also associated in over 75 percent of presenting cases of gallbladder cancer. Colorectal cancer is not usually associated with symptoms that can be clearly identified. Sometimes cramping and a feeling of abdominal fullness are reported by patients. By the time gastrointestinal symptoms such as dysphagia, nausea and vomiting, hematemesis, changes in bowel habits, rectal bleeding, or ascites occur, the malignancy is usually advanced.

Urinary Survey

Most renal cancers occur in children; they comprise only about 2 percent of adult tumors. There are no early signs of renal cancer; the patient usually presents with hematuria, flank mass, and pain. Bladder cancer cannot be assessed in a screening examination either; although changed urine odor may precede hematuria and thus be an early indicator of this malignancy.

Early detection of prostate cancer is by digital examination; there are no early symptoms associated with this malignancy. The patient usually first reports back pain and stiffness from bony metastasis or hesitancy, frequency, and dribbling associated with significant local growth of the prostate gland.

Genital Survey

FEMALES

Cancer of the vulva may be detected by asking the patient about a history of local pruritus or mild soreness. As the cancer progresses, signs such as vaginal discharge, pain, bleeding, dysuria, or a mass may occur and are associated with a poorer prognosis.

Vaginal cancer is uncommon. Physical examination is the best means of establishing an early diagnosis, however patients may report a foul-smelling discharge or dysuria.

There are no early manifestations of ovarian cancer, but a tumor mass may be palpated on a screening physical examination for earlier detection. Endometrial cancer and cervical cancer usually present with a history of bloody discharge or frank bleeding between periods or postmenopausally. Cytologic screening using the Papanicolaou smear technique is useful in detecting these cancers at an early, curable stage, before symptoms have occurred.

MALES

Carcinomas of the penis begin as painless growths; a complaint of pain or bleeding often signals advanced disease. Prostatic symptoms are associated with changes in urinary function, as described earlier. Periodic examination is the best means of early detection. Testicular cancers are very rare and usually present with enlargement of the testis with or without pain.

Musculoskeletal Survey

Weakness has been described earlier as a general, common symptom of malignancies, usually occurring when the cancer is quite advanced. Skeletal pain usually signals bony metastasis of an undiagnosed cancer in the otherwise asymptomatic adult.

If a sarcoma of the bone or soft tissue is present, pain, especially at night, may be the only symptom reported. The pain is often associated with a mass, and the patient will give a history of minor injury to the affected area. These cancers are uncommon, especially in adults.

The Physical Examination

Tests and examinations that should be routinely included in the cancer screening assessment are shown in Table 7.2; the format for the examination is provided in Table 7.3.

The following equipment is needed: assessment recording form,

Table 7.2   Physical Assessment of Asymptomatic Patients

	Procedure	Frequency
Ages 20–40		
Includes:	Papanicolaou test	Every 3 years[a]
	Pelvic examination	Every 3 years
Refer for:	Mammography	Once as baseline after age 34
Ages 40–50		
Includes:	M and F digital rectal examination	Yearly
	Papanicolaou test	Every 3 years[a]
	Pelvic examination	Yearly
Refer for:	Mammography	Once as baseline after age 34
	Endometrial tissue sample	At menopause if high risk[b]
Over age 50		
Includes:	M and F digital rectal examination	Yearly
	Stool guaiac test	Yearly
	Papanicolaou test	Every 3 years[a]
	Pelvic examination	Yearly
Refer for:	Mammography	Yearly
	Sigmoidoscopy	Every 3–5 years[c]

[a]After 2 negative examinations one year apart. Yearly after age 65.
[b]History of infertility, obesity, failure of ovulation, abnormal uterine bleeding, estrogen therapy.
[c]After 2 negative examinations one year apart.
Source: Recommendations of the American Cancer Society, 1982.

Table 7.3 Procedure for Physical Assessment

Position of patient	Procedure
Sitting	Examine hands: skin color and texture, clubbing Examine arms: skin, muscle strength Examine head and neck: skin, cranial nerves, parotid gland, buccal mucosa, tongue, oropharynx, nasopharynx, lips, lymph nodes Examine back: skin, palpate, percuss, and auscultate lungs; assess respiratory function Examine chest: skin, female breasts (arms over head, and hands at small of back, leaning forward)
Supine	Examine breasts: arms at sides and arms over head Examine abdomen: skin; palpate (first lightly), auscultate, percuss all quadrants; liver; spleen; kidneys; inguinal lymph nodes Examine legs and feet: skin, including soles of feet
Standing	Examine buttocks, backs of legs: skin
Females: Lithotomy	Examine genital area and rectum: inspect labia; with speculum, inspect vagina and cervix; take Pap smear; bimanual palpation—vagina, cervix, uterus, and ovaries; vaginal-rectal examination of septum, rectum; digital examination of rectum

Males:
  Supine
  then lateral
  knee-chest
	Examine genital area and rectum: inspect penis, testes
	
	Move patient to lateral knee-chest position—palpate prostate, rectum

penlight, stethoscope, blood pressure cuff, tongue blade, thermometer, pin, reflex hammer, examination gloves, ophthalmoscope, otoscope, lubricant, vaginal speculum, Pap smear kit, occult blood test kit, weighing scales, nasal speculum, laryngeal mirror.

1. Hands

Check for skin cancers, finger clubbing, and general health and fitness.

2. Arms

Check for skin cancer, muscle wasting, and weakness.

3. Head and Neck

Check for skin cancer, oral cancer, nasopharyngeal cancer, lymphomas, and brain cancer.

Include the examination and palpation of the skull in the skin assessment. Palpate frontal and maxillary sinuses for tenderness. Palpate the lymph node chains—preauricular, postauricular, occipital, tonsillar, deep and superficial cervical, posterior cervical, submaxillary, submental, and supraclavicular—for pain or swelling. About 50 perent of all lymphomas present as lymphadenopathy of the supraclavicular or cervical lymph nodes. Assess the neck for masses that may be present besides lymph nodes. Assess for asymmetry in facial grimaces and decreased facial sensation (cranial nerves V, VII). Check extraocular muscle function (CN III, IV, VI) and pupillary response (CN II, III). With the opthalmoscope, observe the optic disk for papilledema (also called choked disk), a sign that eventually occurs in about 75 percent of cancer patients. Evaluate hearing (CN VIII) using the Rinne and Weber tests. Dysfunction of these cranial nerves is frequently associated with brain tumors. Inspect with penlight and perform gloved, digital examination of the mouth. Assess for white or red sores that have persisted over one month; examine under dentures for areas of chronic irritation; check for areas of unusual texture, masses, or bleeding. Assess for tongue movement and lesions (most appear on the lateral tongue surfaces). Use tongue depressor to observe oropharynx and laryngeal mirror to observe hypopharynx and larynx. Inspect lips (most oral cancer occurs on the lower lip) for lesions. Inspection of the nares routinely yields limited information, but should be done if nasal bleeding is a reported symptom or in individuals at high risk for head and neck cancers. Inspect the external ear for skin changes. Palpate thyroid.

4. Back

Check for skin cancer and advanced lung cancer.

Examine skin. Listen to breath sounds. Lung cancer is very difficult to detect in its early stages, even when X-rays and sputum cytology are employed to aid detection. However, because auscultation of the lungs is a painless, easily accomplished assessment tool, it should be included in the cancer screening physical to detect gross areas of diminished breath sounds or pleural effusion that should be further evaluated in otherwise asymptomatic patients or for those exhibiting other signs of advanced lung cancer, such as hemoptysis, wheezing, and chronic cough. Unfortunately, the fact that these signs are also associated with smoking in general complicates differential assessment. Large trials have shown that early detection of lung cancer does not reduce the morbidity or mortality of the disease. As of 1985, the American Cancer Society does not recommend any assessment studies for detecting lung cancer, but recommends that, instead, attention be focused on prevention of this largely incurable disease.

5. Chest

Check for skin cancer and breast cancer.

Examine skin. Perform complete breast examination. Examine all four quadrants and breast tail for lumps, dimpling, edema or skin changes. It has been found that breast cancers are not distributed evenly in breast tissue; most are found in the upper, outer quadrant, and slightly more cancers are found in the right breast rather than the left. Assess the nipple for discharge, retraction, or dermatologic changes. Although breast cancer can present in almost any form, it is usually first seen as a solitary, unilateral, solid, hard, irregular, painless lump. Erythema, edema, or peau d'orange appearance of the skin usually indicate advanced disease.

6. Abdomen

Check for skin cancer and abdominal organ cancers.

There are no early physical signs for stomach cancer; assessment of gastrointestinal symptoms are the most important means of early detection of this cancer and are often vague. In about 25 percent of regionally involved stomach cancers, an epigastric mass is palpable. Pancreatic cancer produces no early signs to detect. A pancreatic mass may be palpable. Liver cancer most frequently presents as a painful mass from hepatomegaly, but splenomegaly, jaundice, ascites, fever, and dependent edema may also be seen with this cancer, and are associated with liver dysfunction. Percuss and palpate liver. Percuss and palpate the spleen for possible splenomegaly associated with lymphomas. Lymphomas usually present as a tumor of the lymph nodes or spleen.

Right colon cancers may be assessed as an abdominal mass. Screening to detect premalignant polyps has not proven easy except when polyps present in the portion of the colon accessible for digital exam. Screening sigmoidoscopy is expensive, does not provide a view of the right colon, and involves patient discomfort. Occult blood testing rarely detects polyps, but does detect ulcerated malignancies. Measurement of carcioembryonic antigen is not a useful screening procedure as it is proportional to the bulk of the tumor. Proportionally more colon cancers are now found in the right colon. During the early 1960s one-third of all colorectal cancers were found in the right half of the colon.

Kidney cancer is not easily detected at an early stage; painless hematuria is the most common presenting symptom. Flank palpation should be done to detect renal masses. Assess inguinal lymph nodes for possible role in metastasizing cancers or lymphomas.

7. *Legs and Feet*

Check for skin cancer and sarcomas of bone and soft tissue.

Examine skin, including soles of the feet. Assess for painless masses. Sarcomas frequently originate in the thigh area and are associated with some previous injury. If severe pain is associated with bone or muscle masses, it may signal a fast-growing tumor.

8. *Buttocks, Backs of Legs*

Check for skin cancer and sarcomas of bone and soft tissue. Examine skin. Assess for painless masses.

9. *Genital Area and Rectum*

FEMALES

Check for uterine (endometrial and cervical) cancers, ovarian, vaginal and colorectal cancers, and cancer of the vulva.

Inspect entire perineum. Invasive vulvar carcinoma has a high mortality rate, so early detection of this accessible tumor is an important part of the cancer screening examination. Vulvar lesions commonly present as white or pink and shiny lesions. Most are found on the anterior labia or around the clitoris.

With a warmed speculum, inspect the entire vagina and cervix. Obtain Papanicolaou smears of the endocervix and portio of the cervix before the manual examination. Perform a bimanual palpation of the pelvic organs and vaginal examination (two fingers in vagina and other hand over abdomen), followed by a rectovaginal examination (index finger in vagina, middle finger in anus) with guaiac testing of any stool encountered. Finally, a rectal examination should be performed to assess any lesions of the rectum or anus.

MALES

Check for cancer of the penis, prostate, and testes.

Examine penis for cancerous lesions. These usually present as painless nodules or wartlike growths. Phimosis may occur with growth of the lesion. Gently palpate the entire scrotum for painless masses, which may indicate testicular cancer. With patient bearing down, insert gloved finger into anus and examine prostate gland. The earliest palpable change is usually a discrete, firm nodule.

DISTRIBUTION OF COLORECTAL TUMORS

In past years, as many as 75 percent of large bowel cancers were present in the rectum and sigmoid colon and could be assessed by digital examination and sigmoidoscopy. Over the past twenty-five years, however, the distribution of colorectal cancer has moved proximally. Now, well over half of large bowel cancers are beyond the reach of the sigmoidoscope and about one-third are in the right colon. Thus, the cancer screening assessment will no longer be able to detect as many early colorectal cancers as previously was possible.

10. Skin Assessment

Although the majority of skin cancer deaths are attributable to malignant melanoma, basal cell and squamous cell carcinomas account for significant morbidity. By performing careful, periodic cutaneous examinations, people can increase the chance of discovering a cutaneous malignant melanoma in its early stages, when cure is possible.

Basal cell carcinomas usually present as pearly gray nodules with the vast majority located on the face, neck and backs of the hands. They are almost 100 percent curable.

Squamous cell carcinomas are usually seen as scaly, keratotic, slightly elevated lesions. They are most likely to spread when arising from a scar, chronically ulcerated area, or radiation-damaged area or in an immunosuppressed patient. Although they are more likely to metastasize than basal cell cancers, they are almost always locally controlled.

Cutaneous malignant melanoma has an excellent prospect for cure by surgical removal when diagnosed at an early stage. Thorough, periodic examination of the entire skin surface is important for early diagnosis. Once a melanoma is at least 3 mm thick, the five-year survival is only 48 percent.

Important features of malignant melanomas include asymmetry, irregular borders and variegated coloration. Colors portending melanoma in brown or black lesions are red, white, and blue. Blue is a particularly ominous shade in a mole. Some melanomas are uniformly colored, however, when they tend to be bluish.

Melanomas are frequently more than 6 mm in diameter when first identified. Pigmented lesions that develop after age forty are frequently melanomas or dysplastic nevi, which have an increased likelihood of developing into melanomas. Any change in a mole or the skin surrounding a mole should signal the examiner to look for melanoma. The average age at which melanoma is identified is fifty.

In the past, practitioners were taught to be suspicious only of pigmented lesions that enlarged, bled, darkened, or ulcerated. Actually, these features occur late in the disease process when metastasis is common. The examiner must be alert for less dramatic changes in preexisting moles and the development of new pigmented lesions with the characteristics of melanomas.

Melanomas can develop anywhere on the skin surface, although worldwide there has been a sharp increase in the incidence of these tumors on the head, neck, and truck of men, and the arms and lower legs of women. Sun-intolerant individuals with pale skin, blue eyes, and blond or reddish hair are more susceptible to developing malignant melanomas than dark-skinned and black individuals. Sunlight is the principle cocarcinogen in the development of melanoma, although a full understanding of the etiology of this disease is not yet known.

Health Counseling

This final portion of the overall assessment process is perhaps the most important. It is at this time that the practitioner can provide information that can influence the future health of the patient, in both a corrective and a preventive manner. The counseling should be organized into four components: an evaluation and discussion of the patient's own cancer risk derived from the data of the preceding assessment process, followed by three educative components (see Fig. 7.5). The seven warning signs of cancer (Fig. 7.6) should be explained or reviewed for all patients at this time. They should be counseled on the process of self-examination of the skin, including how to use a body chart to record the presence and size of moles and skin abnormalities. The practitioner should provide the patient with a copy of a body chart to use annually, or more often if deemed appropriate (see Fig. 7.7). Examination of the body for the presence

1. Patient's cancer risk from data

2. Seven warning signs of cancer

3. Self-examination
   skin
   breast
   testes
   masses

4. Risk reduction
   nutrition
   lifestyle
      tobacco
      alcohol
        sexual practices
   occupational factors
      regular cancer screening check-up
   individual identified factors

Figure 7.5   The Four Components of the Health Counseling Process

CANCER'S 7 WARNING SIGNALS

1. Change in bowel or bladder habits
2. A sore that does not heal
3. Unusual bleeding or discharge
4. Thickening or lump in breast or elsewhere
5. Indigestion or difficulty in swallowing
6. Obvious change in wart or mole
7. Nagging cough or hoarseness

If you have a warning signal, see your doctor

Figure 7.6   Common Signs of Cancer Explained During Health Counseling Phase

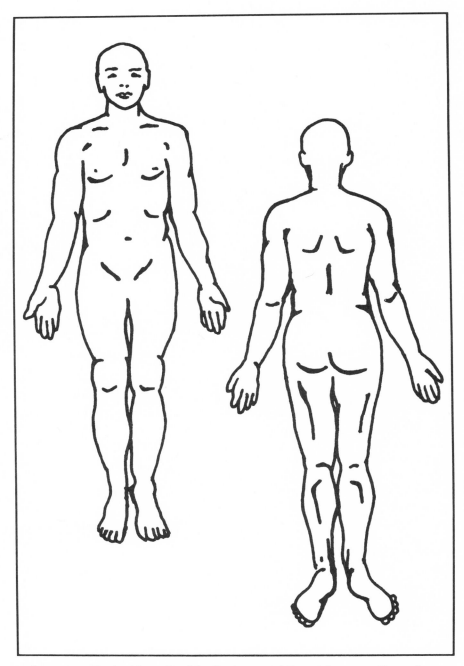

Figure 7.7 Body Chart Used by Patients and Practitioners to Record Skin Abnormalities and Moles during Self-Examination

1. Avoid obesity.

2. Cut down on total fat intake

3. Eat more high fiber foods, including whole grain
    cereals, fruits, and vegetables.

4. Include food rich in vitamins A and C in the daily
    diet.

5. Include cruciferous vegetables, such as cabbage,
    broccoli, brussel sprouts, kohlrabi and cauliflower
    in the diet.

6. Consumption of alcoholic beverages should be moderate.

7. Consumption of salt-cured, smoked and nitrite-cured
    foods should be moderate.

Figure 7.8   Dietary Recommendations for Reducing Cancer Risk
American Cancer Society, 1985

of masses, including enlarged lymph nodes, is another appropriate self-examination technique patients should be taught. Men and women should know how to examine their testes or breasts, respectively. The American Cancer Society's brochures and audiovisual programs, specifically designed to teach these techniques to patients, are available to nurses and others through local American Cancer Society chapters.

The risk reduction component for health counseling is designed to give the patient information on which to base decisions about what changes in life may be appropirate in order to modify cancer risk overall. The practitioner should cover nutrition (Fig. 7.8), lifestyle habits, occupational factors, health check-ups and any other factors deemed important for a specific patient based on the screening assessment. Discussion of how any changes might be made should be part of the counseling.

If the practitioner finds specific abnormalities during the general cancer screening assessment that warrant further consideration, the patient should be referred to a physician who can proceed with more thorough testing and evaluation of the patient's condition. It is useful to have a physician in mind who is willing to accept referred patients for those individuals who will request such a referral. Patients should be encouraged to return for further health teaching as both the practitioner and patient feel is appropriate, and patients should be made aware of the importance of scheduled periodic physical check-ups according to their age and physical condition.

8

Managing Technology of Cancer Care

In recent years, the practice of oncology nursing has been dramatically changed by the development of new technology for the administration of treatments or for symptom control. Included in this chapter are examples of new equipment that requires the expertise of a competent nursing staff. Even if a nurse practices at a center that does not routinely use some of this new technology, he or she should be familiar with the way the devices work and the indications for their use. In our mobile society, patients will arrive at a center with a piece of equipment that they expect to be understood by the oncology nurse, even if the exact protocols for its use are not.

Ambulatory Infusion Pump

This pump system is designed to deliver a continuous ambulatory infusion (CAI) to the patient in any setting. CAI systems are being used with hepatic artery catheters, right atrial catheters, intravenous catheters, Centrasils, Intrasils, and intraperitoneal catheters. Both cancer chemotherapy and analgesia are currently being delivered to cancer patients with these pumps. The Cormed II brand ambulatory infusion pump (see Figs. 8.1 and 8.2) is a prototype of this method of drug delivery. It has been widely available since 1985. The Cormed II permits a flow rate of from 4–5 ml per day from a 60 cc reservoir bag. Very fine adjustments in the flow rate are possible. The unit is approximately 11 cm x 12 cm x 4 cm, which is about the size of a pocketbook. The unit can operate continuously for five days before it needs recharging. An alternate power pack is used while the spent unit is being recharged. The sterile bag and tubing for drug delivery within the casing should be changed as needed or on a regular schedule: bag—every seven days; tubing—every two weeks.

Dennis (1984) has identified procedures for the use of the ambulatory infusion pump with a Hickman brand right atrial catheter for delivery of continuous morphine. Although her procedures are de-

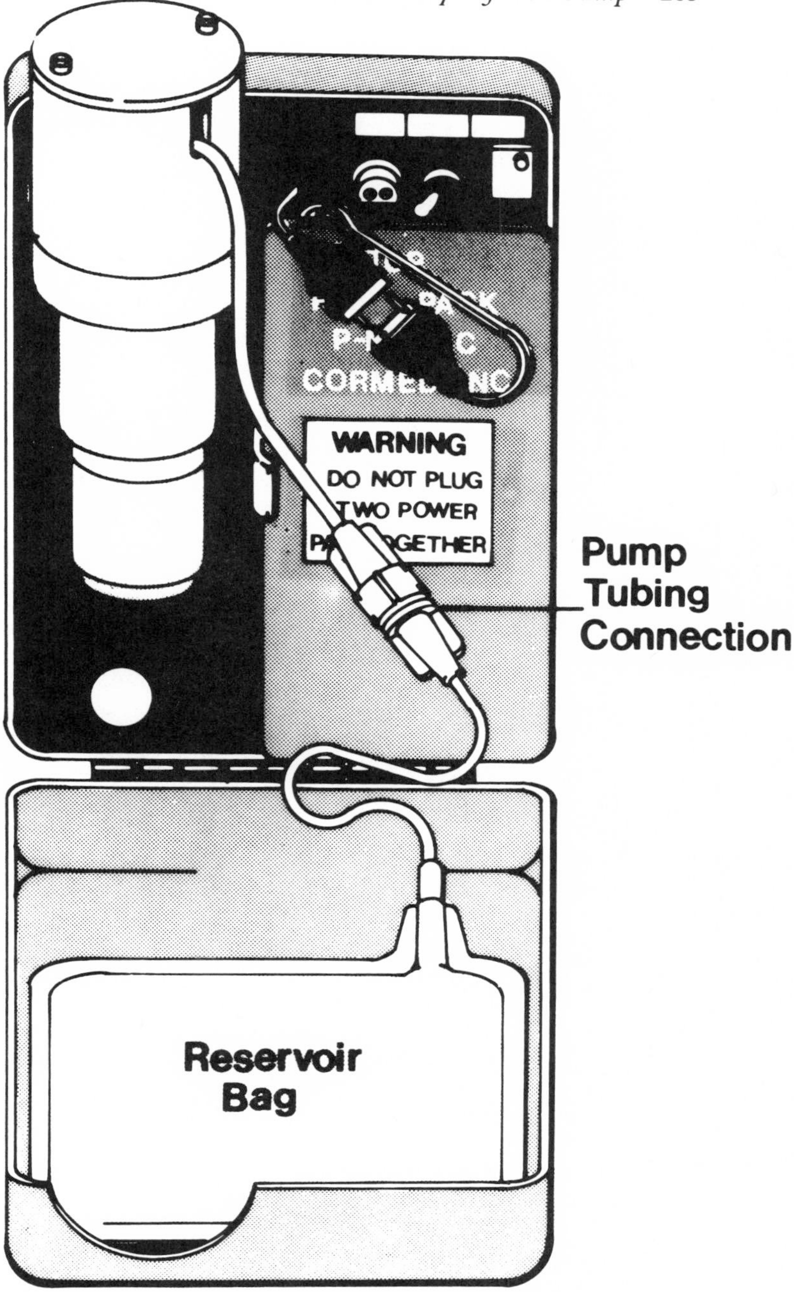

Figure 8.1 Cormed Infusion Pump: Schematic of Pumping Mechanism
Courtesy Cormed, Inc., Medina, New York

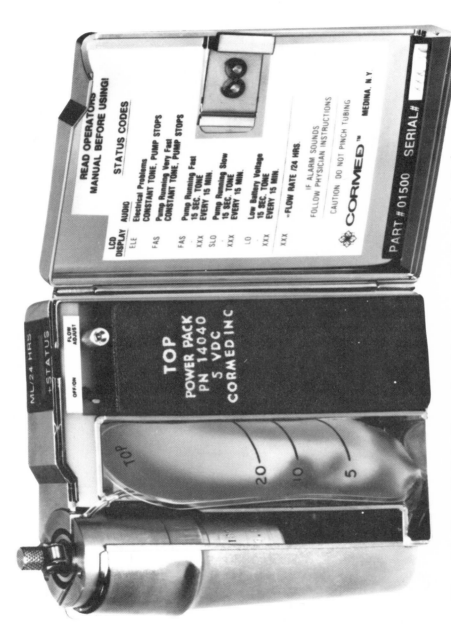

Figure 8.2 Cormed Infusion Pump: Actual Appearance of Inside of Power Pack

Courtesy Cormed, Inc., Medina, New York

signed for an older model of the Cormed pump, they remain relevant, and may be modified as follows to reflect changes in the pump and the expanded uses for this equipment.

Procedures for Use of the Ambulatory Infusion Pump

1. Fill the reservoir bag with the appropriate dilution of drug (using aseptic technique). (Patients are given a supply of pre-filled medication bags for use at home.)
2. Purge and thread the pump tubing through the pump.
3. Calculate the flow rate based on drug strength and hourly dosage desired(mg drug/hr divided by mg drug/cc), and set the machine.
4. Initially flush the intravenous line to the body with saline, as heparin may be incompatible with the drug to be infused (morphine, for example, is incompatible with heparin).
5. By needle and syringe, carefully fill the venous access device or intravenous line to the body with the drug to be infused, according to the capacity of the line (usually 1.5–2.5 cc). This is necessary because these pumps work so slowly that if saline were left in the line, it would be hours before the patient received any of the drug being infused.
6. Attach the pump tubing to the venous access device or intravenous line, and turn on the pump.
7. Check the flow rate and pump function over the next hour. A quiet humming is heard during pump operation.

These procedures are generally applicable for various models of ambulatory infusion pump systems. Patients are able to replace bags, tubing, and batteries, and set the pump on their own with professional help available as a back-up. For patients on continuous chemotherapy or other medications, this allows a measure of independence and control over their cancer treatment.

The pump itself should not be allowed to become wet; if patients wish to shower, they should place the pump in a secure plastic bag. It is all right to get the tubing wet. Bags and tubing used for chemotherapy should be returned to the clinic or hospital for proper disposal as biohazardous waste.

Most insurance companies cover the cost of CAI systems, which are significantly cheaper than in-patient drug therapy. For patients who can themselves manipulate the apparatus involved, or who have family members willing to do so, these pumps can significantly improve quality of life.

Implanted Intra-Arterial Infusion Pumps

This method of drug delivery is being used mainly in the treatment of primary or metastatic liver cancer, although other sites such as the head and neck are being evaluated for use of this infusion system. Implanted pumps are generally replacing hepatic arterial infusions via external catheters. The older technique utilizing an external catheter has been fraught with complications. Arterial thrombi, embolism, infection, and mechanical difficulties with the catheter itself have not been uncommon. The newer system utilizes a better tolerated plastic catheter and is entirely under the skin, factors that lessen the complication rate.

The rationale for treating liver cancer itself should be briefly addressed in this discussion of implanted intra-arterial infusion pumps. Generally, once cancer has been detected in the liver, prognosis is very poor and death may be expected within nine months unless the cancer is entirely resectable. Intra-arterial liver infusions are usually considered only for those patients thought to be curable, as their use in terminal disease has not been found to prolong life. It is now anticipated that direct treatment of the liver with chemotherapy, made possible with regional infusion systems, will result in extended survival time for patients whose cancer is not resectable if the cancer is not generally metastasic.

The Infusaid brand pump system has a catheter that is sutured to an appropriate vessel for perfusion of the entire liver and a pump that is implanted into a subcutaneous pocket in the right upper abdominal wall during a laparotomy. The pump itself has two chambers, one of which is filled with the drug to be delivered and the other, which is called the charging chamber, containing a fluorocarbon fluid. Filling the drug chamber provides passive power that causes the charging chamber to exert pressure on a bellows system, squeezing the drug slowly into the attached catheter and on to the liver. This system permits the continuous infusion of a concentrated drug to the liver with reduced systemic drug circulation, thus causing fewer side effects for the patient. The pump is accessed with huber needles (see page 278) via the main drug chamber or through a sideport that permits bolus injections, perfusion readings, and catheter flushing.

The most common side effect of pump placement is the formation of a seroma (accumulation of sterile fluid) in the pump pocket. This fluid can either be aspirated or allowed to reabsorb over a few weeks. Should infection occur after pump placement, the pump is generally removed, as infections with these systems are difficult to treat.

The two main restrictions on patients who have these pumps

implanted are that they must avoid blunt trauma to the pump site, and that they should avoid activities resulting in a prolonged increase in body temperature, pressure, or altitude. The latter restriction is required because such changes will increase the vapor pressure in the charging chamber and subsequently increase the flow rate of the drug being infused. Patients need to inform their physicians of temperature elevations over two degrees that persist beyond twenty-four hours, or of travel to an area of different elevation, both of which affect drug flow rates. Patients should also report anticipated air travel, as the pump can trigger the metal detectors at airports, and a letter of explanation by a physician may need to be part of travel planning.

An important point in patient teaching regarding these pumps is that patients must keep appointments to have the pump refilled regularly. Should the drug chamber go dry, the resultant cessation of flow through the catheter can cause a clot to form, resulting in permanent blockage. Cycles usually run for two to four weeks with implanted intra-arterial pump systems. Before each refill, a perfusion scan may be performed to ensure that a thrombus is not present in the catheter.

The oncology nurse is essential in the pump protocol for delivery of chemotherapy, as well as teaching and support of the patient. A general knowledge of how the pump works is important for overall oncology nursing competency.

Intraperitoneal Catheter Chemotherapy Infusion System

This modality is most often used to deliver cisplatin in the treatment of different abdominal malignancies, particularly ovarian cancer. It enables greater cell kill while decreasing the major toxic effects associated with systemic administration of the drug. The following explanation of how the intraperitoneal catheter is used for delivery of cisplatin in ovarian cancer can be generalized for an overall appreciation of the catheter's functioning.

A peritoneal catheter is inserted by the physician through the lower abdominal wall of the patient. Any ascitic fluid present is then drained in order to increase the concentration of cisplatin in the peritoneum during the treatment process. The cisplatin dose is mixed in two liters of warmed normal saline and allowed to flow by gravity drainage over ten to twenty minutes into the peritoneum. Once the cisplatin-saline mixture has been delivered, the catheter is clamped for four hours. This allows the cisplatin to bathe the tumor and exert its tumorcidal effect. The patient may be asked to turn from side to side during the treatment period to distribute the cisplatin evenly. After four hours, the catheter is unclamped and the infusion bag is lowered to allow gravity drainage of the fluid. This draining process may take up to two hours. If, as frequently happens, the entire two liters does not return, this fact is recorded, but no treatment is given.

The usual methods employed to prevent toxic effects when delivering high dose cisplatin by the intravenous route are also used with the peritoneal catheter route. Although significant systemic absorption does occur by this method, the direct bathing of an abdominal tumor is considered highly useful.

Patient–Controlled Analgesia System

The patient-controlled analgesia (PCA) system is currently being used in cancer care to allow patients to determine when they will receive a dose of analgesia and to allow them to actually deliver the dose. This is accomplished through the use of a computerized, secured pump system that is set by the nurse according to the physician's orders and is attached to an infusing intravenous line. A syringe of morphine sulfate is housed in a locked pump unit that delivers the drug whenever activated by the patient within the confines of the time intervals and dosage limits preset by the nurse. The patient activates the pump by pushing a button connected by cord to the pump unit. The system has a display function that indicates when the "lock-out" time interval is over and the patient can have another dose of analgesia. Frequently used "lock-out" periods are eight to ten minutes.

By delivering smaller doses of morphine sulfate (MS) over shorter time intervals, the patient does not experience the peaks and troughs of relief that occur with intramuscular administration of MS. Consequently, the patient is more alert and more consistently free from pain with this system than with an injection schedule. Although titrated, continuously infused intravenous MS is most often used for terminally ill patients in pain, the PCA system is a useful alternative in other situations as well, allowing patients to control the drug administration process with excellent pain relief. Many surgical patients on the PCA system use a lesser amount of analgesia to achieve adequate pain control than do those who recieve injections. Because the patient does not need to wait for the nurse who controls the analgesia delivery, the patient using the PCA system does not have the anxiety and pain related to waiting for requested medication. Furthermore, use of the PCA system frees the nurse for other duties.

A disadvantage of the system is that it requires a flowing intravenous line for its operation. Its use is therefore confined to the hospitalized patient for whom a flowing intravenous line is not an unacceptable inconvenience nor contraindicated.

Portable Subcutaneous Infusion Pump

Chemotherapeutic agents that can be safely administered subcutaneously may be candidates for delivery by means of a portable subcutaneous pump that allows for continuous administration of a drug in any setting. Holmes (1985) has described the use of the Auto-Syringe AS–3B pump for delivery of cytosine arabinoside in the treatment of acute leukemia. Cytosine arabinoside is the only antileukemic agent that can safely be administered by the subcutaneous route to date.

The Auto-Syringe pump is battery operated and delivers a prescribed drug at regularly programmed intervals into subcutaneous tissue. Every twenty-four hours the prefilled syringe, tubing, needle, and battery must be changed. The pump is easily loaded and primed by the patient or a nurse. There is no on-off switch with this model, so once the pump is set, it begins working. A red blinking light indicates that the pump is functioning properly. Infusions are completed within twenty-three to twenty-five hours.

The administration procedure for the subcutaneous pump first requires the selection of an appropriate site. For each infusion, a different site is selected, preferably on the abdominal wall, where the patient can easily visualize the area for self-administration of chemotherapy. The site selected is prepped with an alcohol swab, then pinched up in a fold of skin. A 27-gauge needle is inserted at a 15 degree angle to the skin up to its hub. It is secured with a sterile Band-Aid or transparent dressing placed over the insertion site. (If a Band-Aid is used it should be reinforced with tape over the tubing.) Tubing is looped and taped to the abdomen in order to prevent tension on the needle, which could result in dislodgement during the activities of daily living. Finally, the battery is secured and the pump checked for appropriate functioning. Although most normal activities can be undertaken during the infusion period, the patient should not bathe or shower until the infusion is completed. When the infusion is done, the needle is removed from the skin and the disposable equipment used in the infusion, disposed of in a safe manner. The patient or nurse handling the equipment should avoid direct contact of the antineoplastic agent with skin and place all items in a leak-proof container. Thorough hand washing should be done before and after each infusion period.

Microwave Hyperthermic System

The BSD–1000 microwave hyperthermic system is used to provide regional hyperthermia to superficial tumors, or tumors in the chest, abdomen, or pelvis. The system is computer-controlled, and hyperthermia therapy is administered in an electromagnetically screened room, which does allow for visual and verbal communication between the patient and treatment providers. Generally, initial treatments are done on an inpatient basis in order to evaluate patients for possible untoward effects of the hyperthermia. Thereafter, patients may come to the hyperthermia clinic on an outpatient basis for continuing therapy. Treatments are usually given daily for the initial five days, then twice weekly for up to four weeks. Moore (1984a and 1984b) clearly describes these procedures.

When used for internal tumors of the body trunk, the hyperthermia system consists of a cylinder that encloses the body trunk, with water-filled plastic bags creating contact between the cylinder heat source and the body skin surface. Although the water is initially cool, it warms very quickly once power is generated during therapy. In order to monitor internal temperatures, thermal probes penetrate into up to eight parts of the body. The probes are inserted through catheters placed in the body prior to the hyperthermia treatments. The catheters are positioned under local anesthesia directly into tumor masses as well as into adjacent body structures. Deeply placed catheters are positioned using computerized tomography for guidance. These catheters are blind-ended tubes that extend about one-half inch above the body surface and are sutured in place. A simple dry sterile dressing is placed over the catheter entry site. At the time of therapy, the dressings are removed, antiseptic ointment is placed around the catheter insertion point, and thermal probes are threaded through the catheters. During treatments, the patient rests on water bags under the trunk area, with the upper and lower body supported on tables. Water bags are also placed over the superior and medial aspects of the trunk enclosed by the cylinder. Clothing must be removed for direct contact of the water bags with the skin surface. A rectal thermometer catheter is then placed and read continuously by the computer during the treatment. Every ten minutes, therapy is interrupted so that a nurse can take an oral temperature and other vital signs, and attend to any other needs of the patient. Treatment is terminated when the patient can no longer tolerate the heat, or ideally when therapeutic temperatures have been sustained for at least thirty minutes. After treatment, the probes and thermometer are removed, the catheter sites are cleaned and redressed, and the patient evaluated, then returned to the hospital unit or allowed to go home.

The enervating nature of the hyperthermia sessions, the invasive thermometry, catheters, associated laboratory and radiology tests, and fears about the ultimate outcome of this experimental therapy are all aspects of regional microwave hyperthermia with the BSD–1000 that the nurse needs to consider (Moore 1984a and 1984b). Many of the principles and procedures described here can be generalized to other types of hyperthermia units that are beginning to be used throughout the country. Emotional and physical support are important aspects of nursing care during hyperthermia therapy, particularly due to its experimental and physically demanding nature.

In-dwelling Right Atrial Catheters

In 1979, Dr. Robert Hickman published an article describing the modification of a right atrial catheter (Broviac) he had been using with bone marrow transplant patients since 1976. The so-called Hickman in-dwelling right atrial catheter is now routinely used throughout the country for a variety of cancer patients as well as for other chronically ill patients (see Fig. 8.3). There are several manufacturers producing catheters similar to the original Hickman model today. A chief advantage of these silastic catheters over the older Broviac right atrial catheters is that they enable the infusion or sampling of blood through the catheter line.

Hickman-type right atrial catheters have two segments, a thick extravascular component and a thin intravascular tube. On the extravascular segment are one or two Dacron polyester fiber cuffs, usually one near the venous entrance site and one near the skin exit site. They serve as anchors to prevent catheter displacement, and as barriers to infection. The catheter is implanted by use of strict aseptic surgical technique under local anesthesia in a manner described by Heimbach and Ivey (1976). Generally, the intravascular segment is threaded through the cephalic vein to the superior vena cava into the entrance to the right atrium, under fluoroscopic guidance. If the cephalic vein is not viable, the right internal jugular vein is sometimes used. A subcutaneous tunnel is created from the vein entry site to a distal

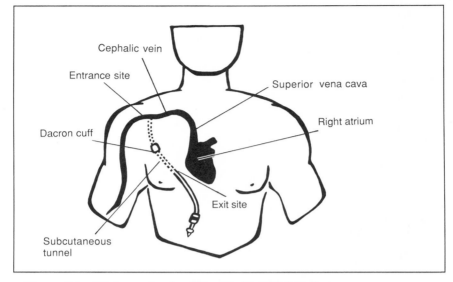

Figure 8.3   Hickman In-dwelling Right Atrial Catheter

point, usually on the chest or abdomen surface. The catheter is pulled through the tunnel so that it exits the body at the site chosen.

These in-dwelling right atrial catheters are useful for patients who will require repetitive blood sampling, or the delivery of a variety of drugs, analgesia, or total parenteral nutrition (TPN) for extended periods of time. Since the catheter does project from the body, a certain degree of caution must be taken to ensure asepsis at the catheter exit point. However, maintenance of the catheter is relatively easy for patients or practitioners, who can easily see and handle the catheter tip. The suggested maintenance of these catheters has changed over the last nine years. Where once masks and sterile gloves were used during catheter irrigations, today patients use a simple cleaning technique to maintain the catheters at home. When not in active use, the catheters must be heparinized at least once daily, usually with 2.5 cc of heparin at a concentration of 100 units per cc. The catheters are also heparinized after any infusions are completed. The exit site is maintained by simple soap and water washing, although if the patient wishes to go swimming, a transparent plastic dressing is recommended for use over the site. Men usually tape the catheter to the chest and women often tuck it into a brassiere.

The most frequent complications with these central venous catheters are clots and infection. Although not common, these complications may require that the catheter be removed, although they can usually be controlled by nursing interventions or the use of antibiotics. If repeated aspiration attempts do not remove a clot, a heparin solution of 1,000 units per cc is injected into the catheter lumen and left for one hour. This usually results in the easy aspiration of the clot. If this measure does not prove successful, a clinical nurse specialist may, on the order of the attending physician, instill a dilute solution of a fibrinolytic drug, such as Streptokinase (250,000 units in 2 cc) into the catheter to dissolve the clot within five to fifteen minutes. This latter procedure is expensive and carries significant side effects such as fever, bleeding, and anaphylaxis. Urokinase, another fibrinolytic drug, is less likely to cause patient reactions, but is more expensive. The manufacturer of one brand of these catheters states that the amount of clotting in these catheters is not enough to cause trouble even if it is flushed into the circulation, but aspriation attempts are the recommended procedure (Hurtubise et al. 1980).

Complications of the use of these catheters that require emergency measures are severing of the catheter or its dislodgement. As long as the catheter is clamped promptly after it is accidently severed (usually by scissors), nurses can temporarily repair the damaged catheter quite easily with no ill effects to the patient. After preparing the damaged catheter end so that it is aseptic and cleanly cut, an angiocath that fits snuggly is completely inserted into the catheter, after which the angiocath stylus is removed and the angiocath capped. The catheter is then splinted with a padded tongue blade and can be used immediately. Permanent repair of these catheters is done by clinical nurse specialists using a repair kit prepared by the catheter manufacturer.

In-dwelling right atrial catheters have occasionally become dislodged into soft tissue. This can be particularly hazardous if vesicants are infused through the catheter. Nurses should watch for swelling in the chest wall during infusions, or leaking at the site of catheter entrance to the chest wall. If blood cannot be withdrawn from the catheter, soft tissue displacement should be considered. There have also been reports of dislodgement into the internal jugular vein, resulting in superior vena cava syndrome. If arm, head, or neck swelling is noted in the patient with an in-dwelling right atrial catheter, further assessment for displacement is warranted.

For patients who prefer to remain independent while on drug therapy, TPN administration, or while requiring frequent or continuous analgesia, these catheters may be very useful. Because they do offer a direct access to the central circulation, patients may feel very vulnerable, particularly when the catheter is first placed, to exsanguination. Sufficient precautionary teaching, without instilling undue fear, is necessary. These catheters have been used successfully in patients for many years, usually remaining in place for about nine months, although some patients have maintained a Hickman-type catheter for eight or more years. These catheters cost about $50 per month to maintain, and third-party payers do not routinely pick up these expenses. Patients should be advised of the financial consequences of catheter placement before it is done.

The removal of these catheters is not difficult and is routinely done by clinical nurse specialists on an outpatient basis. Firm, steady pulling on the catheter for at least one to two minutes without jerking causes the catheter cuffs to loosen from the surrounding tissue, and the catheter slides out of the exit site. Minimal bleeding may be observed from the exit site; the vein entry site closes itself naturally without any interventions.

Small-Gauge Central Venous Catheters

An alternative to in-dwelling right atrial catheters such as the Hickman or Corcath are the small-gauge central venous catheters. Two examples are the Intrasil, which is placed in the basilic vein at the antecubital fossa, and the Centrasil, which is placed into the subclavian vein. These catheters are positioned by specially trained nurses for short-term (ninety-day maximum) use for the delivery of chemotherapy on an outpatient basis. They are not suitable for blood drawing. These catheters are similar to in-dwelling right atrial catheters, but have no subcutaneous tunnel, so are more likely to cause infection, although actual infection rates are very low. They require daily sterile dressing changes, which may be done by the patients themselves at home, and also require heparinization similar to that required for the right atrial catheters. Because of the awkward position of the exit site of these catheters, some patients may have difficulty handling dressing changes and heparinization; these catheters therefore cannot be used for all patients who wish to remain independent. A great advantage in their use, however, is the reduced expense of placement over that of an in-dwelling right atrial catheter. For patients who require short-term chemotherapy and can manipulate the maintenance equipment, they are an excellent resource.

Implanted Infusion Ports

Implanted infusion ports are the most recent vascular access devices on the market (Fig. 8.4). They are placed in a subcutaneous pocket in

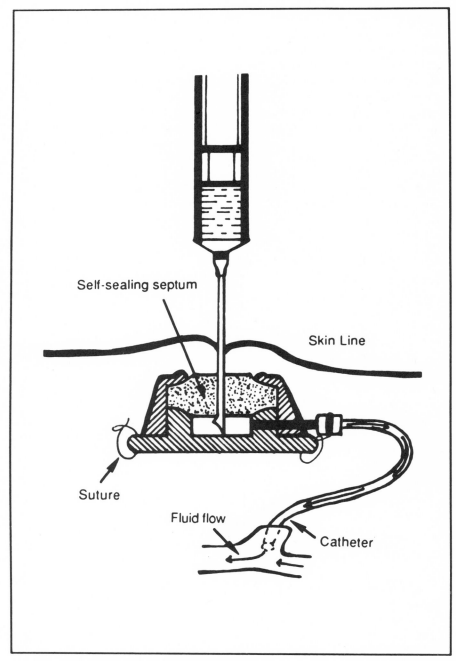

Figure 8.4   An Implanted Infusion Port

the chest wall, sutured into position, and accessed by breaking the skin surface with specially designed Huber needles. The ports consist of a self-sealing silicone septum with an attached catheter which is advanced into the right atrium. They are similar to in-dwelling right atrial catheters in the way in which they are placed, but are unique because the entire system is below the skin's surface. To access the device, the skin over the septum is cleaned and punctured by a Huber needle connected to a stop-cock and tubing for the administration of fluids, antibiotics, total parenteral nutrition, or blood. The catheters may also be used to take blood samples. The Huber needle has a finely deflected point that tears the septum rather than scoring it, so that some 500 to 1,000 punctures are allowed before the septum is considered no longer useful. The septum self-seals after each puncture.

Each time a port is used, it is first flushed with 3 cc of fluid to assure patency and correct positioning. If blood is aspirated or infused through the port, it is flushed with 20 cc of saline to assure that all blood cells are removed from the reservoir prior to heparinizing (3–5 cc of heparin at a concentration of 100 units per cc). When not in use, these implanted venous access devices are irrigated with heparin once every four weeks.

For continuous infusions, a Huber needle that is permanently bent at 90 degrees is placed in the septum. The needle is dressed in a sterile manner and taped securely to the chest wall for the length of the infusion. Afterwards, the septum is heparinized, and the needle may be removed or the tubing capped for later use. These implanted devices are not appropriate for multiple simultaneous infusions, as the double lumen in-dwelling right atrial catheters are, nor are they as easy to draw blood from as the Hickman-type catheters. The implanted devices also necessitate a variably painful needle puncture at each use. However, they do offer the advantages of being maintenance-free for a month at a time when not in active use and of involving a very low risk of infection.

Ommaya Reservoir

The Ommaya reservoir is used primarily to deliver antineoplastic drugs or analgesia into the cerebrospinal fluid (CSF). Resembling a flattened mushroom, it is made of silicone and has a diameter of 3.4 cm. Under local or general anesthesia, the reservoir is placed in the skull at the right frontal region over the coronal suture. A burr hole allows an attached catheter to be placed into a lateral brain ventricle, after which the reservoir is sutured to the pericranium and a scalp flap is sutured over the reservoir. Once placed, the reservoir fills with CSF from the ventricles and remains filled when not in use. These reservoirs are useful for about 200 punctures. To access the reservoir, the nurse places the patient in Trendelenberg position and assures that the hair over the reservoir is shaved and prepped with iodine. The scalp and reservoir are punctured with a 23 or 25-gauge butterfly needle or obliquely by a 25-gauge 1.5 inch straight needle. Initially, 3 cc of cerebral spinal fluid may be withdrawn by gravity drainage for use as a flush after medication instillation. Medications are given slowly in small volumes, after which the system may be flushed with reserved CSF, or alternately, the reservoir may be pumped to distribute the drug to the ventricles. Pumping is done by gently pressing the reservoir several times. Generally, patients are instructed to lie flat for 30 minutes after medication administration. The drugs given must not have preservatives in them that could cause neurotoxic reactions in the patient. Usually a solvent called Elliott's B solution or normal saline is used for mixing with medications. Patients can be maintained at home with the Ommaya reservoir if a family member can successfully handle accessing of the reservoir.

Possible side effects of the use of an Ommaya reservoir include nausea and vomiting, headache, and dizziness. If any of these symptoms lasts beyond a short time, it should be reported. Complications with the Ommaya reservoir include infection, malfunction, and misplacement, but these are rare occurrences. Displacement or malfunction assessment includes pumping the reservoir while keeping a finger on the scalp at the time of release to feel for CSF refill. If the patient complains of unusual neurological symptoms, the reservoir should be checked by a physician. Generally, these reservoirs are left in place permanently unless complications occur.

Patient Teaching

Because patient teaching is an integral part of managing cancer patients, general principles of adult learning are included here for reference by the oncology nurse (see Table 8.1). Implications for learning in a clinical setting are presented so that the nurse can apply the selected principles in a manner conducive to maximum learning for patients who need to become acquainted with technology, learning which usually occurs in a busy clinical environment.

Table 8.1 Guide to Teaching Adults in a Clinical Setting

Characteristics of Adult Learners	Selected Principles of Learning	Implications for Learning in a Clinical Setting
Highly motivated, therefore are ready to learn. Adult students can be anxious and lack self-confidence.	Readiness facilitates learning and presupposes psychological freedom, a freedom from discouragement and/or threat.	Provide a safe learning climate. One that: 1. separates learning from evaluating 2. allows freedom to start, stop, back-up, and start over when necessary. 3. provides for openness between learner and nurse.
Have sense of importance for new learning.	In order for learning to occur goals must be set and organized by the learner, or, the learner must be willing to accept the learning situation.	Provide learning experiences that: 1. will be meaningful to the learner. 2. are suited to learners capabilities. 3. are experienced centered.
Have concrete immediate needs for learning. At the same time have other responsibilities and need for their time. Are self-directed.	Participation in the learning process increases motivation, adaptability and speed of learning.	Discuss immediately. Use small groups if possible. Informal groups most acceptable.
Are more realistic than child learners. By tradition, socialize in small groups. Will progress in a learning situation only as far as is needed to achieve their purpose, or, is satisfying to them.	Learning is more apt to be retained when: 1. recall is used shortly after learning. 2. learned in the "real world" or in a situation much like that in which it is to be used. 3. is immediately preceding the time needed.	Provide the "real world" or simulated facilities, equipment and patient problems. Provide for individual instruction on a one to one basis.
Are unique individuals because of differences in nursing programs, years of practice and inactivity, self-concept and family support.	Practice distributed over time facilitates learning, yet repeated practice beyond achievement does not improve learning.	Repeat information or skills until learning appears to be attained, yet do not assign the same task over and over again. Make room for new learning.
Have the ability to relate new facts to a vast reservoir of experience or	Information concerning progress towards a learning goal facilitates learning.	

Are more rigid in their thinking because of an acquired pattern of behavior and belief system.

They tend to bring all their emotions to the learning experience. The adult student will undoubtedly be anxious and lack self-confidence.

New information that confirms beliefs and attitudes will facilitate learning. Information that contradicts those beliefs will inhibit learning.

Behavior can be changed. Reinforcement of newly learned behaviors will facilitate behavior change.

Treating adult students as dependent persons is conducive to creating conflict. Providing for a series of successes will help students to tolerate failures, and pave the way for learning from mistakes.

Provide immediate feedback on skill performance.

Provide periodic feedback on overall progress.

Build on knowledge from past experiences. Emphasize knowledge that learners have and not what they do not have. (Build on strengths)

Treat adults as co-learners.

Information compiled by Cynthia Mahoney, RN, Ph.D., Continuing Education Coordinator, Pacific Lutheran University

Appendix: Comprehensive Cancer Centers and Cancer Organizations

ALABAMA

Comprehensive Cancer Center
University of Alabama in
   Birmingham
1824 6th Avenue, S., Room 214
Birmingham, AL 35294
(205) 934-5077

CALIFORNIA

Kenneth Norris Jr. Cancer Research
   Institute
University of Southern California
Comprehensive Cancer Center
P.O. Box 33804
1441 Eastlake Avenue
Los Angeles, CA 90033-0804
(213) 224-6416

Jonsson Comprehensive Cancer
   Center
UCLA Medical Center—
   Room 10/247
Louis Factor Health Sciences
   Building
10833 Le Conte Avenue
Los Angeles, CA 90024
(213) 825-1532

CONNECTICUT

Yale University Comprehensive
   Cancer Center
School of Medicine
333 Cedar Street, Room WWW 205
New Haven, CT 06510
(203) 785-4095

DISTRICT OF COLUMBIA

Georgetown University/Howard
   University Comprehensive
   Cancer Center:

Vincent T. Lombardi Cancer
   Research Center
Georgetown University Medical
   Center
3800 Reservoir Road, N.W.
Washington, DC 20007
(202) 625-2042

Cancer Research Hospital
Howard University Hospital
2041 Georgia Avenue, N.W.
Washington, DC 20060
(202) 636-7697

FLORIDA

Comprehensive Cancer Center for
   the State of Florida
University of Miami Hospital and
   Clinics
1475 N.W. 12th Avenue
P.O. Box 016960 (D8-4)
Miami, FL 33101
(305) 548-4810

ILLINOIS

Illinois Cancer Council (includes
   institutions listed and several
   other health organizations):

Illinois Cancer Council
36 S. Wabash Avenue, Suite 700
Chicago, IL 60603
(312) 346-9813

Northwestern University Cancer
  Center
Health Sciences Building
303 E. Chicago Avenue
Chicago, IL 60611
(312) 266-5250

University of Chicago Cancer
  Research Center
5841 S. Maryland Avenue
Box 444
Chicago, IL 60637
(312) 962-6180

MARYLAND

Johns Hopkins Oncology Center
600 North Wolfe Street, Room 157
Baltimore, MD 21205
(301) 955-8822

MASSACHUSETTS

Dana-Farber Cancer Institute
44 Binney Street
Boston, MA 02115
(617) 732-3555

MICHIGAN

Comprehensive Cancer Center of
  Metropolitan Detroit
110 East Warren Street
Detroit, MI 48201
(313) 833-1088

MINNESOTA

Mayo Comprehensive Cancer
  Center
Mayo Clinic
200 First Street, S.W.
Rochester, MN 55905
(507) 284-2511

NEW YORK

Memorial Sloan-Kettering Cancer
  Center
1275 York Avenue
New York, NY 10021
(212) 794-6561

Roswell Park Memorial Institute
666 Elm Street
Buffalo, NY 14263
(716) 845-5770

Columbia University Cancer
  Center
College of Physicians & Surgeons
701 West 168th Street, Room 1208
New York, NY 10032
(212) 694-3647

NORTH CAROLINA

Comprehensive Cancer Center
Duke University Medical Center
227 Jones Building, Research Drive
P.O. Box 3814
Durham, NC 27710
(919) 684-2282

OHIO

Ohio State University
  Comprehensive Cancer Center
410 W. 12th Avenue, Suite 302
Columbus, OH 43210
(614) 422-5022

PENNSYLVANIA

Fox Chase/University of
  Pennsylvania Comprehensive
  Cancer Center:

Fox Chase Cancer Center
7701 Burholme Avenue
Philadelphia, PA 19111
(215) 728-2781

University of Pennsylvania Cancer
  Center
7 Silverstein Pavilion
3400 Spruce Street
Philadelphia, PA 19104
(215) 662-3910

TEXAS

University of Texas System Cancer
  Center
M. D. Anderson Hospital & Tumor
  Institute
6723 Bertner Avenue
Houston, TX 77030
(713) 792-6000

WASHINGTON

Fred Hutchinson Cancer Research
  Center
1124 Columbia Street
Seattle, WA 98104
(206) 467-4302

WISCONSIN

University of Wisconsin Clinical
  Cancer Center
600 Highland Avenue
Madison, WI 53792
(608) 263-8610

ORGANIZATIONS

National Headquarters
American Cancer Society, Inc.
777 Third Avenue
New York, NY 10017
(212) 371-2900

Office of Cancer Communications
National Cancer Institute
Building 31, Room 4B39
Bethesda, MD 20205
(301) 496-6792

Cancer Information Service
  numbers:

CIS: 1-800-4-CANCER
Alaska: 1-800-638-6070
Washington, DC: (202) 636-5700
Oahu: 524-1234 (call collect from
  neighbor islands)

(Spanish-speakers are available for
  callers from California—area
  codes 213, 714, 619,
  805—Florida, Georgia, northern
  New Jersey, New York City,
  and Texas. Daytime hours only.)

Leukemia Society of America, Inc.
733 Third Avenue
New York, NY 10017

United Ostomy Association, Inc.
2001 West Beverly Boulevard
Los Angeles, CA 90057

Make Today Count
P.O. Box 303
Burlington, Iowa 52601
(319) 753-6521

United Cancer Council, Inc.
1803 North Meridian Street
Indianapolis, IN 46202
(317) 923-6490

Bibliography
and References

Chapter One

Amenta, M. 1984. "Hospice USA 1984—Steady and holding." *Oncology Nursing Forum* 11, no. 5: 68–74.

American Cancer Society. 1980. *A Factbook for the Medical and Related Professions.* Professional Education Publication no. 3076-PE.

Anderson, J. L. 1984. "Insurability of Cancer Patients: A Rehabilitation Barrier." *Oncology Nursing Forum* 11, no. 2: 42–47.

Baird, S. B. 1985. "Administrative Support Issues and the Oncology Clinical Nurse Specialist." *Oncology Nursing Forum* 12, no. 2: 51–54.

Brown, H. G. 1983. "Unproven Methods of Cancer Management in the Market Place." Pp. 98–101 in *Proceedings of the 4th National Conference on Cancer Nursing, 1983.* New York: American Cancer Society.

Brown, J. K. 1985. "Ambulatory Services: The Mainstay of Cancer Nursing Care." *Oncology Nursing Forum* 12, no. 1: 57–59.

Burkhalter, P. K., and Donley, D. L. 1978. *Dynamics of Oncology Nursing.* New York: McGraw-Hill.

Davis, C. K. 1985. "Health Care Economic Issues: Projections for Oncology Nurses." *Oncology Nursing Forum* 12, no. 4: 17–23.

Donley, S. R. 1984. "The Effects of Changing Health Care Policy on Cancer Nursing." *Oncology Nursing Forum* 11, no. 4: 64–68.

Dyck, S., and Wright, K. 1985. "Family Perceptions: The Role of the Nurse Throughout an Adult's Cancer Experience." *Oncology Nursing Forum* 12, no. 5: 53–59.

Entmacher, P. S. 1975. "Insurance for the Cancer Patient." *Cancer* 36: 287–89.

Fitzgerald, R. 1981. "Life Insurance after Malignant Disease." *Annals of Internal Medicine* 95: 633–35.

Gallucci, B. B. 1985. "Selected Concepts of Cancer as a Disease: From the Greeks to 1900." *Oncology Nursing Forum* 12, no. 4: 67–71.

Goldberg, R. T. and Habeck, R. 1982. *Vocational Rehabilitation of Cancer Clients: Review and Implications for the Future.* Rehabilitation Counseling Bulletin 26: 18–27.

Grimaldi, P. 1983. "New Medicare DRG Payment Calculations Issued." *Nursing Management* 14, no. 11: 19–23.

Grumet, G. N. 1978. "The Hospice Movement." *Medical Challenge* (September): 18–20.

Hamric, A. B. 1985. "Cancer Nursing Specialist Role Evaluation." *Oncology Nursing Forum* 12, no. 2: 51–57.

Hilkemeyer, R. 1982. "Update on Nursing Issues: A Historical Perspective in Cancer Nursing." *Oncology Nursing Forum* 9, no. 2: 47–54.

Hirctzka, S. 1985. "Knowledge and Attitudes of Persons with Cancer Towards the Use of Unproven Treatment Methods." *Oncology Nursing Forum* 12, no. 1: 36–42.

Holmes, B. C. 1985. "Private Practice in Oncology Nursing." *Oncology Nursing Forum* 12, no. 3: 65–69.

Horton, J., and Hill, G. J. 1977. *Clinical Oncology.* Philadelphia: W. B. Saunders. Pp. 182–87.

Howard-Ruben, J., and Miller, N. 1984. "Unproven Methods of Cancer Management. Part II: Current Trends and Implications for Patient Care." *Oncology Nursing Forum* 11, no. 1: 67–74.

Joel, L. 1983. "DRGs: The State of the Art of Reimbursement for Nursing Services." *Nursing and Health Care* 4, no. 12: 560–63.

Larson, P. J. 1984. "Important Nurse Caring Behaviors Perceived by Patients with Cancer." *Oncology Nursing Forum* 11, no. 6: 46–50.

Levitt, M. M., ed. 1981. *Caring: An Essential Human Need.* Thorofare, N.J.: Slack, Inc.

Martin, M. C., and Brink, G. R. 1980. "Setting Up an In-Hospital Hospice." *Hospital Forum* (January–February): 7–10.

McKenna, R. J. 1984. "Employment and Insurance Issues for the Cancer Patient." Pp. 36–49 in *Proceedings of the 4th National Conference on Cancer Nursing, 1983.* New York: American Cancer Society.

Medicare Regulation: Final Report. 1984. Federal Register 49, no. 1: 234.

Mellette, S. J. 1985. "The Cancer Patient at Work." *CA-A Cancer Journal for Clinicians* 35, no. 6: 360–73.

Meyer, E. L. 1984. "The War Between Doctors and Nurses." *Family Circle* (November 13): 250–55.

Miller, N. J., and Howard-Ruben, J. 1983. "Unproven Methods of Cancer Management. Part I: Background and Historical Perspectives." *Oncology Nursing Forum* 10, no. 4: 46–53.

Mooney, K. H. 1984. "Why People Seek Unproven Methods of Cancer Treatment." Pp. 101–5 in *Proceedings of the 4th National Conference on Cancer Nursing, 1983.* New York: American Cancer Society.

Mortenson, L., and Winn, R. 1983. *The Potential Negative Impact of Prospective Reimbursement on Cancer Treatment and Clinical Research Progress.* Cancer Program Bulletin 9, no. 3: 7–9.

Moseley, J. R., and Brown, J. S. 1985. "The Organization and Operation of Oncology Units." *Oncology Nursing Forum* 12, no. 5: 17–24.

Nevidjon, B., and Warren, B. 1984. "Documenting the Activities of the Oncology Clinical Nurse Specialist." *Oncology Nursing Forum* 11, no. 3: 54–55.

Ogle, M. E. 1983. "States of Burnout Among Oncology Nurses in the Hospital Setting." *Oncology Nursing Forum* 10, no. 1: 31–34.

Oncology Nursing Forum. 1985. A report from the First National Invitational Conference. 12, no. 2: 35–62.

Orsolits, M. 1984. "Effects of Organizational Characteristics on the Turn-over in Cancer Nursing." *Oncology Nursing Forum* 11, no. 1: 59–63.

Outcome Standards for Cancer Nursing Practice, 1979. Kansas City, Mo.: American Nurses' Association.

Rogers, J. 1985. "You're Leaving When? Looking at Recruitment and Retention in Today's Economy." *Oncology Nursing Forum* 12, no. 4: 72–75.

Schmitt, D. 1984. "Caring for Patients Who Seek Unproven Methods." Pp. 106–9 in *Proceedings of the 4th National Conference on Cancer Nursing, 1983.* New York: American Cancer Society.

Spross, J., and Donoghue, M. 1984. "The Future of the Oncology Nursing Specialist." *Oncology Nursing Forum* 11, no. 1: 74–78.

Stanfill, P. H., and McDonnell, J. W. 1985. "Determining Nursing Costs: A Strategy for Professional Survival." *Oncology Nursing Forum* 12, no. 5: 79–84.

Tillman, Michael C. 1984. "A Comparison of Nursing Care Requirements of Patients on General Medical-Surgical Units and on an Oncology Unit in a Community Hospital." *Oncology Nursing Forum* 11, no. 4: 42–45.

U.S. Dept. of Health and Human Services. 1985. *Taking Time.* NIH Publication no. 85-2059.

Yasko, Joyce M., and Fleck, A. 1984. "Prospective Payment (DRGs): What Will Be the Impact on Cancer Care?" *Oncology Nursing Forum* 11, no. 3: 63–72.

Weisman, A. D. 1979. *Coping with Cancer.* New York: McGraw-Hill.

Chapter Two

American Cancer Society (ACS). 1978. *Proceedings of the American Cancer Society and National Cancer Institute National Conference on Nutrition in Cancer.* Professional Education Publication no. 3025-PE. New York: American Cancer Society.

———. 1984. Second National Conference on Diet, Nutrition and Cancer, September 5–7. Houston.

———. 1985. *Cancer Facts and Figures—1985.* New York: American Cancer Society.

Brady, J.; Laimins, L. A.; and Khoury, G. 1984. "Stimulation of Gene Expression by Viral Transforming Proteins." Pp. 105–10 in *Cancer Cells*. New York: Cold Spring Harbor Laboratory.

Cameron, E. 1983. "Vitamin C and Cancer: An Overview." *International Journal of Nutritional Research* 23 (suppl): 115–27.

Cochran, B. H.; Reffel, A. C.; Callahan, J. N.; et al. 1984. "Cell-Cycle Genes Regulated by Platelet-Derived Growth Factor." Pp. 51–56 in *Cancer Cells*. New York: Cold Spring Harbor Laboratory.

DeWys, W. D. 1985. "Dietary Prevention of Cancer." Paper at Conference on Dietary Prevention of Cancer and Nursing Management of Bowel Cancer, Tacoma General Hospital, Tacoma, Washington. November 1.

Doll, R., and Peto, R. 1981. *The Causes of Cancer*. New York: Oxford University Press.

Ernster, V. L.; Sacks, S. T.; Holly, S. A.; et al. 1985. *U.S. Cancer Incidence Rates by Sex, Race, and Age: Graphics of SEER Program Data*. American Cancer Society, Professional Education Publication no. 3392-PE. New York.

Fat and Cancer: How Fat in Diet Affects Cancer Risk. 1984. American Institute for Cancer Research Newsletter 5 (Fall): 1–6.

Freedman, A. E.; Gilden, R. V.; Vernon, M. L.; et al. 1973. "5-Bromo-2'-deoxyuridine Potentiation of Transformation of Rat-Embryo Cells Induced in Vitro by 3-Methylcholanthrene." *Proceedings of the National Academy of Science U.S.A.* 70: 2415–19.

Greenvald, P. 1984. "Manipulation of nutrients to prevent cancer." *Hospital Practice* 19, no. 5: 119–34.

Higginson, J. 1983. "The Face of Cancer Worldwide." *Hospital Practice* 18, no. 11: 145–57.

Kamata, T., and Feramisco, J. R. 1984. "Is the Ras Oncogene Protein a Component of the Epidermal Growth Factor Receptor System?" Pp. 11–16 in *Cancer Cells*. New York: Cold Spring Harbor Laboratory.

Larson, E. 1983. "Epidemiologic Correlates of Breast, Endometrial, and Ovarian Cancer." *Cancer Nursing* 6, no. 4: 295–362.

McClure, D. B.; Dermody, M.; and Topp, W. C. 1984. "In Vitro Correlates of Tumorigenicity of REF52 Cells Transformed by Simian Virus 40." Pp. 19–24 in *Cancer Cells*. New York: Cold Spring Harbor Laboratory.

McDonald, J. 1985. "Understanding Carcinogenesis—Its Mechanism and Causes." *Issues in Oncology* 2, no. 3: 2–3.

National Institute of Health (NIH). 1979. "Estrogen Use and Post-menopausal Women." Consensus Development Conference Summary. Washington, D.C.

Office of Technology Assessment. 1982. *Cancer Risk*. Boulder, Colo.: Westview Press.

Pines, M. 1981. *Medicine and You*. National Institute of Health Publication no. 81-2140. Washington, D.C.: U.S. Department of Health and Human Services.

Pitot, H. C. 1981. *Fundamentals of Oncology,* 2d ed. New York: Marcel Dekker.

Rensberger, B. 1984. "Cancer—the New Synthesis." *Science 84* (September): 28–40.

Schottenfeld, D., and Fraumeni, J. F., ed. 1982. *Cancer Epidemiology and Prevention.* Philadelphia: W. B. Saunders.

Shamberger, R. J. 1984. "Genetic Toxicology of Ascorbic Acid." *Mutation Research* 133: 135–59.

Stolley, P. D. 1982. "Drugs." In *Cancer Epidemiology and Prevention,* ed. D. Schottenfeld and J. F. Fraumeni. Philadelphia: W. B. Saunders.

Thomas, D. 1985. "Cancer Epidemiology, EPI 524." University of Washington Graduate Course Syllabus, spring semester. Seattle, Washington.

U.S. Department of Health and Human Services. 1985. *Diet, Nutrition and Cancer Prevention.* National Institute of Health Publication no. 85-2711. Washington, D.C.

Wynder, E. L., and Rose, D. P. 1984. "Diet and Breast Cancer." *Hospital Practice* 19, no. 4: 73–88.

Zeigler, R. G.; Morris, L. E.; Blot, W. J.; et al. 1981. "Esophageal Cancer Among Black Men in Washington, D.C. II. Role of Nutrition." *Journal of the National Cancer Institute* 67: 1199–1206.

Chapter Three

American Cancer Society. 1983. *Cancer Manual.* 6th ed. Boston: ACS, Massachusetts Division.

American Society of Clinical Oncologists. 1985. *Interferon Research Continuing at Various Institutions.* Report No. 4. Richmond, Va.: A. H. Robins Co.

Barry, L., and Booher, R. 1985. "Promoting the Responsible Handling of Antineoplastic Agents in the Community." *Oncology Nursing Forum* 12, no. 5: 41–46.

Boehringer Ingelheim Pharmaceuticals, Inc. 1985a. "Interferon May Help in Hairy-cell Leukemia." *Oncology Update* 12: 4–5.

———. 1985b. "Some Lymphomas Respond to Monoclonal ABs." *Oncology Update* 12: 4.

Borden, E. 1984. "Progress Toward Therapeutic Application of Interferons, 1979–1983." *Cancer* 54: 2770–76.

Bull, J. M. 1982. "Whole Body Hyperthermia as an Anticancer Agent." *Cancer* 32, no. 2: 123–26.

Cady, B. 1983. "Surgery." Pp. 47–71 in *Cancer Manual.* Boston: American Cancer Society, Massachusetts Division.

Capizzi, R. L. 1985. "Schedule-Dependent Drug Interactions in Cancer Therapy." *Mediguide to Oncology* 4, no. 3: 2–6.

Cavaliere, R.; Ciocatto, E. C.; Giovanella, B. C.; and Ada, P. C. 1967. "Selective Heat Sensitivity of Cancer Cells: Biochemical and Clinical Studies." *Cancer* 20: 1351–81.

Chabner, B. A.; Fine, R.; Allegra, B. C.; Yeh, G. W.; and Curt, G. C. 1984. "Cancer Chemotherapy." *Cancer* 54: 2599–2608.

Champagne, E. E., and Kane, N. E. 1980. "Teaching Program for Patients Receiving Interstitial Radioactive Iodine-125 for Cancer of the Prostate." *Oncology Nursing Forum* 7, no. 1; 12–16.

Cloak, M. M.; Connor, T. H.; Stevens, K. R.; Theiss, J. C.; Alt, J. M.; Matney, T. S.; and Anderson, R. W. 1985. "Occupational Exposure of Nursing Personnel to Antineoplastic Agents." *Oncology Nursing Forum* 12, no. 5: 33–40.

DiJulio, J. E., and Bedigian, J. S. 1983. "Hybridoma Monoclonal Antibody Treatment of T-cell Lymphomas: Clinical Experience and Nursing Management." *Oncology Nursing Forum* 10, no. 2: 24–28.

"Experts Urge Care in Handling Chemotherapeutic Drugs." 1983. *Cancer Nursing News* 2, no. 6: 1–3.

Farris, J. S., and Mayer, D. 1983. "Patient Education: A Guide to Interferon for Patients and Nurses." *Oncology Nursing Forum* 10, no. 4: 65–69.

Garvey, E. 1984. "Care of the Patient Undergoing Interferon Treatment." *Cancer Nursing* 6, no. 4: 303–6.

Grady, E. D.; McLaren, J.; Auda, S. P.; McGinley, P. H. 1983. "Combination of Internal Radiation Therapy and Hyperthermia to Treat Liver Cancer." *Southern Medical Journal* 76, no. 9: 1101–6.

Gross, L. 1983. *Oncogenic Viruses.* New York: Pergamon Press.

Hart, C. N., and Rasmussen, D. 1982. "Patient Care Evaluation: A Comparison of Current Practice and Nursing Literature for Oral Care of Persons Receiving Chemotherapy." *Oncology Nursing Forum* 9, no. 2: 22–27.

Harwood, K. V. 1984. "Extravasation of Chemotherapeutic Agents." *Issues in Oncology* 1, no. 2: 6–8.

Hassey, K. 1985. "Demystifying Care of Patients with Radioactive Implants." *American Journal of Nursing* 85, no. 7: 788–92.

Haus, E.; Halberg, F.; and Schewing, L. E. 1972. "Increased Tolerance of Leukemia Mice to Ara-binosyl Cytosine with Schedule Adjusted to Circadian System." *Science* 177:80–82.

Hilderley, L. 1983. "Clinical Reviews: Skin Care in Radiation Therapy, a Review of the Literature." *Oncology Nursing Forum* 10, no. 1: 51–57.

Hrushesky, W. J. 1984. "The Effect of Anticancer Drug Timing on Therapeutic Index." *Mediguide to Oncology* 4, no. 2: 1–5.

Hughes, C. B. 1986. "Giving Cancer Drugs: Some Guidelines." *American Journal of Nursing* 86, no. 1: 34–38.

Hyland, S.; Loughner, J.; and Bonnett, J. 1979. *University of Rochester Cancer Center Chemotherapy Handbook*. Rochester: University of Rochester.

Jeffs, C., and Laszlo, J. 1983. "A Coordinating Role for the Nursing Clinician in a Phase I Interferon Study." *Cancer Nursing* 6, no. 6: 379–84.

Jones, R. B.; Frank, R.; and Mass, T. 1983. "Safe Handling of Chemotherapeutic Agents: A Report from the Mt. Sinai Medical Center." *CA-A Cancer Journal for Clinicians* 33, no. 5: 35–42.

Kapp, J. A.; Pierce, C. W.; and Sorensen, C. M. 1984. "Antigen-Specific Suppressor T-cell Factors." *Hospital Practice* (August): 85–98.

Kreamer, K. M. 1982. "Anaphylaxis Resulting from Chemotherapy." *Oncology Nursing Forum* 8, no. 4: 13–16.

Laughlin, R. A.; Landeen, J. M.; and Habal, N. B. 1979. "The Management of Inadvertent Sub-cutaneous Adriamycin Infiltration." *American Journal of Surgery* 137: 408–12.

Levene, M. B., and Harris, J. R. 1982. "Radiation Therapy." Pp. 27–71 in *Cancer Manual*. Boston: American Cancer Society, Massachusetts Division.

Mayer, D. K.; Hetrick, K.; Riggs, C.; et al. 1984. "Weight Loss in Patients Receiving Recombinant Leukocyte A Interferon." *Cancer Nursing* 7, no. 1: 53–56.

Mayer, D. K., and Smalley, R. 1983. "Interferon: Current Status." *Oncology Nursing Forum* 10, no. 4: 14–19.

Moore, C. L. 1984a. "Hyperthermia: A Modern Experiment in Cancer Treatment." *Oncology Nursing Forum* 11, no. 2: 31–36.

———. 1984b. "Nursing Management of the Patient Receiving Local or Regional Hyperthermia." *Oncology Nursing From* 11, no. 3: 40–44.

Nguyen, T. V.; Theiss, J. C.; and Matney, T. S. 1982. "Exposure of Pharmacy Personnel to Mutogenic Antineoplastic Drugs." *Cancer Research* 42, no. 11: 4792–96.

Oldham, R. K.; Thurman, G.; Talmadge, J.; Stevenson, H. C.; and Foon, K.A. 1984. "Lymphokines, Monoclonal Antibodies and Other Biological Response Modifiers in the Treatment of Cancer." *Cancer* 54: 2795–2806.

Oncology Nursing Society. 1984. Cancer chemotherapy: Guidelines and recommendations for nursing education and practice. Philadelphia: ONS.

Pitot, H. C. 1981. *Fundamentals of Oncology*. New York: Marcel Dekker.

Quesada, J., Stevenson, H. C.; and Poste, G. 1984. "Alpha Interferon for Induction of Remission in Hairy-cell Leukemia." *New England Journal of Medicine* 310, no. 1: 15–18.

Richter, M. P.; Laramore, G.; Griffin, T.; and Goodman, R. L. 1984. "Current Status of High Linear Energy Transfer Irradiation." *Cancer* 54: 2814–22.

Rogers, J. E. 1983. "Catching Cancer Strays." *Science* 83 (July–August): 42–48.

Schlom, J.; Greiner, J.; Hand, P.; Colcher, D.; Inghirami, G.; Weeks, M.; Pestka, S.; Fisher, P. B.; Noguchi, P.; and Kufe, D. 1984. "Monoclonal AB to Breast Cancer—Associated Antigens as Potential Reagents in the Management of Breast Cancer." *Cancer* 54: 2777–94.

Scogna, D. M., and Schoenberger, C. S. 1982. "Biological Response Modifiers: An Overview and Nursing Implications." *Oncology Nursing Forum* 9, no. 1: 45–49.

Skeel, R. T., ed. 1982. *Manual of Cancer Chemotherapy.* Boston: Little, Brown.

Stevenson, D.; Emmrich, B.; and Lucas, V. 1985. "Preventing Extravasation During Administration of Antineoplastic Drugs." *Oncology Nursing Forum* (Letter to Practice Corner) 12, no. 2: 83.

Stewart, J. R., and Gibbs, F. 1984. "Hyperthermia in the Treatment of Cancer." *Cancer* 54: 2823–30.

Storm, F. K., and Morton, D. L. 1983. "Localized Hyperthermia in the Treatment of Cancer." *CA-A Cancer Journal for Clinicians* 33, no. 1: 44–47.

Suppers, V., and McClamrock, E. 1985. "Biologicals in Cancer Treatment: Future Effects in Nursing." *Oncology Nursing Forum* 12, no. 3: 27–32.

Teta, J., and O'Conner, L. 1984. "Local Tissue Damage from 5-fluorouracil Extravasation." *Oncology Nursing Forum* 11, no. 4: 54.

Tyson, L. B., and Grossano, D. 1984. "Handling Antineoplastic Agents—Potential Hazards." *Issues in Oncology* 1, no. 4: 4–5.

U.S. Department of Health and Human Services. 1983. *Recommendations for the Safe Handling of Parenteral Antineoplastic Drugs.* National Institute of Health Publication no. 83-2621. Washington, D.C.

———. 1984. *Cancer Treatment Reports.* National Institute of Health Publication no. 84-22. Washington, D.C.

———. 1985. *Radiation Therapy and You: A Guide to Self-help During Treatment.* National Institute of Health Publication no. 85-2227. Washington, D.C.

Venitt, S.; Crofton-Sleigh, C.; et al. 1984. "Monitoring Exposure of Nursing and Pharmacy Personnel to Cytotoxic Drugs." *Lancet* 1, no. 8368: 74–77.

Vincent, B. J. 1985. "Investigational Chemotherapy." Paper presented in January in Seattle through Medical Media Associates.

Vrevevoe, D. L.; Derdiarian, A.; Sarna, L. P.; et al. 1981. *Concepts of Oncology Nursing.* Englewood Cliffs, N.J.: Prentice-Hall.

Weiss, R. B., and Trush, D. M., 1982. "A Review of the Pulmonary Toxicity of Cancer Chemotherapeutic Agents." *Oncology Nursing Forum* 9, no. 1: 16–21.

Wilson, R. E. 1984. "Surgical Oncology." *Cancer* 54: 2595–98.

Wood, H., and Ellerhorst-Ryan, J. 1984. "Delayed Adverse Skin Reactions Associated with Mitomycin-C Administration." *Oncology Nursing Forum* 11, no. 4: 14–19.

Yasko, J. M. 1983. *Guidelines for Cancer Care: Symptom Management.* Reston, Va.; Reston.

Chapter Four

Academy of Professional Information Services. 1982. "Two Newer Antiemetic Agents Seen Promising in Cancer Chemotherapy." *Symposium Highlights.* (September). New York.

Arnold, C. 1984. "The Macrobiotic Diet: A Question of Nutrition." *Oncology Nursing Forum* 11, no. 3: 50–54.

Baldwin, P. D. 1983. "Epidural Spinal Cord Compression Secondary to Metastatic Disease: A Review of the Literature." *Cancer Nursing* 6, no. 6: 441–46.

Beck, S. 1979. "Impact of a Systemic Oral Protocol on Stomatitis After Chemotherapy." *Cancer Nursing* 2, no. 3: 185–99.

Berstein, I. 1985. "Etiology of Anorexia in Cancer." Paper read at American Cancer Society Conference on Diet and Cancer, January, Houston.

Biomedical Information Corp. 1982. *Cancer Chemotherapy: Controlling Side Effects.* (November) New York.

Brandt, B. 1984. "A Nursing Protocol for the Client with Neutropenia." *Oncology Nursing Forum* 11, no. 2: 24–30.

Carlson, A. C. 1985. "Infection Prophylaxis in the Patient with Cancer." *Oncology Nursing Forum* 12, no. 3: 56–64.

Cleeland, C. S. 1984. "The Impact of Pain on the Patient with Cancer." *Cancer* 54: 2635–41.

Cohen, D. G. 1984. "Metabolic Complications of Induction Therapy for Leukemia and Lymphoma." *Cancer Nursing* 6, no. 4: 307–10.

Cotanch, P. 1985. "Self-hypnosis Has Anti-emetic Effect in Youth." *Oncology Update* 2: 8–9.

Cotanch, P.; Hockenberry, M.; and Herman, S. 1985. "Self-hypnosis as Antiemetic Therapy in Children Receiving Chemotherapy." *Oncology Nursing Forum* 12, no. 4: 41–48.

Cronin, C. 1982. *The Clinical Management of Emesis in the Cancer Patient.* Symposium Highlights, Academy of Professional Information Services, Inc. (September).

Donoghue, M.; Nunnally, C.; and Yasko, J. 1982. *Nutritional Aspects of Cancer Care.* Reston, Va.: Reston.

Foley, K. M. 1985. "The Treatment of Cancer Pain." *New England Journal of Medicine* 313: 84–95.

Foltz, A. T. 1980. "Nursing Care of Ulcerating Metastatic Lesions." *Oncology Nursing Forum* 7, no. 2: 8–13.

Gannon, C. T. 1983. "Bleeding Due to Thrombocytopenia." In *Guidelines for Cancer Care,* ed. J. Yasko. Reston, Va.: Reston.

Gralla, R. 1982. "Cancer Chemotherapy: Controlling Side Effects." *Oncology Information* (Biomedical Information Corp.) (September–October).

Graze, P. 1980. "Bone Marrow Failure: Management of Anemia, Infections, and Bleeding in the Cancer Patient." Pp. 961–83 in *Cancer Treatments,* ed. C. Haskell. Philadelphia: W. B. Saunders.

Hart, C. N., and Rasmussen, D. 1982. "Patient Care Evaluation: A Comparison of Current Practice and Nursing Literature for Oral Care of Persons Receiving Chemotherapy." *Oncology Nursing Forum* 9, no. 2: 56–61.

Hogan, C. 1983. "Nausea and Vomiting." In *Guidelines for Cancer Care,* ed. J. Yasko. Reston, Va.: Reston.

———. 1984. "Vitamin E for Stomatitis." *Oncology Nursing Forum* (Letter in Practice Corner) 11, no. 2: 36.

Ingle, R. J.; Burish, T. G.; and Wallston, K. A. 1984. "Conditionability of Cancer Chemotherapy Patients." *Oncology Nursing Forum* 11, no. 4: 97–103.

Kaempfer, S. H. 1982. "Relaxation Training Reconsidered." *Oncology Nursing Forum* 9, no. 2: 15–18.

Kempen, A. J. 1981. *Nursing Care of the Cancer Patient with Nutritional Problems,* 4. Report of the Ross Oncology Nursing Round-Table. Columbus: Ross Laboratories.

Kennedy, M.; Parkard, R.; Grant, M.; Padilla, G.; Presant, C.; and Chillar, R. 1983. "The Effects of Using Chemocap on Occurrence of Chemotherapy-induced Alopecia." *Oncology Nursing Forum* 10, no. 1: 19–24.

Keyes, N. A. "Role of the Health Care Professional in Nutrition." 1981. Paper read at Cancer 1981/Cancer 2001: An International Colloquium. University of Texas, M. D. Anderson Hospital.

Knobf, M. K.; Fischer, O. S.; and Welch-McCaffrey, D. 1984. *Cancer Chemotherapy: Treatment and Care.* Boston: G. K. Hall.

Kubler-Ross, E. 1959. *On Death and Dying.* New York: Macmillan.

Larson, D. 1985. "What's the Appropriate Management of Tissue Extravasation by Antitumor Agents?" *Plastic and Reconstructive Surgery* 75: 397–402.

Lindquist, S. F.; Hickey, A. M.; and Drane, J. B. 1978. "Effect of Oral Hygiene on Stomatitis in Patients Receiving Cancer Chemotherapy." *Journal of Prosthetic Dentristry* 40: 312–14.

Lindsey, A. M. 1985a. "Building the Knowledge Base for Practice, Part 1: Nausea and Vomiting." *Oncology Nursing Forum* 12, no. 1: 49–56.

———. 1985b. "Building the Knowledge Base for Practice, Part 2: Alopecia, Breast Self-examination and Other Human Responses." *Oncology Nursing Forum* 12, no. 2: 27–34.

Lindsey, A. M.; Piper, B.; and Stotts, N. 1982. "Clinical Reviews: The Phenomena of Cancer Cachexia." *Oncology Nursing Forum* 9, no. 2: 38–42.

Lucas, S. M. 1980. "Grief—the Healing Pain of Profound Loss." *Hospital Forum* (January–February): 12–16.

Metroclopramide Studies Focus of Antiemetic Session. 1985. American Society of Clinical Oncologists Reports (September). Richmond, Va.: Robins.

Miner, S. 1985. "Sulfadiazide for Fungating Breast Wounds." *Oncology Nursing Forum* (Letter to Practice Corner) 12, no. 4: 83.

Myers, J. S. 1985. "Cancer Pain: Assessment of Nurses' Knowledge and Attitudes." *Oncology Nursing Forum* 12, no. 4: 62–66.

Nunnally, C., and Yasko, J. 1983. "Infection." In *Guidelines for Cancer Care,* ed. J. Yakso. Reston, Va.: Reston.

Nursing Care of the Cancer Patient with Nutritional Problems. 1981. Report of the Ross Round-Table on Oncology Nursing. Columbus: Ross Laboratories.

Paice, J. A. 1983. "Metoclopramide Therapy for Chemotherapy-Induced Nausea and Vomiting." *Oncology Nursing Forum* 10, no. 3: 28–31.

Pizzo, P. A. 1984. "Granulocytopenia and Cancer Therapy." *Cancer* 54: 2649–61.

Powell, E. 1985. "Combining Ativan and Decadron for CMF Patients." *Oncology Nursing Forum* (Letter in Practice Corner) 12, no. 2: 84.

Quesada, J., and Lowder, J. M. 1985. "Some Lymphomas Respond to Monoclonal AB." *Oncology Update* 2: 3.

Rankin, M., and Snider, B. 1984. "Nurses' Perceptions of Cancer Patients' Pain." *Cancer Nursing* 7, no. 2: 23–29.

Rooney, A., and Hawley, C. 1985. "Nursing Management of Disseminated Intravascular Coagulation." *Oncology Nursing Forum* 12, no. 1: 15–22.

Schwittman, R. S.; Shoham, S.; and Cleeland, C. S. 1983. "Relating Cancer Pain to the Physical Basis of Cancer Pain." Paper presented at the American Pain Society, Chicago.

Shell, J. A.; Stanutz, F.; and Grimm, J. 1986. "Comparison of Moisture Vapor Permeable Dressings to Conventional Dressings for Management of Radiation Skin Reactions." *Oncology Nursing Forum* 13, no. 1: 11–16.

Smith, S. A. 1982. "Theories and Interventions of Nutritional Deficits in Neoplastic Disease." *Oncology Nursing Forum,* 9, no. 2: 43–46.

Stapczynski, J. S. "1984. Dealing with Life-Threatening Complications of Cancer." *Consultant* (October): 207–23.

Stickney, S. K., and Gardner, E. R. 1984. "Companions in Suffering." *American Journal of Nursing* 84, no. 12: 1491–94.

Strum, S. B. 1985. "Management of Chemotherapy-Induced Nausea and Vomiting." *Issues in Oncology* 2, no. 1 (April).

Waldenstrom, J. G. 1978. *Paraneoplasia: Biological Signals in the Diagnosis of Cancer*. New York: John Wiley & Sons.

Welch-McCaffrey, D. 1984. "Nursing Management of Chemotherapy-Related Emesis." *Issues in Oncology* 1, no. 2: 6.

Wood, L. 1985. "Vitamin E's Effect on Adriamycin-Induced Alopecia." *New England Journal of Medicine* (April 18): 1060.

"Wound Care Forum." 1985. *American Journal of Nursing* 85, no. 6: 715–18.

Yarbro, C. H. 1985. "Cancer Pain." *Seminars in Oncology* 1, no. 2.

Yasko, J. M. 1982. *Care of the Client Receiving External Radiation Therapy*. Reston, Va.: Reston.

——, ed. 1983. *Guidelines for Cancer Care*. Reston, Va.: Reston.

Zook, D., and Yasko, J. 1983. "Psychological Factors: Their Effect on Nausea and Vomiting Experienced by Clients Receiving Chemotherapy." *Oncology Nursing Forum* 10, no. 3: 76–81.

Chapters Five and Six

"AIDS—the Growing Threat and What's Being Done." 1985. *Time* Magazine (August 12): 40–47.

American Cancer Society. 1981. *A Cancer Source Book for Nurses*. Professional Educational Publication no. 3010-PE.

—— 1982. *Cancer Manual*. 6th ed. Boston: American Cancer Society, Massachusetts Division.

—— 1984. *Third International Symposium on Colorectal Cancer—1983*. Professional Education Publication no. 3438-PE.

—— 1985a. *Cancer Facts and Figures*. New York: American Cancer Society.

—— 1985b. "Hereditary Colon Cancer: Polyposis and Nonpolyposis Variants." *CA-A Cancer Journal for Clinicians* 35, no. 2: 16–23.

Appelbaum, F. R. 1984. "The Potential Role of Autologous Marrow Transplantation in the Treatment of Malignant Disease." Pp. 46–55 in *Proceedings of the 4th National Conference on Cancer Nursing, 1983*. New York: American Cancer Society.

American Society of Clinical Oncologists. 1985a. *CMF Adjuvant Therapy Efficacious in Breast Cancer Patients*. A. H. Robins Co. (September).

—— 1985b. *ECOG Reports CMFP of No Benefit in Preventing Recurrence of Breast Cancer in Postmenopausal Women*. A. H. Robins Co. (September).

——. 1985c. *Hormonal Treatment for Prostate Cancer Tested at Various Institutions*. A.H. Robins Co. (May).

Baum, M., et al. 1985. "Controlled Trial of Tamoxifen as Single Adjuvant in Management of Early Breast Cancer." *Lancet* (April 13): 836.

Bennett, J. 1985. "AIDS Epidemiology Update." *American Journal of Nursing* 85, no. 9: 35–42.

Blot, W. J.; Fraumeni, J. F.; and Stone, B. J. 1976. "Geographic Patterns of Large Bowel Cancer in the United States." *Journal of the National Cancer Institute* 57: 1225–31.

———. 1978. "Geographic Correlates of Pancreas Cancer in the United States." *Cancer* 42: 373–80.

Bonadonna, G.; Brusamolino, P.; and Valagussa, P. 1976. "Combination Chemotherapy as an Adjuvant Treatment in Operable Breast Cancer." *New England Journal of Medicine* 294: 405–10.

Bonadonna, G., and Valagussa, P. 1983. "Chemotherapy of Breast Cancer: Current Issues and Results." *International Journal of Radiation Oncology, Biology and Physics* 9: 279–97.

Burkitt, D. P. 1984. "Etiology and Prevention of Colorectal Cancer." *Hospital Practice* 19, no. 2: 67–77.

Cody, H. S.; Bretsky, S. S.; and Urban, J. A. 1982. "The Continuing Importance of Adequate Surgery for Operable Brain Cancer." *CA-A Cancer Journal for Clinicians* 32, no. 4: 242–48.

Cooper, R. A. 1979. "Winning the War on Cancer: A Conversation." *Rochester Review* (October): 11–18.

Cramer, D. W. 1982. "Uterine Cervix." Pp. 881–890 in *Cancer Epidemiology and Prevention*, ed. D. Schottenfeld and J. F. Fraumeni. Philadelphia: W. B. Saunders.

DeWaard, F. 1982. "Uterine Corpus." Pp. 901–9 in *Cancer Epidemiology and Prevention*, ed. D. Schottenfeld and J. F. Fraumeni. Philadelphia: W. B. Saunders.

Donna, A.; Betta, P.; and Robutti, F. 1984. "Ovarian Mesothelial Tumors and Herbicides." *Carcinogenesis* 5, no. 7: 941–42.

Dugan, K. K. 1985. "The Bleak Outlook on Ovarian Cancer." *American Journal of Nursing* 85, no. 2: 144–50.

Faulkenberry, J. E. 1984. "Cancer Prevention and Detection: Colorectal Cancer." *Cancer Nursing* 7, no. 5: 415–23.

Feinstein, A. 1985. "The Will Rogers Phenomena: Stage Migration and New Diagnosis Techniques as a Source of Misleading Statistics for Survival of Cancer." *New England Journal of Medicine* 312: 1604–10.

Fetsch, S. H. 1984. "The 7-to-10 Year-Old Child's Conceptualization of Death." *Oncology Nursing Forum* 11, no. 6: 52–62.

Fraumeni, J. F. 1983. "The Face of Cancer in the U.S." *Hospital Practice* 18, no. 12: 81–96.

Fraumeni, J. F., and W. J. Blot. 1982. "Lung and Pleura." Pp. 564–682 in *Cancer Epidemiology and Prevention*, ed. J. F. Schottenfeld and J. F. Fraumeni. Philadelphia: W. B. Saunders.

Frenkel, E. P., and M. S. Graham. 1984. "Clinical Forms of Chronic Lymphocytic Leukemia." *Postgraduate Medicine* 75, no. 4: 101–9.

Gallo, N. 1981. "Good-bye Halsted, hello . . ." *View* (April/May): 18–24.

Garnick, M. B. 1984. "Novel Endocrine Approaches in the Management of Prostate Cancer." *Mediguide to Oncology* 5, no. 1: 1–4.

Goldsmith, H. S., and Alday, E. S. 1972. "Role of the Surgeon in the Rehabilitation of the Breast Cancer Patient." *Cancer* 28: 1659–63.

Greene, M. H. 1982. "Non-Hodgkin's Lymphoma and Mycosis Fungoides." Pp. 754–78 in *Cancer Epidemiology and Prevention,* ed. D. Schottenfeld and J. F. Fraumeni. Philadelphia: W. B. Saunders.

Greenwald, P. 1982. Prostate. Pp. 938–46 in *Cancer Epidemiology and Prevention,* ed. D. Schottenfeld and J. F. Fraumeni. Philadelphia: W. B Saunders.

Grufferman, S. 1982. "Hodgkin's Disease." Pp. 739–53 in *Cancer Epidemiology and Prevention,* ed. D. Schottenfeld and J. F. Fraumeni. Philadelphia: W. B. Saunders.

Hamilton, H. K., ed. *Nurse's Clinical Library: Neoplastic Disorders.* 1985. Springhouse, Pennsylvania: Springhouse.

Health, C. W. 1982. "The Leukemias." Pp. 728–39 in *Cancer Epidemiology and Prevention,* ed. D. Schottenfeld and J. F. Fraumeni. Philadelphia: W. B. Saunders.

Henderson, W. J.; Josolin, C. A.; and Turnvull, A. C. 1971. "Talc and Carcinoma of the Ovary and Cervix." *Journal of Obstetrics and Gynecology of the British Commonwealth* 78: 266–72.

Horton, J., and Hill, G. J. 1977. *Clinical Oncology.* Philadelphia: W. B. Saunders.

Huang, A. T. 1984. "Bone Marrow Transplant—Present Status and Prospects." *Issues in Oncology* 1, no. 2: 1–8.

Hughes, W. T. 1984. "Infections in Children with Cancer." *Primary Care and Cancer* (October): 66–69.

Kirkpatrick, C. S. 1980. "Receptivity to Breast Reconstruction after Mastectomy." Masters thesis, University of Rochester (Unpublished).

Klemm, P. 1985. "Cyclosporin A: Use in Preventing Graft Versus Host Disease." *Oncology Nursing Forum* 12, no. 5: 25–32.

Knobf, M. K. 1984. "Breast Cancer—The Treatment Evolution." *American Journal of Nursing* (September): 1110–28.

Kramer, R. F. 1984. "Living with Childhood Cancer: Impact on the Healthy Siblings." *Oncology Nursing Forum* 11, no. 6: 44–56.

Kushner, R. 1984. "Is Aggressive Adjuvant Chemotherapy the Halsted Radical of the 80s?" *CA-A Cancer Journal for Clinicians* 34, no. 6: 345–50.

Lahane, D. 1984. "Non-small-cell Lung Cancer." *Issues in Oncology* 1, no. 2: 4.

Lane, C. 1985. Quoted in "AIDS: The Growing Threat and What's Being Done." *Time* Magazine (August 12): 42.

Lovejoy, N. 1983. "The Leukemic Child's Perceptions of Family Behaviors." *Oncology Nursing Forum* 10, no. 4: 20–25.

Mack, T. M. 1982. "Pancreas." Pp. 638–67 in *Cancer Epidemiology and Prevention,* ed. D. Schottenfeld and J. F. Fraumeni. Philadelphia: W. B. Saunders.

Marino, L. B. 1981. *Cancer Nursing.* St. Louis: C. V. Mosby.

Markham, M. J. 1984. "Progress in Managing of Breast Cancer." *Mediguide to Oncology* 4, no. 1: 1–6.

Maxwell, M. B. 1985. "Dyspnea During Lung Cancer." *American Journal of Nursing* 85, no. 6: 672.

McKinney, F., and DeCuir-Whalley, S. 1983. "Allogeneic Bone Marrow Transplant for Children with Acute Leukemia." *Oncology Nursing Forum* 10, no. 3: 49–53.

Medical Publishing Enterprises, Inc. 1985. "Self-care After Mastectomy Seems Feasible." *Oncology Update* 1: 7–8.

Mueller, S. 1982. "Patient Education: Bone Marrow Transplant Teaching and Documentation Tool." *Oncology Nursing Forum* 9, no. 2: 57–63.

Murphy, W. 1984. "Small-cell Lung Cancer." *Issues in Oncology* 1, no. 2: 3–5.

National Cancer Institute, 1984a. *Advanced Cancer: Living Each Day.* Publication no. 84-856. Washington, D.C.

———. 1984b. *After Breast Cancer: A Guide to Followup Care.* Publication no. 84-2400. Washington, D.C.

———. 1984c. *When Cancer Recurs: Meeting the Challenge Again.* Publication no. 85-2709. Washington, D.C.

Nelson, J. H.; Averette, H. E.; and Richart, R. M. 1982. "Dysplasia, Cancer in Situ, and Early Invasive Cervical Cancer." *CA-A Cancer Journal for Clinicians* 34, no. 6: 306–11.

Paietta, L. 1985. "WBC Receptor Status May Predict Clinical Response." *Oncology Update* (September): 8.

Perloff, M. 1981. "Treatment of Breast Cancer." *Mediguide to Oncology* 1, no. 3: 1–7.

Petersen, O. 1956. "Spontaneous Course of Cervical Precancerous Conditions." *American Journal of Obstetrics and Gynecology* 72: 1065–71.

Petrakis, N. L.; Ernster, V. L.; and King, M. 1982. "Breast." Pp. 855–70 in *Cancer Epidemiology and Prevention.* Philadelphia: W. B. Saunders.

Piver, S. 1984. "Ovarian Cancer: A Decade of Progress." *Cancer* 54: 2706–15.

Richart, R. M., and Barron, B. A. 1969. "A Follow-up Study of Patients with Cervical Dysplasia." *American Journal of Obstetrics and Gynecology* 105: 386–93.

Rogers, T. F.; Bauman, L. J.; and Metzher, L. 1985. "An Assessment of the Reach to Recovery Program." *CA-A Cancer Journal for Clinicians* 35, no. 2: 116–121.

Rowbotham, J. L. 1981. *Managing Colostomies.* American Cancer Society Professional Education Publication no. 3422-PE. New York.

Sandler, R. S.; Freund, D. A.; and Herbst, C. A. 1984. "Cost Effectiveness of Post-operative Carcinoembryonic Antigen Monitoring in Colorectal Cancer." *Cancer* 53: 193–98.

Santos, G. 1984. "Bone Marrow Transplantation in Leukemia." *Cancer* 54: 2737–40.

Sauter, G. 1984. "Acute Myelogenous Leukemia: Maintenance Chemotherapy After Early Consolidation Treatment Does not Prolong Survival." *Lancet* 1: 379–82.

Schottenfeld, D., and Fraumeni, J. F. 1982. *Cancer Epidemiology and Prevention.* Philadelphia: Saunders.

Schottenfeld, D., and Winawer, S. J. 1982. "Large Intestine." Pp. 703–26 in *Cancer Epidemiology and Prevention,* ed. D. Schottenfeld and J. F. Fraumeni. Philadelphia: W. B. Saunders.

Shealey, T. 1985. "A Lifesaver Called Sigmoidoscopy." *Prevention* 37, no. 9: 84–91.

Sischy, B.; Graney, M. J.; and Hinson, E. J. 1984. "Endocavitary Irradiation for Adenocarcinoma of the Rectum." *CA-A Cancer Journal for Clinicians* 34, no. 6: 340–46.

Ultman, J. E., and Jacobs, R. H. 1985. "The Non-Hodgkin's Lymphomas." *CA-A Cancer Journal for Clinicians* 35, no. 2: 66–87.

U.S. Department of Health, Education and Welfare. 1979. *The Leukemic Child.* National Institutes of Health Publication no. 79-863.

———. 1984. *The Breast Cancer Digest.* National Institutes of Health Publication no. 84-1691.

Viele, C.; Dodd, M.; and Morrison, C. 1984. "Caring for Acquired Immune Deficiency Syndrome Patients." *Oncology Nursing Forum* 11, no. 3: 56–60.

Weiss, N. S. 1982. "Ovary." Pp. 871–80 in *Cancer Epidemiology and Prevention,* ed. D. Schottenfeld and J. D. Fraumeni. Philadelphia: W. B. Saunders.

Wynder, E. L. 1973. "A Case Control Study of Cancer of the Pancreas." *Cancer* 31: 641–48.

Wynder, E. L., and Rose, D. P. 1984. "Diet and Breast Cancer." *Hospital Practice* 19, no. 4: 73–88.

Chapter Seven

American Cancer Society. 1982. *Cancer Manual.* Boston: American Cancer Society, Massachusetts Division.

———. 1983. *Mammography: Two statements of the American Cancer Society.* Professional Education Publication no. 3431-PE.

Bowers, A. C., and Thompson, J. M. 1984. *Clinical Manual of Health Assessment.* St. Louis: C. V. Mosby.

Dotz, W., and Berman, B. 1984. "Signs That Indicate Internal Malignancies." *Consultant* (October): 268–80.

Faulkenberry, J. E. 1983. "Cancer Prevention and Detection: Risk Assessment: The Medical History." *Cancer Nursing* 6, no. 5: 389–401.

———. 1984. "Cancer Prevention and Detection: Colorectal Cancer." *Cancer Nursing* 7, no. 5: 415–22.

Friedman, R. J., Rigel, D. S.; and Kopf, A. W. 1985. "Early Detection of Malignant Melanoma: The Role of Physician Exams and Self-examination of the skin." *CA-A Cancer Journal for Clinicians* 35, no. 3: 4–26.

Griffiths, M. J.; Murray, K. H.; and Russo, P. C. 1984. *Oncology Nursing.* New York: Macmillan.

Gusberg, S. B. 1984. "Guidelines for Cancer Screening." Pp. 60–65 in *Proceedings of the 4th National Conference on Cancer Nursing, 1983.* New York: American Cancer Society.

Nash, J. A. 1984. "Cancer Prevention and Detection: Breast Cancer." *Cancer Nursing* 7, no. 2: 163–78.

Newell, G. R. ed. 1983. *Cancer Prevention in Clinical Medicine.* New York: Raven.

Sargis, W. M. 1983. "Detecting Ovarian Cancer." *Oncology Nursing Forum* 10, no. 2: 48–52.

Schleper, J. R. 1984. "Cancer Prevention and Detection: Skin Cancer." *Cancer Nursing* 7, no. 1: 67–77.

Scotto, J. 1985. "Melanoma Among Caucasians in the U.S.—Incidence Predicted for the 1980's." *The Skin Cancer Foundation Journal:* 17–22.

Senie, R. T.; Rosen, P. P.; and Lesser, M. L. 1981. "Breast Self-examination and Medical Examination Related to Breast Cancer Stages." *American Journal of Public Health* 71, no. 6: 583–87.

"Teaching Self-examination Helps Detect Breast Cancer." 1985. *Oncology Update* 2, no. 2.

White, L. H. 1984. "Cancer Prevention and Detection: Cervical Cancer." *Cancer Nursing* 7, no. 4: 335–43.

Chapter Eight

Anderson, M. 1985. "Drug Administration: Update in Techniques." Paper read at conference at Seattle, Washington, January 18. Medical Media Associates.

Anderson, M. A.; Aker, S. N.; and Hickman, R. O. 1982. "The Double-Lumen Hickman Catheter." *American Journal of Nursing* 82: 272–74.

Bender, C. M.; Bast, J.; and Draper, D. 1984. "Patient Teaching in Hepatic Artery Infusion." *Oncology Nursing Forum* 11, no. 2: 61–65.

Bjeletich, J., and Hickman, R. O. 1980. "The Hickman Indwelling Catheter." *American Journal of Nursing* 80: 62–65.

Boehringer Ingelheim Pharmaceuticals, Inc. 1985. "Infusion Therapy at Home Cuts Costs." *Oncology Update* 2: 5–6.

Bottino, J. 1979. "Continuous Intravenous Cytosine Arabinoside Infusions Delivered by a New Portable Infusion System." *Cancer* 43 (June): 2197–2201.

Bull, J. M. 1982. "Whole Body Hyperthermia as an Anticancer Agent." *Cancer* 32, no. 2: 123–26.

Cormed, Inc. 1984. "Cormed Model ML6-6." In *Nursing Manual*. Medina, N.Y.: Cormed.

Cozzi, E.; Hagle, M.; and McGregor, M. L. 1984. "Nursing Management of Patients Receiving Hepatic Arterial Chemotherapy Through an Implanted Infusion Pump." *Cancer Nursing* 7, no. 3: 229–34.

Daeffler, R. J., and Lewinski, J. 1982. "Patient Education: Home Care of the Hickman/Broviac Catheter." *Oncology Nursing Forum* 9, no. 4: 59–63.

Dangel, R. B. 1985. "How to Use an Implantable Infusion Pump." *R.N.* (September): 40–43.

Dennis, E. 1984. "An Ambulatory Infusion Pump for Pain Control." *Cancer Nursing* 7, no. 4: 34–39.

Ellerhorst-Ryan, J. 1985. "Troubleshooting the Venous Access System." *American Journal of Nursing* 85, no. 7: 795–98.

Ensminger, W. D., and Niederhuber, J. E. 1981. "A Totally Implanted Drug Delivery System for Hepatic Arterial Chemotherapy." *Cancer Treatment Reports* 65: 393–400.

Esparza, D. M., and Weyland, J. B. 1982. "Nursing Care for the Patient with an Ommaya Reservoir." *Oncology Nursing Forum* 9, no. 4: 17–20.

Fiscus, J. 1984. *Continuous Ambulatory Chemotherapy*. Columbia, Ohio, Hospital (booklet).

Fraser, D. 1980. "Intravenous Morphine Infusion for Chronic Pain." *Annals of Internal Medicine* 93: 781–82.

Garvey, E., and Kramer, R. 1983. "Improving Cancer Patients' Adjustment to Infusion Chemotherapy: Evaluation of a Patient Education Program." *Cancer Nursing* 6, no. 5: 373–78.

Goodman, M. S. 1984. "Teaching Strategies for an Ambulatory Chemotherapy Program." *Oncology Nursing Forum* 11, no. 5: 23–25.

Goodman, M. S., and Wickham, R. 1984. "Venous Access Devices: An Overview." *Oncology Nursing Forum* 11, no. 5: 16–23.

Gyves, J.; Ensminger, W.; and Niederhuber, J. 1982. "Totally Implanted System for Intravenous Chemotherapy in Patients with Cancer." *American Journal of Medicine* 73: 841–45.

Haylock, P. 1984. "Intraperitoneal Cisplatin with Systemic Thiosulfate Protection." *Oncology Nursing Forum* (Letter in Practice Corner) 11, no. 2: 65.

Heimbach, D. M., and Ivey, T. D. 1976. "Technique for Replacement of a Permanent Home Hyperalimentation Catheter." *Surgery, Gynecology, and Obstetrics* 143: 635–37.

Hickman, R. O. 1979. "A Modified Right Atrial Catheter for Access to the Venous System in Marrow Transplant Recipients." *Surgery, Gynecology, and Obstetrics* 148: 871–75.

Holmes, W. 1985. "SQ Chemotherapy at Home." *American Journal of Nursing* 85, no. 2: 168–70.

Howell, S. B., and Pfeifle, C. L. 1982. "Intraperitoneal Cisplatin with Systemic Thiosulfate Protection." *Annals of International Medicine* 97: 845–51.

Hughes, C. B. 1985. "Venous Access in Chemotherapy Patients." *Issues in Oncology* 2, no. 3: 4–6.

Hurtubise, M. R.; Bottino, J. C.; and Lawson, M. 1980. "Restoring Patency of Occluded Central Venous Catheters." *Archives of Surgery* 115: 212–13.

Jacobs, A.; Clifford, P.; and Kay, H. E. 1981. "The Ommaya Reservoir in Chemotherapy for Malignant Disease in the CNS." *Clinical Oncology* 7: 123–29.

Koga, S. 1983. "Effects of Hyperthermia in Cancer Therapy." *Cancer* (October 1): 1173.

Kowolenko, M. 1980. "Additional Comment on Morphine Infusion." *Drug Intelligence and Clinical Pharmacology* 14: 296–97.

Leavens, M. E.; Beards, S.; and Kowolenko, M. 1982. "Intrathecal and Intraventricular Morphine for Pain in Cancer Patients: Initial Study." *Journal of Neurosurgery* 56: 241–45.

Medvec, B. R. 1984. "Implantable Infusion Systems and Regionally Directed Chemotherapy Approaches—An Overview." Pp. 129–34 in *Proceedings of the 4th National Conference on Cancer Nursing*. New York: American Cancer Society.

Moore, C. L. 1984a. "Hyperthermia: A Modern Experiment in Cancer Treatment." *Oncology Nursing Forum* 11, no. 2: 31–36.

———. 1984b." Nursing Management of the Patient Receiving Local or Regional Hyperthermia." *Oncology Nursing Forum* 11, no. 3: 45–49.

Niederhuber, J. E.; Ensminger, W.; and Gyves, J. W. 1982. "Totally Implanted Venous and Arterial Access to Replace External Catheters in Cancer Treatment." *Surgery:* 706–12.

O'Laughlin, K. 1984. *The Care and Feeding of Your Cormed Pump.* University of Chicago (booklet).

Oncology Nursing Society Clinical Practice Committee. 1983. "Guidelines for Nursing Care of Patients with a Knowledge Deficit." *Oncology Nursing Forum* 10, no. 3: 64–66.

Pharmacia Nu Tech. 1984. *Nursing Protocol for Port-a-Cath System.* Pharmacia, Inc., Piscataway, N.J. (booklet).

Pituk, T. L.; DeYoung, J. L.; and Levin, H. J. 1983. "Volumes of

Selected Central Venous Catheters—Implications for Heparin Fluid Use." *National Intravenous Therapists Association* 6: 98–100.

Pollack, P. F.; Kadden, M.; and Byrne, W. J. 1981. "100 Patient Years' Experience with the Broviac Silastic Catheter for Central Venous Nutrition." *Journal of Parenteral and Enteral Nutrition* 5, no. 1: 32–36.

"Resistant Tumors Yield to Regional Therapy." 1984. *Oncology Update* (Toronto convention issue): 2–4.

Riella, M. C., and Scribner, B. H. 1976. "Five Years' Experience with a Right Atrial Catheter for Prolonged Parenteral Nutrition at Home." *Surgery, Gynecology and Obstetrics* 143 (August): 205–8.

Ruebusch, C. L. 1984. "Hickman Catheter Displacement into Soft Tissue." *Oncology Nursing Forum* (Letter) 11, no. 3: 85–86.

Storm, F. K., and Morton, D. L. 1983. "Localized Hyperthermia in the Treatment of Cancer." *CA-A Cancer Journal for Clinicians* 33, no. 1: 44–47.

Teich, C. J., and Raia, K. 1984. "Teaching Strategies for an Ambulatory Chemotherapy Program." *Oncology Nursing Forum* 11, no. 5: 24–29.

Wilkes, A. M.; Vannicola, P.; and Starck, P. 1985. "Long-term Venous Access." *American Journal of Nursing* 85, no. 7: 793–95.

Winters, V. 1984. "Implantable Vascular Access Devices." *Oncology Nursing Forum* 11, no. 6: 25–30.

Index

Page numbers in italics signify illustrations.